TEST BANK

Pamela Langley
New Hampshire Technical Institute

PRINCIPLES OF ANATOMY AND PHYSIOLOGY

NINTH EDITION

Gerard J. Tortora
Bergen Community College

Sandra Reynolds Grabowski
Purdue University

JOHN WILEY & SONS, INC.
NEW YORK • CHICHESTER • WEINHEIM • BRISBANE • SINGAPORE • TORONTO

To order books or for customer service call 1-800-CALL-WILEY (225-5945).

ISBN 0-471-37469-5

Printed in the United States of America

10 9 8 7 6 5 4 3 2 1

Printed and bound by Bradford & Bigelow, Inc.

PREFACE

This test bank is designed to accompany *Principles of Anatomy and Physiology,* Ninth Edition, by Gerard J. Tortora and Sandra Reynolds Grabowski. There are approximately 3,625 questions in a variety of formats: multiple choice, true/false, matching, short answer, and essay.

Although this printed test bank can be used alone, the maximum benefit and flexibility are afforded the instructor if the test bank is used with the electronic testing file. This user-friendly test generator enables the instructors to view and edit existing test bank questions and to easily add questions to customize the test bank to meet their own course requirements. The built-in question editor allows instructors to create questions in six different formats and to import graphics. On-screen tools allow you to choose and transfer questions to tests and print tests in a variety of fonts and forms. The test bank together with the testing software thus provides you with a ready-to-use powerful instrument for creating a variety of classroom tests, ranging from short, subject-specific quizzes to final comprehensive examinations.

Additional resources are available to instructors using *Principles of Anatomy and Physiology,* Ninth Edition. To find out more, please visit our website at **www.wiley.com/college/bio/tortora.**

Comments and suggestions on this test bank are welcome and may be sent to the author c/o John Wiley & Sons, Inc., 605 Third Avenue, New York, New York 10158-0412.

Pamela Langley
New Hampshire Technical Institute

CONTENTS

CHAPTER 1   An Introduction to the Human Body

MULTIPLE CHOICE. Choose the one alternative that best completes the statement or answers the question.

1) Which of the following correctly lists the levels of organization from **least** complex to **most** complex?
   A) cellular, tissue, chemical system, organ, organism
   B) chemical, cellular, tissue, organ, system, organism
   C) tissue, cellular, chemical, organ, system, organism
   D) chemical, tissue, cellular, system, organ, organism
   E) organism, system, organ, tissue cellular, chemical

   Answer: B
   Page Ref: 3

2) An **organ** is defined as a structure that has a specific structure and is composed on two or more different types of
   A) molecules.
   B) cells.
   C) systems.
   D) tissues.
   E) membranes.

   Answer: D
   Page Ref: 4

3) The sum of all chemical reactions that occur in the body is known as
   A) growth.
   B) reproduction.
   C) metabolism.
   D) differentiation.
   E) responsiveness.

   Answer: C
   Page Ref: 4

4) Tom has been lifting weights. As a result of the physical work, his muscle cells have added proteins and become larger. Which of the following terms best describes this increase in size?

   A) metabolism

   B) growth

   C) responsiveness

   D) differentiation

   E) reproduction

   Answer: B
   Page Ref: 6

5) The cranial cavity is

   A) where the brain is located.

   B) lined by the meninges.

   C) part of the ventral body cavity.

   D) A and B only are correct.

   E) A, B, and C are all correct.

   Answer: D
   Page Ref: 16

6) A plane or section that divides an organ such that you could view an **inferior** surface of the section of that organ would be a

   A) coronal section.

   B) medial section.

   C) sagittal section.

   D) transverse section.

   E) oblique section.

   Answer: C
   Page Ref: 12

7) Interstitial fluid is the fluid

   A) inside blood vessels.

   B) inside cells.

   C) between the cells in a tissue.

   D) inside lymph vessels.

   E) that is consumed as part of the diet.

   Answer: C
   Page Ref: 6

8) A transverse plane divides the body into
   A) superior and inferior portions.
   B) right and left halves.
   C) anterior and posterior portions.
   D) ventral and dorsal body cavities.
   E) quadrants.

   Answer: A
   Page Ref: 12

9) The two body systems that regulate homeostasis are the
   A) cardiovascular and respiratory systems.
   B) cardiovascular and urinary systems.
   C) cardiovascular and endocrine systems.
   D) nervous and cardiovascular systems.
   E) nervous and endocrine systems.

   Answer: E
   Page Ref: 7

10) The word **axillary** refers to the
    A) groin.
    B) armpit.
    C) upper arm.
    D) neck.
    E) back of the knee.

    Answer: B
    Page Ref: 11

11) The word **popliteal** refers to the
    A) groin.
    B) armpit.
    C) upper arm.
    D) neck.
    E) back of the knee.

    Answer: E
    Page Ref: 11

12) Which of the following best describes the relationship between the urinary bladder and the stomach?

   A) The urinary bladder is **distal** to the stomach.

   B) The urinary bladder is **proximal** to the stomach.

   C) The urinary bladder is **inferior** to the stomach.

   D) The urinary bladder is **superior** to the stomach.

   E) The urinary bladder is **anterior** to the stomach.

   Answer: C
   Page Ref: 14

13) Which of the following best describes the relationship between the right plantar region and the right femoral region?

   A) The right plantar region is **distal** to the right femoral region.

   B) The right plantar region is **proximal** to the right femoral region.

   C) The right plantar region is **inferior** to the right femoral region.

   D) The right plantar region is **superior** to the right femoral region.

   E) The right plantar region is **anterior** to the right femoral region.

   Answer: A
   Page Ref: 14

14) The region of the abdominopelvic cavity that is inferior and medial to the left lumbar region is the

   A) left hypochondriac region.

   B) left inguinal region.

   C) umbilical region.

   D) hypogastric region.

   E) epigastric region.

   Answer: D
   Page Ref: 19

15) Which of the following most correctly describes the relationship between the visceral pleura and the parietal pleura?

   A) The visceral pleura is **anterior** to the parietal pleura.

   B) The visceral pleura is **posterior** to the parietal pleura.

   C) The visceral pleura is **superficial** to the parietal pleura.

   D) The visceral pleura is **deep** to the parietal pleura.

   E) The visceral pleura is **medial** to the parietal pleura.

   Answer: D
   Page Ref: 14

16) Which of the following most correctly describes the relationship between the spine and the lungs?

A) The spine is **lateral** and **posterior** to the lungs.

B) The spine is **medial** and **posterior** to the lungs.

C) The spine is **lateral** and **anterior** to the lungs.

D) The spine is **medial** and **posterior** to the lungs.

E) The spine is **medial** and **deep** to the lungs.

Answer: B
Page Ref: 14

17) A plane or section that divides an organ such that you would be looking at a **medial** surface of the section would be a(n)

A) coronal section.

B) horizontal section.

C) sagittal section.

D) transverse section.

E) oblique section.

Answer: C
Page Ref: 12

18) Which of the following best describes the endocrine system?

A) It regulates homeostasis by means of nerve impulses.

B) It absorbs nutrients.

C) It contains hair, skin, and nails.

D) It produces blood cells that transport oxygen.

E) It is made up of glands that secrete hormones.

Answer: E
Page Ref: 5

19) The term **cephalic** refers to the

A) head.

B) neck.

C) back of the lower leg.

D) chest.

E) spinal column.

Answer: A
Page Ref: 11

20) Which of the following best describes the relationship between the ears and the tip of the nose?

    A) The ears are **medial** and **posterior** to the tip of the nose.

    B) The ears are **lateral** and **posterior** to the tip of the nose.

    C) The ears are **medial** and **anterior** to the tip of the nose.

    D) The ears are **lateral** and **posterior** to the tip of the nose.

    E) The ears are **superior** and **medial** to the tip of the nose.

Answer: D
Page Ref: 14

21) Which of the following best describes the relationship between the right shoulder and the navel?

    A) The right shoulder is **inferior** and **medial** to the navel.

    B) The right shoulder is **inferior** and **lateral** to the navel.

    C) The right shoulder is **superior** and **medial** to the navel.

    D) The right shoulder is **superior** and **lateral** to the navel.

    E) The right shoulder is **superior** and **proximal** to the navel.

Answer: D
Page Ref: 14

22) During the process of development of the skeletal system, embryonic cells, known as mesenchyme cells, may develop into either osteoblasts or chondroblasts, which, in turn, may develop into osteocytes and chondrocytes (respectively). This process is an example of

    A) growth.

    B) metabolism.

    C) differentiation.

    D) responsiveness.

    E) movement.

Answer: C
Page Ref: 6

23) The body system that distributes oxygen and nutrients to cells and carries carbon dioxide and wastes away from cells is the

    A) respiratory system.

    B) cardiovascular system

    C) endocrine system.

    D) urinary system.

    E) integumentary system.

Answer: B
Page Ref: 5

24) The system that plays the major role in regulating the volume and chemical composition of blood, eliminating wastes, and regulating fluid and electrolyte balance is the
   A) respiratory system.
   B) cardiovascular system.
   C) endocrine system.
   D) urinary system.
   E) integumentary system.

   Answer: D
   Page Ref: 5

25) Which of the following body parts would be considered **ipsilateral** to each other?
   A) heart and diaphragm
   B) right arm and right leg
   C) left lung and right lung
   D) collar bones and shoulder blades
   E) vertebral column and digestive organs

   Answer: B
   Page Ref: 14

26) Which of the following lines the abdominal cavity?
   A) peritoenum
   B) pericardium
   C) pleura
   D) meninges
   E) mediastinum

   Answer: A
   Page Ref: 16

27) **ALL** of the following are primarily studies of anatomy (as opposed to physiology) **EXCEPT**:
   A) observing the arrangement of cells in the adrenal gland
   B) describing the process by which nerve impulses are transmitted
   C) exploring the embryonic origins of endocrine cells
   D) finding the location of the biceps femoris muscle
   E) identifying types of tissues present in the walls of the intestinal tract

   Answer: B
   Page Ref: 1

28) **ALL** of the following are primarily studies of physiology (as opposed to anatomy) **EXCEPT**:

   A) describing the process by which glucose molecules are broken down

   B) explaining how substances are secreted from cells

   C) describing the process by which nerve impulses are transmitted

   D) identifying the types of tissues present in the walls of the intestinal tract

   E) identifying the factors that affect blood pressure

   Answer: D
   Page Ref: 1

29) Which of the following are considered part of the integumentary system?

   A) liver, stomach, and intestines

   B) brain and spinal cord

   C) hormone-secreting glands

   D) kidneys and urinary bladder

   E) hair, skin, and nails

   Answer: E
   Page Ref: 5

30) Generation of heat (thermogenesis) is a function of the

   A) integumentary system.

   B) muscular system.

   C) cardiovascular system.

   D) digestive system.

   E) nervous system.

   Answer: B
   Page Ref: 5

31) Osmometer cells sense changes in the concentration of blood plasma; therefore, they must be

   A) receptors.

   B) control centers.

   C) stimulators.

   D) part of the cardiovascular system.

   E) effectors.

   Answer: A
   Page Ref: 7

32) Osmometer cells in the brain sense an increase in the concentration of the blood plasma. They then notify the pituitary gland to release the hormone, ADH. This hormone causes the kidney to save water, which lowers the concentration of the plasma. **ALL** of the following are **TRUE** for this scenario **EXCEPT**:

A) The kidney acts as an effector in this feedback loop.

B) The osmometer cells acts as receptors in this feedback loop.

C) The stimulus in this feedback loop is an increase in the plasma concentration.

D) The controlled condition regulated by this feedback loop is constant ADH secretion.

E) This is an example of a negative feedback loop.

Answer: D
Page Ref: 7

33) Which of the following is an example of a **positive** feedback loop?

A) A neuron is stimulated, thus opening membrane channels to allow sodium ions to leak from the extracellular fluid to the intracellular fluid. This causes more membrane channels to open, thus allowing more sodium ions to enter the intracellular fluid.

B) Baroreceptors notify the brain that the blood pressure has increased. The brain then notifies the blood vessels to dilate, thus lowering the blood pressure.

C) Low levels of glucose in the blood cause the pancreas to release less insulin (a hormone that lowers blood glucose).

D) Elevated body temperature is sensed by cells in the brain. As a result, sweat is produced, and heat is lost as the water in the sweat evaporates.

E) An auto factory produces 1000 cars per week. The sales office could sell 1200 cars per week. Extra production personnel are added at the factory to meet the sales demand.

Answer: A
Page Ref: 9

34) You are eating a hot fudge sundae. The pleasant taste information is sensed by your taste buds, which notify your brain. Your brain releases endorphins, which make you feel very good. You now associate the good feeling with hot fudge sundaes, so you eat another hot fudge sundae. Now you feel even better. Which of the following statements is **TRUE** regarding this scenario?

A) This is a negative feedback loop because two hot fudge sundaes will make you sick.

B) This is a positive feedback loop because the results make you feel good.

C) This is a negative feedback loop because you were doing something bad for your health in the first place, and the result makes the situation worse.

D) This is a positive feedback loop because the stimulus (eating a hot fudge sundae) and the effect (eating another hot fudge sundae) are the same.

E) This is a negative feedback loop because the stimulus (eating a hot fudge sundae) and the effect (eating another hot fudge sundae) are the same.

Answer: D
Page Ref: 7

35) Which of the following best defines **tissue**?

    A) the basic structural and functional unit of an organism

    B) the molecules that form the body's structure

    C) a group of cells and the surrounding materials that work together to perform a particular function

    D) a group of related organs with a common function

    E) the membranes that cover organs

Answer: C
Page Ref: 4

36) **ALL** of the following would be considered **signs** of infection **EXCEPT**:

    A) skin lesions of chicken pox

    B) elevated body temperature

    C) swollen lymph nodes

    D) dull pain localized in the back of the neck

    E) enlargement of the liver

Answer: D
Page Ref: 10

37) Which of the following body systems provides protection against disease and returns proteins and plasma to the cardiovascular system?

    A) respiratory

    B) urinary

    C) endocrine

    D) lymphatic

    E) integumentary

Answer: D
Page Ref: 5

38) Assessment of body structure and function by touching body surfaces with the hands is called

    A) auscultation.

    B) percussion.

    C) palpation.

    D) autopsy.

    E) epidemiology.

Answer: C
Page Ref: 2

39) Which of the following structures is located in the mediastinum?

A) heart

B) lungs

C) brain

D) liver

E) Both A and B are correct.

Answer: A
Page Ref: 16

40) Which of the following is **TRUE** regarding the skeletal system?

A) It provides support and protection.

B) It stores minerals.

C) It assists in body movements.

D) It houses cells that give rise to blood cells.

E) All of the above are true.

Answer: E
Page Ref: 5

41) Which of the following is located in the pelvic cavity?

A) uterus

B) spleen

C) gallbladder

D) stomach

E) Both A and C are correct.

Answer: A
Page Ref: 16

42) **ALL** of the following are found in the thoracic cavity **EXCEPT** the

A) thymus.

B) lungs.

C) trachea.

D) larynx.

E) esophagus.

Answer: D
Page Ref: 16

43) Which of the following is considered to be the body's "internal environment" when discussing homeostasis?

 A) intracellular fluid

 B) plasma

 C) interstitial fluid

 D) hormones

 E) lymph

Answer: C
Page Ref: 6

44) A person in **anatomical position** will exhibit **ALL** of the following **EXCEPT**:

 A) standing erect

 B) facing observer

 C) feet flat on floor

 D) arms at sides

 E) palms against the lateral sides of the thighs

Answer: E
Page Ref: 10

45) A sonogram is produced by

 A) the response of protons to a pulse of radio waves while they are being magnetized.

 B) comparison of an x-ray of a body organ before and after a contrast dye has been injected into a blood vessel.

 C) an x-ray beam moving in an arc around the body.

 D) high-frequency sound waves transmitted to a video monitor.

 E) computer interpretation of radioactive emissions from injected substances.

Answer: D
Page Ref: 20

46) Ginny is six years old and has grown 12 inches during the last year. Her family physician has referred her to an **endocrinologist**. This is because he suspects there is a problem with her

 A) blood flow to the bones.

 B) bone tissue structure.

 C) hormone balance.

 D) nerve impulse transmission.

 E) ability to absorb nutrients.

Answer: C
Page Ref: 5

47) Ginny has grown 12 inches during the last year. Her endocrinologist has ordered an **MRI**, possibly because he suspects a

    A) problem with the growth plates of the bones.

    B) tumor growing on a gland.

    C) problem with blood flow to the bones.

    D) malfunction of the metabolisms in part of her brain.

    E) problem with her heart valves.

Answer: B
Page Ref: 5

48) Which of the following would be considered a **symptom** of disease?

    A) tremors in the hands

    B) excessive urine output

    C) a skin rash

    D) dizziness

    E) diarrhea

Answer: D
Page Ref: 10

49) In order to discuss the details of the metabolism of a cell, which level of structural organization would it be most helpful to understand?

    A) chemical

    B) tissue

    C) system

    D) organ

    E) organism

Answer: A
Page Ref: 4

50) When dividing the abdominopelvic cavity into quadrants, a transverse plane and a midsagittal plane are passed through the

    A) tops of the hip bones.

    B) heart.

    C) nipples.

    D) diaphragm.

    E) umbilicus.

Answer: E
Page Ref: 18

MATCHING. Choose the item in column 2 that best matches each item in column 1.

Choose the item from column 2 that best matches each item in column 1.

1) Column 1: brachial
   Column 2: arm

   Answer: arm
   Page Ref: 11

2) Column 1: cervical
   Column 2: neck

   Answer: neck
   Page Ref: 11

3) Column 1: otic
   Column 2: ear
           Foil: eye

   Answer: ear
   Page Ref: 11

4) Column 1: crural
   Column 2: lower leg
   Answer: lower leg
   Page Ref: 11

5) Column 1: cephalic
   Column 2: head
   Answer: head
   Page Ref: 11

6) Column 1: carpal
   Column 2: wrist
           Foil: hand
   Answer: wrist
   Page Ref: 11

7) Column 1: calcaneal
   Column 2: heel of foot
   Answer: heel of foot
   Page Ref: 11

8) Column 1: plantar
   Column 2: sole of foot
   Answer: sole of foot
   Page Ref: 11

9) Column 1: popliteal
   Column 2: hollow behind knee
       Foil: knee cap
   Answer: hollow behind knee
   Page Ref: 11

10) Column 1: axillary
    Column 2: armpit
    Answer: armpit
    Page Ref: 11

MATCHING. Choose the item in column 2 that best matches each item in column 1.

Choose the item from column 2 that best matches each item in column 1.

1) Column 1: integumentary system
   Column 2: provides protection from
           external stresses; helps
           regulate body temperature
   Answer: provides protection from external stresses; helps regulate body temperature
   Page Ref: 5

2) Column 1: skeletal system
   Column 2: provides support and
           protection; stores minerals
           and lipids
   Answer: provides support and protection; stores minerals and lipids
   Page Ref: 5

3) Column 1: muscular system
   Column 2: produces movement;
           generates heat; stabilizes body
           position
   Answer: produces movement; generates heat; stabilizes body position
   Page Ref: 5

4) Column 1: nervous system
   Column 2: detects, interprets, and
             responds to changes in the
             environment; regulates
             homeostasis
   Answer: detects, interprets, and responds to changes in the environment; regulates homeostasis
   Page Ref: 5

5) Column 1: cardiovascular system
   Column 2: transports oxygen, carbon
             dioxide, nutrients, and wastes
             to and from cells
   Answer: transports oxygen, carbon dioxide, nutrients, and wastes to and from cells
   Page Ref: 5

6) Column 1: endocrine system
   Column 2: regulates body activities via
             hormone secretion
   Answer: regulates body activities via hormone secretion
   Page Ref: 5

7) Column 1: lymphatic system
   Column 2: returns proteins and fluids to
             blood and transports fats from
             gastrointestinal tract to blood
   Answer: returns proteins and fluids to blood and transports fats from gastrointestinal tract to
           blood
   Page Ref: 5

8) Column 1: respiratory system
   Column 2: transfers oxygen and carbon
             dioxide between air and
             blood; helps regulate acid-
             base balance
   Answer: transfers oxygen and carbon dioxide between air and blood; helps regulate acid-base
           balance
   Page Ref: 5

9) Column 1: digestive system
   Column 2: breaks down food, absorbs
             nutrients, and eliminates
             wastes
   Answer: breaks down food, absorbs nutrients, and eliminates wastes
   Page Ref: 5

10) Column 1: urinary system
   Column 2: regulates volume and
      chemical composition of
      blood; helps regulate red
      blood cell production;
      eliminates wastes

   Answer: regulates volume and chemical composition of blood; helps regulate red blood cell
      production; eliminates wastes
   Page Ref: 5

TRUE/FALSE. Write 'T' if the statement is true and 'F' if the statement is false.

1) When a new cell differs in structure and function from the ancestor cell that gave rise to it,
   growth has occurred.

   Answer: FALSE
   Page Ref: 6

2) Interstitial fluid is an extracellular fluid filling the spaces between the cells of tissues.

   Answer: TRUE
   Page Ref: 6

3) The effector is the part of a feedback loop that notifies the control center of changes in the
   environment.

   Answer: FALSE
   Page Ref: 7

4) Negative feedback loops are so–called because they cause harm to the body.

   Answer: FALSE
   Page Ref: 7

5) The endocrine system helps regulate homeostasis via the secretion of hormones.

   Answer: TRUE
   Page Ref: 5

6) A positive feedback loop reverses a change in a controlled condition.

   Answer: FALSE
   Page Ref: 9

7) A person in the anatomical position is also in a prone position.

   Answer: FALSE
   Page Ref: 10

8) The diaphragm separates the abdominal cavity from the pelvic cavity.

Answer: FALSE
Page Ref: 16

9) A body lying face down is said to be in the prone position.

Answer: TRUE
Page Ref: 10

10) A sagittal plane divides the body (or an organ) into anterior and posterior portions.

Answer: FALSE
Page Ref: 12

11) The dorsal body cavity is lined by the peritoneum.

Answer: FALSE
Page Ref: 16

12) There are two pleural cavities, each surrounding a lung.

Answer: TRUE
Page Ref: 16

13) Radiography (x-ray) is better than magnetic resonance imaging (MRI) for showing the fine details of bony structures.

Answer: TRUE
Page Ref: 21

14) Plasma is a type of intracellular fluid.

Answer: FALSE
Page Ref: 6

15) The parietal layer of the pericardium is superficial to the visceral layer of the pericardium.

Answer: TRUE
Page Ref: 16

SHORT ANSWER. Write the word or phrase that best completes each statement or answers the question.

1) Groups of cells (and the substance surrounding them) that usually arise from common ancestor cells and work together to perform a particular function comprise a _____.
Answer: tissue
Page Ref: 4

2) The study of functional changes associated with disease and aging is called _____.
Answer: pathophysiology
Page Ref: 2

3) Listening to body sounds to evaluate the functioning of certain organs is called _____.
Answer: auscultation
Page Ref: 2

4) _____ is the ability of an organism to detect and react to changes in the external or internal environment.
Answer: Responsiveness
Page Ref: 6

5) _____ is a condition of equilibrium in the body's internal environment produced by the interplay of all the body's regulatory processes.
Answer: Homeostasis
Page Ref: 6

6) Any disruption that changes a controlled condition is called a(n) _____.
Answer: stimulus
Page Ref: 7

7) The chemicals produced by the endocrine system that help regulate homeostasis are called _____.
Answer: hormones
Page Ref: 7

8) In a feedback loop, the control center provides output to and elicits a response from a(n) _____.
Answer: effector
Page Ref: 7

9) The stimulus in a feedback loop is an increase in blood sugar. If this is a positive feedback loop, then the effector will cause blood sugar to _____.
Answer: increase
Page Ref: 9

10) When different kinds of tissues are joined together, they form the structures of the next level of organization called _____.
Answer: organs
Page Ref: 4

11) The anatomical term used to describe a structure that is nearer to the point of origin than another structure is the term _____.
Answer: proximal
Page Ref: 14

12) Ancestor cells that can divide and give rise to progeny that undergo differentiation are called _____.
Answer: stem cells
Page Ref: 6

13) The fluid within cells is called _____.
Answer: intracellular fluid
Page Ref: 6

14) The body's "internal environment" is the fluid that surrounds cells, which is called _____.
Answer: interstitial fluid
Page Ref: 6

15) The body system that eliminates wastes, regulates the volume and composition of blood, and helps regulate red blood cell production is the _____ system.
Answer: urinary
Page Ref: 5

16) The study of the causes, transmission, and distribution of diseases within a community is called _____.
Answer: epidemiology
Page Ref: 10

17) If the body is lying face up, it is in the _____ position.
Answer: supine
Page Ref: 10

18) The study of structure and the relationship between structures is called _____.
Answer: anatomy
Page Ref: 1

19) The study of the function of body parts is called _____.
Answer: physiology
Page Ref: 1

20) The basic structural and functional unit of an organism is the _____.
Answer: cell
Page Ref: 4

21) The body is divided into anterior and posterior portions by a _____ plane.
Answer: frontal (coronal)
Page Ref: 12

22) The heart, esophagus, trachea, and thymus are all located in a subdivision of the thoracic cavity known as the _____.

Answer: mediastinum

Page Ref: 16

23) The cranial cavity is a subdivision of the _____ body cavity.

Answer: dorsal

Page Ref: 16

24) The abdominopelvic region that is superior and ipsilateral to the right lumbar region is the _____ region.

Answer: right hypochondriac

Page Ref: 19

25) A plane or section that divides an organ such that you would be looking at a medial surface of that organ would be a _____ section.

Answer: sagittal

Page Ref: 16

26) Homeostasis is regulated by the endocrine system and the _____ system.

Answer: nervous

Page Ref: 7

27) The component of a feedback loop that senses changes in the environment and notifies the control center of the changes is called the _____.

Answer: receptor

Page Ref: 7

28) The location of the right brachial region is _____ to the right carpal region.

Answer: proximal

Page Ref: 14

29) The location of the pericardial cavity is _____ to the pleural cavities.

Answer: medial

Page Ref: 14

30) Histology is the study of the microscopic structure of _____.

Answer: tissues

Page Ref: 2

ESSAY. Write your answer in the space provided or on a separate sheet of paper.

1) Define the term **differentiation**. Use your textbook to find and describe an example of this process other than the example given in Chapter One.

 Answer: Differentiation is the process a cell undergoes to develop from an unspecialized to a specialized state. Students presumably will be able to find several suitable examples, such as the development of osteocytes or gametes. (note: The example in Chapter One involved blood cells.)

 Page Ref: 6

2) Identify and briefly define the six important life processes of the human body described in Chapter One.

 Answer: **Metabolism** is the sum of all chemical processes that occur in the body. **Responsiveness** is the ability to detect and respond to environmental changes. **Movement** is the motion of the body or its parts. **Growth** is an increase in the size and/or number of cells. **Differentiation** is the development of specialized from unspecialized cells. **Reproduction** is the formation of new cells or a new individual.

 Page Ref: 6

3) Mr. Barry is experiencing pain in his left hypochondriac and left lumbar regions. He has just been admitted to the emergency room following a construction accident in which he was pulled from beneath the rubble of a collapsed wall. One intern yells, "Get him to X–Ray now!" Yet another intern orders him to CT scanning. What would each intern hope to determine from the procedure ordered?

 Answer: X–rays (radiography) will give good clear indications of broken bones (such as ribs), while a CT scan would give a better indication of soft organ damage (such as a ruptured spleen).

 Page Ref: 20–21

4) Define the term **homeostasis**. Identify the components of a typical feedback loop, and describe the role of each.

 Answer: Homeostasis is a condition of equilibrium in the body's internal environment produced by the interplay of all the body's regulatory processes. Homeostasis is regulated by feedback loops, which typically consist of a receptor, a control center, and an effector. The receptor monitors changes (stimuli) in controlled conditions, and sends this information to the control center. The control center compares this input with other information from other receptors, and notifies and effector to make an appropriate change. The effector makes the appropriate response, as dictated by the control center.

 Page Ref: 6–7

5) Explain how a positive feedback loop differs from a negative feedback loop.

 Answer: In a positive feedback loop, the response of the effector enhances or amplifies the original stimulus, that is, the condition is moved further away from homeostasis. In a negative feedback loop, the response of the effector is the opposite of the original stress, and tends to move the controlled condition back toward homeostasis.

 Page Ref: 7–9

6) Identify and describe the locations of the major body fluid compartments. Which is most often called the body's "internal environment?"

Answer: Intracellular fluid (ICF) is the fluid within cells. Extracellular fluid (ECF) is the fluid outside of cells. Plasma is the ECF within blood vessels. Interstitial fluid is the fluid surrounding cells, and is considered the internal environment.

Page Ref: 6

7) Osmometer cells in the brain sense and increase in the concentration of plasma. This information is sent to the hypothalamus, which notifies the pituitary gland to release the hormone, ADH. ADH causes the kidney to save water, which lowers the concentration of the plasma.
Identify the elements of a feedback loop in this scenario. Is this a positive or a negative feedback loop? Explain your answer.

Answer: The controlled condition is plasma concentration, and increased plasma concentration is the stimulus. Osmometer cells are the receptors because they sense the increased concentration. The hypothalamus is the control center, which receives the input from the receptors and notifies the effector of the appropriate response. The pituitary gland and the kidneys act as effectors, since both are required to carry out the response. This is a negative feedback loop because the original stimulus (increased plasma concentration) is reversed.

Page Ref: 7–9

8) Consider the following situation as a feedback loop: Tuition at a small college has been $1000 per semester for many years, and the student enrollment has remained constant at 1000 students for an equal number of years. This income exactly covers the expenses of faculty/staff salaries. The college administrators voted this year to fund a raise for the faculty and staff by raising tuition to $2000 per semester. Now only 300 students are enrolled at the college.
Continue this story as a **negative** feedback loop.

Answer: There are many possible answers to this questions, but the usual answer is to forget the raise and lower tuition so that the students come back.

Page Ref: 7–9

9) Consider the following situation as a feedback loop: Tuition at a small college has been $1000 per semester for many years, and the student enrollment has remained constant at 1000 students for an equal number of years. This income exactly covers the expenses of faculty/staff salaries. The college administrators voted this year to fund a raise for the faculty and staff by raising tuition to $2000 per semester. Now only 300 students are enrolled at the college.
Continue this story as a **positive** feedback loop.

Answer: There are several correct answers to this question, but the usual answer is that the administrators raise tuition again, enrollment drops further, and the school closes.

Page Ref: 7–9

10) One of the members of your study group is insisting that a feedback loop is a positive feedback loop because it is "doing good for the body." What is wrong, if anything, with this student's thinking?

Answer: This student is confusing the terms **positive** and **negative** with **good** and **bad**. When describing feedback loops, the terms **positive** and **negative** are used in a more quantitative way to describe whether the effects of a loop amplify (increase) or reverse (decrease) a change in a controlled condition.

Page Ref: 9

CHAPTER 2   The Chemical Level of Organization

MULTIPLE CHOICE. Choose the one alternative that best completes the statement or answers the question.

1) Which of the following is **TRUE** regarding this situation: Solution A has a pH of 7.38 and Solution B has a pH of 7.42:

A) Solution B is more acidic than Solution A.

B) The pH of Solution A falls within the homeostatic pH range for extracellular body fluids, but the pH of Solution B does not.

C) Solution A contains a higher concentration of hydrogen ions that Solution B.

D) Solution B contains a higher concentration of hydrogen ions than Solution A.

E) Both B and C are correct.

Answer: C
Page Ref: 41

2) An object's mass is determined by:

A) the amount of matter it contains.

B) its weight.

C) the type of chemical bonds present in it.

D) its state (solid, liquid, or gas).

E) Both B and D are correct.

Answer: A
Page Ref: 26

3) The chemical symbol for sodium is:

A) S

B) So

C) Sd

D) K

E) Na

Answer: E
Page Ref: 27

4) The four elements making up about 96% of the body's mass are represented by the symbols:

   A) O, Ca, H, Na

   B) O, C, H, N

   C) O, C, He, Na

   D) O, H, K, N

   E) O, Ca, H, Ni

   Answer: B
   Page Ref: 26

5) Which of the following carry a negative charge?

   A) protons only

   B) neutrons only

   C) electrons only

   D) both protons and electrons

   E) both electrons and neutrons

   Answer: C
   Page Ref: 27

6) Peptide bonds are found in:

   A) carbohydrates.

   B) lipids.

   C) proteins.

   D) inorganic compounds.

   E) any type of molecule.

   Answer: C
   Page Ref: 48

7) The smallest unit of matter that retains the properties and characteristics of an element is the:

   A) atom.

   B) molecule.

   C) proton.

   D) nucleus.

   E) electron.

   Answer: A
   Page Ref: 27

8) Atom A has 17 protons and 20 neutrons in its nucleus. Atom B has 17 protons and 18 neutrons in its nucleus. What can you tell about these two atoms?

   A) Both atoms have 17 electrons.

   B) They are atoms of different elements.

   C) They are isotopes of the same element.

   D) Atom A has a neutral charge, and Atom B is a free radical.

   E) Both A and C are correct.

Answer: E
Page Ref: 27–28

9) To produce lactose:

   A) two amino acids must form a peptide bond.

   B) pairing of nitrogenous bases must occur between nucleotides.

   C) glucose and galactose must undergo a dehydration reaction.

   D) glucose and fructose must undergo a hydrolysis reaction.

   E) at least two fatty acids must bind to glycerol.

Answer: C
Page Ref: 44

10) The biological function of a protein is determined by its:

   A) primary structure.

   B) secondary structure.

   C) tertiary structure.

   D) quaternary structure.

   E) denatured structure.

Answer: C
Page Ref: 50

11) A **dalton** is:

   A) a special type of high–energy phosphate bond.

   B) a measure of atomic electrical charge.

   C) another name for an isotope.

   D) a unit of measurement for atomic mass.

   E) a measure of the amount of energy contained in a chemical bond.

Answer: D
Page Ref: 28

12) The function of ATP is to:

A) act as a template for production of proteins.

B) store energy.

C) act as a catalyst.

D) determine the function of the cell.

E) hold amino acids together in a protein.

Answer: B
Page Ref: 54

13) What can you tell from the molecular formula $C_6H_{12}O_6$?

A) It easily forms free radicals.

B) It is an organic compound.

C) The formula represents six molecules of the substance.

D) It contains six carbon atoms.

E) Both B and D are correct.

Answer: E
Page Ref: 29, 42

14) What can you tell from the chemical formula SO_4^{2-}?

A) This substance would have to bond with a free radical containing two more protons than electrons to form an uncharged molecule.

B) This group of atoms has two "extra" electrons.

C) This group of atoms has "lost" two electrons.

D) Both A and B are correct.

E) Both A and C are correct.

Answer: D
Page Ref: 29

15) **ALL** of the following are organic molecules **EXCEPT**:

A) ATP.

B) glucose.

C) DNA.

D) enzymes.

E) water.

Answer: E
Page Ref: 39

16) The most abundant inorganic substance in the human body is:
   A) glucose.
   B) fat.
   C) ATP.
   D) water.
   E) iron.

   Answer: D
   Page Ref: 39

17) Which of the following is considered to be neutral on the pH scale?
   A) urine
   B) pure water
   C) blood plasma
   D) cytoplasm
   E) interstitial fluid

   Answer: B
   Page Ref: 41

18) **ALL** of the following are compounds **EXCEPT**:
   A) H_2O
   B) CO_2
   C) H_2
   D) $CaCl_2$
   E) H_2CO_3

   Answer: C
   Page Ref: 30

19) Superoxide is considered dangerous to the body because it:
   A) is too large to enter cells for use in metabolic reactions.
   B) occupies carrier sites on hemoglobin so "normal" oxygen can't be transported.
   C) causes radical shifts in pH.
   D) causes formation of heavier-than-normal water, thus comprising its effectiveness as a solvent.
   E) readily gives up its unpaired electrons, thus breaking apart important body molecules.

   Answer: E
   Page Ref: 29

20) The "octet rule" states that:

A) a minimum of eight atoms is required to form a molecule.

B) two or more atoms interact in ways that produce a chemically stable arrangement of eight valence electrons for each atom.

C) eight different elements make up 96% of the body's mass.

D) all atoms contain eight electrons or some multiple of eight.

E) the most stable atoms are those that have eight valence shells.

Answer: B
Page Ref: 30

21) An atom in a polar covalent bond that attracts electrons more strongly is said to have greater:

A) ionization efficiency.

B) pH.

C) heat capacity.

D) activation energy.

E) electronegativity.

Answer: E
Page Ref: 33

22) The term referring to all the chemical reactions occurring in the body is:

A) metabolism.

B) oxidation–reduction.

C) hydrolysis.

D) growth.

E) electronegativity.

Answer: A
Page Ref: 34

23) The two factors that most influence the chance that a collision will occur between atoms of chemical reactants are:

A) atomic mass and temperature.

B) atomic mass and concentration.

C) concentration and temperature.

D) electrical charge and temperature.

E) concentration and the types of chemical bonds that will form.

Answer: C
Page Ref: 35

24) An inorganic acid dissociates in water into:

    A) one or more hydroxide ions and one or more cations.

    B) one or more hydrogen ions and one or more anions.

    C) one or more hydroxide ions and one or more anions.

    D) one or more hydrogen ions and one or more cations.

    E) cations and anions other than hydroxide and hydrogen ions.

Answer: B
Page Ref: 38

25) An inorganic base dissociates in water into:

    A) one or more hydrogen ions and one or more anions.

    B) one or more hydroxide ions and one or more cations.

    C) one or more hydrogen ions and one or more cations.

    D) one or more hydroxide ions and one or more anions.

    E) cations and anions other than hydroxide and hydrogen ions.

Answer: B
Page Ref: 38

26) An inorganic salt dissociates in water into:

    A) one or more hydrogen ions and one or more anions.

    B) one or more hydroxide ions and one or more cations.

    C) one or more hydrogen ions and one or more cations.

    D) one or more hydroxide ions and one or more anions.

    E) cations and anions other than hydroxide and hydrogen ions.

Answer: E
Page Ref: 38

27) Which of the following is most likely a description of an exergonic reaction?

    A) Three fatty acids form ester bonds with glycerol.

    B) A molecule of pyruvic acid is oxidized into water and carbon dioxide.

    C) A hydrogen ion gains an electron.

    D) A third phosphate is added to ADP.

    E) Both B and C are correct.

Answer: B
Page Ref: 34

28) The function of a catalyst is to:

    A) convert strong acids and bases into weak acids and bases.

    B) store energy released during exergonic reactions.

    C) act as the chemical link between atoms in a covalent bond.

    D) lower the activation energy needed for a chemical reaction to occur.

    E) keep particles in a colloid from settling out.

Answer: D
Page Ref: 36

29) Which of the following represents accurate base-pairing in DNA molecules?

    A) adenine to adenine and guanine to guanine

    B) adenine to uracil and cytosine to guanine

    C) adenine to cytosine and guanine to thymine

    D) adenine to thymine and cytosine to guanine

    E) adenine to guanine and cytosine to thymine

Answer: D
Page Ref: 53

30) In the body, synthesis reactions are:

    A) anabolic reactions.

    B) redox reactions.

    C) catabolic reactions.

    D) usually endergonic reactions.

    E) Both A and D are correct.

Answer: E
Page Ref: 36

31) In the body, decomposition reactions are:

    A) anabolic reactions.

    B) exchange reactions.

    C) catabolic reactions.

    D) usually endergonic reactions.

    E) Both C and D are correct.

Answer: C
Page Ref: 37

32) In cells, a molecule from which two hydrogen atoms have been removed has been:
    A) oxidized.
    B) reduced.
    C) ionized.
    D) denatured.
    E) hydrolyzed.

    Answer: A
    Page Ref: 37

33) The atom of one element is distinguished from an atom of another element by the number of:
    A) neutrons in the nucleus.
    B) electrons in the nucleus.
    C) protons in the nucleus.
    D) electrons orbiting the nucleus.
    E) electrons it can lose when bonding.

    Answer: C
    Page Ref: 27

34) The **atomic number** of an atom is the:
    A) sum of the numbers of subatomic particles.
    B) number of electrons in the outer orbital shell.
    C) number of neutrons in the nucleus.
    D) number of protons in the nucleus.
    E) sum of the numbers of protons and neutrons only.

    Answer: D
    Page Ref: 27

35) A molecule which has gained electrons has been:
    A) oxidized.
    B) reduced.
    C) neutralized.
    D) denatured.
    E) hydrolyzed.

    Answer: B
    Page Ref: 37

36) Solutes that are **hydrophilic** are those that:

A) have been reduced by addition of hydrogen atoms.

B) dissolve easily in water because they contain polar covalent bonds.

C) dissolve easily in water because they contain nonpolar covalent bonds.

D) dissolve poorly because they contain polar covalent bonds.

E) dissolve poorly because they contain nonpolar covalent bonds.

Answer: B
Page Ref: 39

37) The special kind of decomposition reaction that is the opposite of a dehydration synthesis reaction is a(n):

A) oxidation reaction.

B) reduction reaction.

C) polymerization reaction.

D) denaturation reaction.

E) hydrolysis reaction.

Answer: E
Page Ref: 36

38) A compound that is a sugar is:

A) also a carbohydrate.

B) one that contains peptide bonds.

C) named using the suffix *-ase*.

D) most often seen as a part of structural units in the body.

E) All of these are correct.

Answer: A
Page Ref: 42

39) Which of the following is a carbohydrate?

A) acetone

B) formaldehyde

C) creatine kinase

D) erythrose

E) There is no way of knowing which is a carbohydrate.

Answer: D
Page Ref: 44

40) Glycerol is the backbone molecule for:

   A) disaccharides.

   B) DNA.

   C) peptides.

   D) triglycerides.

   E) ATP.

   Answer: D
   Page Ref: 45

41) An atom of oxygen has 8 protons, 8 neutrons, and 8 electrons. What is its atomic number?

   A) 8, because it has 8 protons.

   B) 8, because it has 8 neutrons.

   C) 8, because it has 8 electrons.

   D) 16, because it has 8 protons plus 8 electrons.

   E) 16, because it has 8 protons plus 8 neutrons.

   Answer: A
   Page Ref: 27

42) An atom of oxygen has 8 protons, 8 electrons, and 8 neutrons. Which of the following is the mass number of oxygen?

   A) 8, because it has 8 protons.

   B) 8, because it has 8 electrons.

   C) 8, because it has 8 neutrons.

   D) 16, because it has 8 protons plus 8 electrons.

   E) 16, because it has 8 protons plus 8 neutrons.

   Answer: E
   Page Ref: 28

43) An atom of oxygen has 8 protons, 8 electrons, and 8 neutrons. How would you expect the electrons to be "arranged" in this atom?

   A) All electrons are located in the nucleus of the atom.

   B) All 8 electrons are located in the outermost electron shell.

   C) All 8 electrons are located in the electron shell nearest the nucleus.

   D) Two electrons are in the electron shell nearest the nucleus, and six are in the second shell.

   E) Six electrons are in the electron shell nearest the nucleus, and two are in the second shell.

   Answer: D
   Page Ref: 27

44) An atom of oxygen has 8 protons, 8 electrons, and 8 neutrons. In order to achieve stability, the oxygen atom will:

A) donate two electrons from its outer shell to another atom.

B) accept two electrons into its outer electron shell from another atom.

C) donate two protons to another atom.

D) accept two protons from another atom.

E) do nothing, because the outer electron shell is already stable.

Answer: B
Page Ref: 30

45) The pH scale measures:

A) total electrolyte concentration.

B) ATP levels.

C) the level of enzyme activity.

D) hydrogen ion concentration.

E) total hydrogen content of all organic compounds in the body.

Answer: D
Page Ref: 40

46) A fatty acid with only single covalent bonds is said to be:

A) oxidized.

B) reduced.

C) saturated.

D) denatured.

E) hydrolyzed.

Answer: C
Page Ref: 45

47) Which of the following provides the most energy per gram?

A) acids

B) bases

C) carbohydrates

D) fats

E) proteins

Answer: D
Page Ref: 45

48) A molecule that is **amphipathic** is one that:

A) has been damaged by a free radical.

B) has at least two isomeric forms.

C) can act as both an acid and a base.

D) has both polar and nonpolar portions.

E) contains both a carbohydrate portion and a protein portion.

Answer: D
Page Ref: 46

49) The nonprotein portion of an enzyme is the:

A) apoenzyme.

B) active site.

C) cofactor.

D) substrate.

E) holoenzyme.

Answer: C
Page Ref: 51

50) **ALL** of the following are **TRUE** regarding DNA and RNA **EXCEPT**:

A) Both contain pentose sugars.

B) Both contain adenine and guanine.

C) Both contain purines and pyrimidines.

D) Both have a double helix structure.

E) Three types of RNA act to carry out the instructions coded in DNA.

Answer: D
Page Ref: 54

MATCHING. Choose the item in column 2 that best matches each item in column 1.

Choose the item from column 2 that best matches each item in column 1.

1) Column 1: made up of amino acids

Column 2: proteins

Answer: proteins

Page Ref: 48

2) Column 1: glucose, fructose, and ribose are examples

Column 2: monosaccharides

Answer: monosaccharides

Page Ref: 44

3) Column 1: double helix structure
   Column 2: DNA

   Answer: DNA
   Page Ref: 54

4) Column 1: the cell's "energy currency"
   Column 2: ATP

   Answer: ATP
   Page Ref: 54

5) Column 1: starch and glycogen are
             examples
   Column 2: polysaccharides

   Answer: polysaccharides
   Page Ref: 44

6) Column 1: sucrose and lactose are
             examples
   Column 2: disaccharides

   Answer: disaccharides
   Page Ref: 44

7) Column 1: steroids and triglycerides are
             examples
   Column 2: lipids

   Answer: lipids
   Page Ref: 45

8) Column 1: electrolytes that are hydrogen
             ion donors
   Column 2: acids

   Answer: acids
   Page Ref: 38

9) Column 1: electrolytes that are hydrogen
             ion acceptors
   Column 2: bases

   Answer: bases
   Page Ref: 38

10) Column 1: acts as a solvent for ionic
            compounds in body fluids
    Column 2: water
    Answer: water
    Page Ref: 39

MATCHING. Choose the item in column 2 that best matches each item in column 1.

Choose the item from column 2 that best matches each item in column 1.

1) Column 1: substances that cannot be
            split into simpler substances
            by ordinary chemical means
    Column 2: elements
    Answer: elements
    Page Ref: 26

2) Column 1: found in the valence shells of
            an atom
    Column 2: electrons
        Foil: protons plus electrons
    Answer: electrons
    Page Ref: 27

3) Column 1: their number determines the
            atomic number of an element
    Column 2: protons
        Foil: neutrons
    Answer: protons
    Page Ref: 27

4) Column 1: atoms having the same
            number of protons, but
            different numbers of neutrons
            in their nuclei
    Column 2: isotopes
    Answer: isotopes
    Page Ref: 28

5) Column 1: their number determines the
            mass number of an element
    Column 2: protons plus neutrons
        Foil: neutrons plus electrons
    Answer: protons plus neutrons
    Page Ref: 28

6) Column 1: substances in which two or
             more atoms share electrons
   Column 2: molecules
   Answer: molecules
   Page Ref: 29

7) Column 1: electrically charged atoms or
             groups of atoms
   Column 2: free radicals
   Answer: free radicals
   Page Ref: 29

8) Column 1: substances that can be broken
             down into two or more
             different elements
   Column 2: compounds
   Answer: compounds
   Page Ref: 30

9) Column 1: ionic compounds that
             dissociate into cations and
             anions in solution
   Column 2: electrolytes
   Answer: electrolytes
   Page Ref: 31

10) Column 1: compounds that speed up
              chemical reactions by
              lowering the activation energy
    Column 2: catalysts
    Answer: catalysts
    Page Ref: 36

TRUE/FALSE. Write 'T' if the statement is true and 'F' if the statement is false.

1) The monomers of nucleic acids are nucleotides.

   Answer: TRUE
   Page Ref: 53

2) A molecule that has gained electrons has been oxidized.

   Answer: FALSE
   Page Ref: 37

3) In a solution, the solvent dissolves the solute.

Answer: TRUE
Page Ref: 38

4) All decomposition reactions that occur in the body are collectively called anabolic reactions.

Answer: FALSE
Page Ref: 36

5) The electrons of an atom are located within the atom's nucleus.

Answer: FALSE
Page Ref: 27

6) An acid is a proton acceptor.

Answer: FALSE
Page Ref: 38

7) When a covalent bond forms, neither of the combining atoms loses or gains electrons.

Answer: TRUE
Page Ref: 31

8) Molecules containing mainly nonpolar covalent bonds are hydrophilic.

Answer: FALSE
Page Ref: 39

9) The pH scale of 0 to 14 is based on the concentration of hydrogen ions in a solution.

Answer: TRUE
Page Ref: 40

10) Hydrolysis reactions are those reactions in which water molecules are added to large molecules to split them apart.

Answer: TRUE
Page Ref: 40

11) Carbonic acid is considered an example of a strong acid.

Answer: FALSE
Page Ref: 41

12) The atomic number of an atom represents the number of protons in the nucleus of the atom.

Answer: TRUE
Page Ref: 27

13) A solution with a pH of 3 contains ten times more hydrogen ions than a solution with a pH of 4.

Answer: TRUE
Page Ref: 40

14) A solution with a pH of 3 contains three moles of hydrogen ions.

Answer: FALSE
Page Ref: 40

15) Molecules that have the same molecular formula but different structures are called isotopes.

Answer: FALSE
Page Ref: 42

SHORT ANSWER. Write the word or phrase that best completes each statement or answers the question.

1) The smallest units of matter that retain the properties and characteristics of an element are

_____ .

Answer: atoms
Page Ref: 27

2) Anything living or nonliving that occupies space and has mass is known as _____ .

Answer: matter
Page Ref: 26

3) Different atoms of an element that have the same number of protons but different numbers of neutrons are called _____ .

Answer: isotopes
Page Ref: 28

4) A substance that can be broken down into two or more different elements is a _____ .

Answer: compound
Page Ref: 30

5) All organic compounds contain the elements _____ and _____ .

Answer: carbon; hydrogen
Page Ref: 42

6) Substances that can speed up chemical reactions without being altered themselves are known

as _____ .

Answer: catalysts
Page Ref: 36

7) The element that "saturates" a saturated fat is _____.
   Answer: hydrogen
   Page Ref: 45

8) The complete hydrolysis of proteins yields _____.
   Answer: amino acids
   Page Ref: 48

9) The pentose sugar found in DNA is _____.
   Answer: deoxyribose
   Page Ref: 54

10) The most abundant elements making up the human body are carbon, hydrogen, oxygen, and
    _____.
    Answer: nitrogen
    Page Ref: 26

11) In RNA, the nitrogenous bases found in the molecule can include adenine, cytosine, guanine, and _____.
    Answer: uracil
    Page Ref: 54

12) Homeostatic mechanisms maintain the pH of blood between _____ and 7.45.
    Answer: 7.35
    Page Ref: 41

13) A molecule that gains hydrogen atoms during chemical reactions in the body is said to be
    _____.
    Answer: reduced
    Page Ref: 37

14) The suffix –*ose* on a chemical name indicates that the compound is a(n) _____.
    Answer: sugar
    Page Ref: 44

15) The two factors that most influence the chance that a collision will occur between atoms are the concentration and the _____.
    Answer: temperature
    Page Ref: 36

16) Energy that travels in waves, such as light, is known as _____ energy.
    Answer: radiant
    Page Ref: 34

17) The most abundant inorganic compound in the human body is _____.
    Answer: water
    Page Ref: 39

18) The type of energy present in the bonds between atoms is known as _____ energy.
    Answer: chemical
    Page Ref: 34

19) In a solution, the substance that is dissolved is the _____.
    Answer: solute
    Page Ref: 38

20) The sum of the number of protons and neutrons in an atoms is known as the _____.
    Answer: mass number
    Page Ref: 28

21) Macromolecules are broken down into monomers by the addition of water in a reaction known as _____.
    Answer: hydrolysis
    Page Ref: 40

22) The electron shell nearest the nucleus of an atom holds a maximum of _____ electrons.
    Answer: two
    Page Ref: 30

23) An atom that has given up electrons from its outermost electron shell has become a(n) _____.
    Answer: cation (positive ion)
    Page Ref: 30

24) An atom that has accepted electrons into its outermost electron shell has become a(n) _____.
    Answer: anion (negative ion)
    Page Ref: 30

25) Triglycerides are made up of fatty acids and _____.
    Answer: glycerol
    Page Ref: 45

26) An element that is always present in protein molecules that is not necessarily present in carbohydrate molecules is _____.

Answer: nitrogen

Page Ref: 48

27) The major type of subatomic particle **NOT** found within the nucleus of an atom is the _____.

Answer: electron

Page Ref: 27

28) The standard unit for measuring the mass of atoms is the _____.

Answer: dalton (amu)

Page Ref: 28

29) An electrically charged atom or group of atoms with an unpaired electron in its outermost shell is called a(n) _____.

Answer: free radical

Page Ref: 29

30) The outermost electron shell of an atom is also called the _____ shell.

Answer: valence

Page Ref: 30

31) The protein portion of an enzyme is called the _____, and the nonprotein portion is called the _____.

Answer: apoenzyme; cofactor

Page Ref: 51

32) The reactant molecules upon which enzymes act are called _____.

Answer: substrates

Page Ref: 41

33) The process by which a protein loses its characteristic shape, and thus loses it biological function, is called _____.

Answer: denaturation

Page Ref: 41

34) A mixture in which the solute particles scatter light but do not settle out is called a(n) _____.

Answer: colloid

Page Ref: 38

35) A "water-loving" polar covalent solute is said to be _____.
    Answer: hydrophilic
    Page Ref: 39

ESSAY. Write your answer in the space provided or on a separate sheet of paper.

1) Describe/discuss the structural arrangement of the subatomic particles of an atom.
   Answer: The positively charged protons and the uncharged neutrons are located in the nucleus of the atom. Negatively charged electrons, equal in number to the protons, orbit the nucleus in various energy levels, depending on the total number of electrons.
   Page Ref: 27

2) Compare and contrast ionic vs. covalent chemical bonds.
   Answer: Chemical bonding involves either donating/receiving electrons or sharing electrons between atoms. In an ionic bond, atoms are held together by the opposite electrical charges created by donating or receiving electrons. In a covalent bond, two atoms share electrons to stabilize their outer electron orbitals without loss or gain of electrons. Most organic compounds are held together by covalent bonds. Electrolytes are held together by ionic bonds.
   Page Ref: 30–33

3) Explain the role of water in maintenance of body temperature.
   Answer: Because water has such a high heat capacity, it can absorb and release large amounts of heat with only a modest change in its own temperature, thus lessening the impact of changes in environmental temperatures on the body. Also, because of the high heat of vaporization of water, the evaporation of sweat acts as an important cooling mechanism.
   Page Ref: 40

4) Explain the relationship between water's polar covalent molecular structure and its role as a solvent in the body.
   Answer: Water's "bent" shape allows interaction with four or more other ions or molecules. Because it has positive and negative regions, solutes with polar covalent bonds (and so, also with positive and negative regions) will dissolve easily, as positive regions of the solute molecules are attracted to negative regions of the water molecules, and vice versa.
   Page Ref: 39

5) Explain the role of water in the formation and breakdown of triglycerides and proteins.
   Answer: Ester linkages result from the removal of water molecules from between each of three fatty acids and each of the three carbon atoms in glycerol. If water molecules are added to ester linkages in hydrolysis reactions, triglycerides are broken down. Similarly, the dehydration synthesis between the carboxyl group of one amino acid and the amine group of another amino acid results in the peptide bond, the characteristic bond of proteins. Hydrolysis reactions break peptide bonds via the addition of water, and thus proteins are broken down into amino acids.
   Page Ref: 45–49

6) Compare and contrast the structures of DNA and RNA.

Answer: DNA and RNA are both formed from smaller units, known as nucleotides. DNA nucleotides contain a phosphate group, deoxyribose, and a nitrogenous base —either adenine, thymine, guanine, or cytosine. RNA nucleotides contain a phosphate group, ribose, and a nitrogenous base —either adenine, uracil, guanine, or cytosine. DNA molecules are made of two strands of nucleotides joined by complementary base pairing (A–T and C–G). RNA molecules are a single strand of nucleotides, and are much shorter than DNA molecules, having been formed from a fraction of a DNA molecule.

Page Ref: 52–54

7) Describe the roles of ATP and ADP in living systems.

Answer: ATP temporarily stores energy liberated by exergonic catabolic reactions (especially the catabolism of glucose) for cellular activities that require energy. Energy is liberated from ATP when its terminal phosphate group is hydrolyzed. The liberated energy can then be used to fuel cellular activities. The "leftover" ADP then remains available to acquire a third phosphate group, and energy can be stored in the bonding of the phosphate group to form ATP.

Page Ref: 54

8) In the carbonic acid–bicarbonate buffer system, carbonic acid acts as a weak acid and bicarbonate ion acts as a weak base.
A) What does the term *weak acid* mean?
B) How can bicarbonate ion be considered a weak base, if it does not contain a hydroxide ion?
C) How could this buffer system compensate for an excess of hydrogen ions?

Answer: A) A weak acid does not ionize completely, and so, has a smaller effect on the pH of a solution than does a strong acid.
B) Bicarbonate ion acts as a hydrogen ion acceptor —another definition of a base.
C) hydrogen ions will combine with bicarbonate ion to form carbonic acid, which will dissociate into water and carbon dioxide; thus the hydrogen ion is unavailable to have an impact on pH.

Page Ref: 41

9) What are hydrogen bonds, and what is their importance to protein structure?

Answer: Hydrogen bonds form when the hydrogen atom in a polar covalent bond develops a partial positive charge that attracts the partial negative charge of neighboring electronegative atoms. Hydrogen bonds are important for stabilizing the secondary structure of proteins.

Page Ref: 33–34

10) Consider the following situation: At 8:00 PM, Patient X, a diabetic, is found to have a blood pH of 7.33. His brain tells his diaphragm to contract more frequently so that his respiratory (breathing) rate increases. At midnight, his blood pH is found to be 7.38, and his breathing rate is normal.

A) State the range of pH that is considered to be homeostatic balance for extracellular fluids.

B) Did this patient have more hydrogen ions in his blood at 8:00 PM or at midnight? How can you tell?

C) Does this illustrate a positive or a negative feedback loop? How can you tell?

Answer: A) 7.35–7.45

B) more at 8:00 PM—lower pH indicates higher hydrogen ion concentration (more acidic)

C) negative feedback loop—homeostasis is restored

Page Ref: 7, 40–41

CHAPTER 3   The Cellular Level of Organization

MULTIPLE CHOICE. Choose the one alternative that best completes the statement or answers the question.

1) The predominant lipids in the lipid bilayer of human plasma membranes are:
   A) phospholipids.
   B) glycolipids.
   C) cholesterols.
   D) lipoproteins.
   E) steroids.

   Answer: A
   Page Ref: 62

2) The term *chromatin* refers to:
   A) the color of certain cells.
   B) uncoiled DNA.
   C) highly coiled DNA.
   D) the fluid within the nucleus.
   E) the protein that makes up the mitotic spindle fibers.

   Answer: B
   Page Ref: 86

3) Organelles that contain enzymes that destroy material engulfed by phagocytes are:
   A) mitochondria.
   B) lysosomes.
   C) ribosomes.
   D) nucleoli.
   E) centrioles.

   Answer: B
   Page Ref: 83

4) Organelles that contain enzymes for production of ATP are:
   A) mitochondria.
   B) lysosomes.
   C) ribosomes.
   D) nucleoli.
   E) centrioles.

   Answer: A
   Page Ref: 84

5) How are phospholipid molecules arranged within the lipid bilayer of the plasma membrane?
   A) Phospholipid molecules are arranged randomly.
   B) The polar lipid tails are oriented toward the ECF and the ICF because they are hydrophobic.
   C) The polar phosphate heads are oriented toward the ECF and the ICF because they are hydrophilic.
   D) The nonpolar lipid tails are oriented toward the ECF and the ICF because they are hydrophobic.
   E) The nonpolar phosphate heads are oriented toward the ECF and the ICF because they are hydrophobic.

Answer: C
Page Ref: 62

6) The reason the lipid bilayer of a plasma membrane is asymmetric is that:
   A) the phospholipids are randomly arranged.
   B) glycolipids make up the outer layer, while phospholipids make up the inner layer.
   C) cholesterol molecules line up on the inner surface of the membrane.
   D) the phospholipids in the outer layer are larger molecules than those of the inner layer.
   E) glycolipids appear only on the extracellular side of the membrane.

Answer: E
Page Ref: 63

7) The glycocalyx of a cell is:
   A) a type of organelle unique to phagocytic cells.
   B) the carbohydrate portion of membrane glycolipids and glycoproteins that identifies the cell as "self."
   C) the part of a mitochondrion in which glucose is oxidized for ATP production.
   D) all of the glucose channels in a plasma membrane.
   E) a glucose storage site within a cell.

Answer: B
Page Ref: 63

8) The cell does not need to expend energy (ATP) in order to perform:
   A) osmosis.
   B) pinocytosis.
   C) facilitate diffusion.
   D) active transport.
   E) Both A and C are correct.

Answer: E
Page Ref: 67, 69

9) Carrier molecules within the plasma membrane are required in order to transport a substance across a membrane via:

   A) osmosis.

   B) filtration.

   C) facilitated diffusion.

   D) simple diffusion.

   E) exocytosis.

   Answer: C
   Page Ref: 69

10) The term *mediated transport* refers to:

   A) transport of materials into the nucleus, which is in the middle of the cell.

   B) passage of materials into the space in the middle of the two layers of the lipid bilayer.

   C) passive transport of materials at an average rate.

   D) passage of materials across a membrane with the assistance of a transporter protein.

   E) passage of materials across a membrane that requires the hydrolysis of ATP.

   Answer: D
   Page Ref: 66

11) Solutes move "down" a concentration gradient in:

   A) primary active transport.

   B) secondary active transport.

   C) osmosis.

   D) facilitated diffusion.

   E) phagocytosis.

   Answer: D
   Page Ref: 65

12) Which of the following is a form of vesicular transport?

   A) primary active transport

   B) secondary active transport

   C) osmosis

   D) pinocytosis

   E) Both B and D are correct.

   Answer: D
   Page Ref: 74

13) Symporters are transporters that:

   A) move two substances in the same direction across a membrane.

   B) move two substances in opposite directions across a membrane.

   C) can move a substance both into and out of a cell.

   D) move materials into the nucleus.

   E) move materials over the surface of a cell.

   Answer: A
   Page Ref: 66

14) Cells try to move sodium ions from the cytoplasm to the outside of the cell where the sodium concentration is 14 times higher than in the cytoplasm. This means sodium ions are moved out of the cells by:

   A) simple diffusion.

   B) facilitated diffusion.

   C) osmosis.

   D) active transport.

   E) exocytosis.

   Answer: D
   Page Ref: 70

15) Nonmotile fingerlike projections of the plasma membrane that are supported by microfilaments are called:

   A) aquaporins.

   B) cisterns.

   C) cristae.

   D) cilia.

   E) microvilli.

   Answer: E
   Page Ref: 77

16) The advantage of the presence of microvilli on cell membranes is:

   A) such cells can move.

   B) materials can be pushed across the cell surface.

   C) the membrane has a greater surface area for an increased rate of diffusion.

   D) the microvilli can extend out to engulf solid particles.

   E) the membrane is more permeable to polar substances.

   Answer: C
   Page Ref: 77

17) Which of the following would decrease the rate of diffusion across a membrane?

   A) increasing the rate of exergonic chemical reactions

   B) adding folds in the plasma membrane

   C) adding more solute to the fluid on the side of the membrane that has the greater concentration of solute

   D) splitting the diffusing substance into smaller units

   E) adding a layer of cells to the membrane

   Answer: E
   Page Ref: 67

18) Which of these substances would diffuse the fastest (assuming no inhibitions to diffusion)?

   A) a hydrogen molecule

   B) a glucose molecule

   C) DNA

   D) an oxygen molecule

   E) All substances diffuse at the same rate.

   Answer: A
   Page Ref: 67

19) Osmosis is considered a special case of diffusion because:

   A) a solute moves against its gradient.

   B) it is the net movement of solvent down its own gradient.

   C) water is moving against its own gradient.

   D) water requires a transporter protein to get through the lipid bilayer.

   E) Both C and D are correct.

   Answer: B
   Page Ref: 67

20) Aquaporins are:

   A) the places where receptors bind to ligands.

   B) the "rivers" of water flow throughout the cytosol.

   C) sites of hydrolysis within the cytoplasm.

   D) water channels in a plasma membrane.

   E) the sugar molecules that attract a fluid layer to the cell's surface.

   Answer: D
   Page Ref: 67

21) The shrinking of cells when placed in a hypertonic solution is called:

A) autophagy.

B) cytokinesis.

C) cytolysis.

D) denaturation.

E) crenation.

Answer: E
Page Ref: 69

22) The end result of mitosis is:

A) two diploid cells identical to the parent cell.

B) two haploid cells identical to the parent cell.

C) sperm cells and egg cells.

D) two cells with twice as much DNA as the parent cell.

E) one cell with twice as many organelles as the parent cell.

Answer: A
Page Ref: 91

23) Facilitated diffusion is said to have a transport maximum because:
A) when all the transporters are occupied, the rate of facilitated diffusion cannot be increased further.

B) there is a maximum size of particle that can be transported by facilitated diffusion.

C) the concentration gradient has to be of a certain steepness for facilitated diffusion to "kick in."

D) a cell can only make sufficient ATP up to a certain maximum rate to fuel facilitated diffusion.

E) once electrical charges equalize, facilitated diffusion shuts down.

Answer: A
Page Ref: 69

24) The Na^+/K^+ATPase transports:

A) both sodium and potassium ions into a cell.

B) both sodium and potassium ions out of a cell.

C) sodium ions into a cell and potassium ions out of a cell.

D) sodium ions out of a cell and potassium ions into a cell.

E) ATP across a plasma membrane.

Answer: D
Page Ref: 71

25) Energy stored in concentration gradients is used to fuel:

    A) primary active transport.

    B) secondary active transport.

    C) osmosis.

    D) receptor–mediated endocytosis.

    E) Both B and C are correct.

Answer: B
Page Ref: 72

26) Invagination of a membrane to form a vesicle in receptor–mediated endocytosis is triggered by:

    A) the hydrolysis of ATP by Na^+/K^+ ATPase.

    B) alterations in the integrity of the glycocalyx as the ligand passes through.

    C) interaction between the protein *clathrin* and the receptor-ligand complex.

    D) a reversal in the head/tail orientation of the phospholipids in the membrane.

    E) an increase in tRNA production.

Answer: C
Page Ref: 73

27) Cells that can perform phagocytosis include:

    A) red blood cells.

    B) certain white blood cells.

    C) endothelial cells lining blood vessels.

    D) neurons.

    E) Any cell can perform phagocytosis.

Answer: B
Page Ref: 74

28) During the process of translation, the code carried by mRNA is:

    A) turned into DNA.

    B) decoded into a protein.

    C) decoded into a pentose.

    D) produced by copying the DNA template.

    E) used to manufacture RNA.

Answer: B
Page Ref: 89

29) Most microfilaments are composed of:

   A) actin.

   B) tubulin.

   C) rRNA.

   D) histones.

   E) cholesterol.

   Answer: A
   Page Ref: 77

30) Cilia and flagella are made mostly of:

   A) microfilaments.

   B) intermediate filaments.

   C) microtubules.

   D) rRNA.

   E) phospholipids.

   Answer: C
   Page Ref: 78

31) The process of transcription involves production of:

   A) mRNA from a DNA template.

   B) two new DNA strands from the two original strands.

   C) DNA from an mRNA template.

   D) an amino acid chain from an mRNA template.

   E) new amino acids.

   Answer: A
   Page Ref: 87

32) The structure which plays an important role in microtubule formation in nondividing cells is the:

   A) nucleolus.

   B) Golgi complex.

   C) centrosome.

   D) glycocalyx.

   E) endoplasmic reticulum.

   Answer: C
   Page Ref: 78

33) What can you tell about the following nucleotide (nitrogenous base) sequence: ADENINE-URACIL-GUANINE?

   A) It could be part of DNA.

   B) It could be part of RNA.

   C) A complementary strand of RNA nucleotides (nitrogenous bases) would be THYMINE-ADENINE-CYTOSINE.

   D) The bases are linked by peptide bonds.

   E) Both A and C are correct.

   Answer: B
   Page Ref: 87

34) The subunits of a ribosome are produced in the:

   A) nucleolus.

   B) Golgi complex.

   C) centrosome.

   D) glycocalyx.

   E) endoplasmic reticulum.

   Answer: A
   Page Ref: 79

35) If this nitrogenous base sequence (CYTOSINE-CYTOSINE-ADENINE) represents the nucleotides of a codon, then:

   A) the anticodon would be GUANINE-GUANINE-URACIL.

   B) the complementary sequence on the sense strand of DNA is the same.

   C) it is part of tRNA.

   D) it can code for any amino acid.

   E) Both A and C are correct.

   Answer: A
   Page Ref: 87

36) Secretory proteins and membrane molecules are synthesized mainly by the:

   A) mitochondria.

   B) rough ER.

   C) centrosome.

   D) Golgi complex.

   E) nucleolus.

   Answer: B
   Page Ref: 80

37) The Golgi complex is most extensive in cells that:

   A) do not reproduce.

   B) have many mitochondria.

   C) move fluids across their surfaces.

   D) secrete proteins into the ECF.

   E) frequently change shape.

   Answer: D
   Page Ref: 81

38) The major type of storage vesicles produced by the Golgi complex is the:

   A) centrosome.

   B) nucleosome.

   C) glycocalyx.

   D) lysosome.

   E) clathrin pit.

   Answer: D
   Page Ref: 83

39) Recycling of worn out organelles is accomplished by autophagy, which is carried out by:

   A) mitochondria.

   B) the Golgi complex.

   C) ribosomes.

   D) smooth ER.

   E) lysosomes.

   Answer: E
   Page Ref: 83

40) Toxic hydrogen peroxide resulting from oxidation reactions is broken down by an enzyme in peroxisomes called:

   A) ATPase

   B) kinesin.

   C) catalase.

   D) kinase.

   E) polymerase.

   Answer: C
   Page Ref: 84

41) An electrical gradient, or membrane potential, exists across a cell membrane because in most cells the inside surface of the membrane is:

A) more negatively charged than the outside surface.

B) more positively charged that the outside surface.

C) more hydrophilic that the outside surface.

D) more hydrophobic that the outside surface.

E) richer in lipid molecules.

Answer: A
Page Ref: 65

42) The reactions of cellular respiration occur in:

A) ribosomes.

B) mitochondria.

C) smooth ER.

D) the nucleolus.

E) Both A and B are correct.

Answer: B
Page Ref: 84

43) Solution A and Solution B are separated by a selectively permeable membrane. Solution A contains 5% sodium chloride dissolved in water. Solution B contains 10% sodium chloride dissolved in water. Which of the following statements is TRUE regarding this situation?

A) Solution A has the higher osmotic pressure, because it has the greater concentration of solute.

B) Solution B has the higher osmotic pressure, because it has the greater concentration of solute.

C) Solution A has the higher osmotic pressure, because it has the greater concentration of solvent.

D) Solution B has the higher osmotic pressure, because it has the greater concentration of solvent.

E) There is no way of knowing the relative osmotic pressures of these solutions.

Answer: B
Page Ref: 68

44) Solution A contains 5% NaCl dissolved in water. Solution B contains 10% NaCl dissolved in water. Which of the following best describes the relative concentrations of these solutions?

A) Solution A is hypertonic to Solution B.

B) Solution B is hypertonic to Solution A.

C) Solutions A and B are isotonic to each other.

D) Solution B is hypotonic to Solution A.

E) Both A and D are correct.

Answer: B
Page Ref: 68

45) Red blood cell membranes are not normally permeable to NaCl, and maintain an intracellular concentration of NaCl of 0.9% If these cells are placed in a solution containing 9% NaCl, what would happen?

A) Nothing, because the membrane is not permeable to NaCl.

B) Water will enter the cell, because the intracellular fluid has a higher osmotic pressure.

C) The cell will undergo hemolysis due to membrane damage from the 9% NaCl solution.

D) The cell will undergo crenation, because the extracellular solution has a higher osmotic pressure.

E) The cell will start to generate NaCl to make up the difference in concentrations.

Answer: D
Page Ref: 69

46) Which of the following are known to be self-replicating?

A) ribosomes

B) peroxisomes

C) mitochondria

D) the Golgi complex

E) Both B and C are correct.

Answer: E
Page Ref: 84

47) Cells maintain the proper gradient to favor facilitated diffusion of glucose into cells by:

A) breaking down the transporters when the internal concentration of glucose rises too high.

B) inserting insulin into the membrane channel until internal glucose concentrations fall to proper levels.

C) attaching a phosphate group onto the glucose, thus converting it to a different compound.

D) making more ATP to help the transporters.

E) reversing the pressure gradient to close the membrane channels until glucose levels fall.

Answer: C
Page Ref: 70

48) The membranes of lysosomes contain active transport pumps to pump hydrogen ions into the lysosomes because:

A) hydrogen ions need to be destroyed.

B) the hydrogen ions will raise the pH inside the lysosome so the lysosomal enzymes can work more efficiently.

C) the hydrogen ions will lower the pH inside the lysosome so the lysosomal enzymes can work more efficiently.

D) they need to pump sodium ions out by secondary active transport.

E) the lysosomal enzymes need to be alternately reduced and oxidized to function.

Answer: C
Page Ref: 83

49) The process of meiosis results in:

A) gametes.

B) haploid cells.

C) sperm cells or oocytes.

D) cells with 23 chromosomes.

E) All of these are correct.

Answer: E
Page Ref: 91

50) Which of the following lists the phases of the cell cycle in the correct sequence?

A) S-phase, G_1-phase, G_2-phase, cytokinesis, S-phase

B) mitosis, cytokinesis, G_1-phase, G_2-phase, mitosis

C) cytokinesis, G_1-phase, S-phase, G_2-phase, mitosis

D) G_1-phase, G_2-phase, mitosis, S-phase, cytokinesis

E) G_1-phase, S-phase, G_2-phase, mitosis, cytokinesis

Answer: E
Page Ref: 91

MATCHING. Choose the item in column 2 that best matches each item in column 1.

Choose the item from column 2 that best matches each item in column 1.

1) Column 1: contains an anticodon

Column 2: tRNA

Answer: tRNA
Page Ref: 88

2) Column 1: the end result of translation

Column 2: protein

Answer: protein
Page Ref: 89

3) Column 1: the component of a ribosome made in the nucleolus

Column 2: rRNA

Answer: rRNA
Page Ref: 88

4) Column 1: template for RNA synthesis

Column 2: sense strand of DNA

Answer: sense strand of DNA
Page Ref: 89

5) Column 1: parts of sense strand that do
   not code for synthesis of part
   of a protein
   Column 2: introns
   Answer: introns
   Page Ref: 89

6) Column 1: parts of sense strand that do
   code for parts of proteins
   Column 2: exons
   Answer: exons
   Page Ref: 89

7) Column 1: contains codons
   Column 2: mRNA
   Answer: mRNA
   Page Ref: 87

8) Column 1: part of DNA that connects
   nucleosomes
   Column 2: linker DNA
   Answer: linker DNA
   Page Ref: 86

9) Column 1: double–stranded DNA
   wrapped around histones
   Column 2: nucleosome
   Answer: nucleosome
   Page Ref: 86

10) Column 1: proteins that help organize
    the coiling and folding ability
    of DNA
    Column 2: histones
    Answer: histones
    Page Ref: 86

MATCHING. Choose the item in column 2 that best matches each item in column 1.

Choose the item from column 2 that best matches each item in column 1.

1) Column 1: controls what enters and
   leaves the cell
   Column 2: plasma membrane
   Answer: plasma membrane
   Page Ref: 62

2) Column 1: provide mechanical support
   responsible for strength and
   shapes of cells
   Column 2: microfilaments
   Answer: microfilaments
   Page Ref: 77

3) Column 1: site of mRNA synthesis
   Column 2: nucleus
   Foil: cytosol
   Answer: nucleus
   Page Ref: 85

4) Column 1: wave to ensure steady fluid
   movement along a cell's
   surface
   Column 2: cilia
   Answer: cilia
   Page Ref: 79

5) Column 1: function to move an entire cell
   Column 2: flagella
   Answer: flagella
   Page Ref: 79

6) Column 1: sites of protein synthesis
   Column 2: ribosomes
   Answer: ribosomes
   Page Ref: 79

7) Column 1: organizing center for mitotic spindle

Column 2: centrosome

Answer: centrosome

Page Ref: 78

8) Column 1: synthesizes phospholipids, fats, and steroids

Column 2: smooth ER

Answer: smooth ER

Page Ref: 81

9) Column 1: responsible for the modification, sorting, and packaging of secreted products

Column 2: Golgi complex

Answer: Golgi complex

Page Ref: 81

10) Column 1: vesicular structures that contain many types of enzymes to break down a wide variety of molecules

Column 2: lysosomes

Answer: lysosomes

Page Ref: 83

11) Column 1: vesicular structures that contain enzymes, such as catalase, that oxidize toxic substances

Column 2: peroxisomes

Answer: peroxisomes

Page Ref: 84

12) Column 1: double–membrane–bound organelle containing enzymes for cellular respiration

Column 2: mitochondria

Answer: mitochondria

Page Ref: 84

TRUE/FALSE. Write 'T' if the statement is true and 'F' if the statement is false.

1) The rupture of red blood cells due to their placement into a hypotonic solution is known as crenation.

   Answer: FALSE
   Page Ref: 69

2) Transcription is the process by which the genetic information found in DNA is copied onto messenger RNA.

   Answer: TRUE
   Page Ref: 87

3) The DNA strand which serves as a template for RNA synthesis is referred to as the antisense strand.

   Answer: FALSE
   Page Ref: 89

4) Cilia are responsible for moving entire cells.

   Answer: FALSE
   Page Ref: 79

5) The cristae of mitochondria increase the surface area available for chemical reactions.

   Answer: TRUE
   Page Ref: 84

6) The chemical reactions of cellular respiration occur on ribosomes.

   Answer: FALSE
   Page Ref: 79

7) Haploid cells result from the process of mitosis.

   Answer: FALSE
   Page Ref: 91

8) Regions within a gene that code for protein synthesis are called exons.

   Answer: TRUE
   Page Ref: 89

9) Cells that do not have a nucleus cannot reproduce.

   Answer: TRUE
   Page Ref: 85

10) Chromatid pairs are lined up on the equator of the spindle apparatus during metaphase of mitosis.

Answer: TRUE
Page Ref: 94

11) DNA replication occurs during the S phase of interphase.

Answer: TRUE
Page Ref: 92

12) The major compound making up plasma membranes is cholesterol.

Answer: FALSE
Page Ref: 62

13) Transporters that move two substances in the same direction across a membrane are called symporters.

Answer: TRUE
Page Ref: 72

14) Osmosis does not require the expenditure of ATP by a cell.

Answer: TRUE
Page Ref: 67

15) The larger the molecule, the faster the rate of diffusion.

Answer: FALSE
Page Ref: 67

SHORT ANSWER. Write the word or phrase that best completes each statement or answers the question.

1) If Solution A has proportionally more solutes and less water than Solution B, then Solution A is considered to be _____ to Solution B.

Answer: hypertonic
Page Ref: 69

2) A group of nucleotides on a DNA molecule whose purpose is to serve as the "directions" for manufacturing a specific protein is a _____.

Answer: gene
Page Ref: 86

3) Distribution of two sets of chromosomes into two separate and equal nuclei is known as _____.

Answer: mitosis
Page Ref: 91

4) The cytosol and the organelles are the two components of the _____.
Answer: cytoplasm
Page Ref: 60

5) Because phospholipids have both polar and nonpolar parts, they are said to be _____.
Answer: amphipathic
Page Ref: 62

6) The part of a phospholipid molecule that is hydrophilic is the _____.
Answer: head (polar end or phosphate-containing end)
Page Ref: 62

7) Chromosome number does not double with each generation of cell division because of a special nuclear division called _____.
Answer: meiosis
Page Ref: 91

8) Membrane proteins that extend across the entire lipid bilayer are known as _____ proteins.
Answer: integral
Page Ref: 63

9) The sugar coat that provides a means of cellular recognition is known as the _____.
Answer: glycocalyx
Page Ref: 63

10) The property of membranes that allows some substances to pass more readily than others is called _____.
Answer: selective permeability
Page Ref: 64

11) The fluid mosaic model describes the structure of the _____.
Answer: plasma membrane
Page Ref: 61

12) Transmembrane proteins that function as water channels are called _____.
Answer: aquaporins
Page Ref: 67

13) The part of a phospholipid molecule that lines up facing away from the intracellular and the extracellular fluids is the _____.
Answer: tail (hydrophobic, nonpolar, lipid part)
Page Ref: 62

14) In facilitated diffusion, once all the transporters are occupied, it is said that the _____ has been reached.

Answer: transport maximum

Page Ref: 70

15) The peripheral protein lining pits involved in the binding phase of receptor–mediated endocytosis is called _____.

Answer: clathrin

Page Ref: 73

16) Projections of the plasma membrane and cytoplasm of a phagocytic cell toward its target are called _____.

Answer: pseudopods

Page Ref: 74

17) The cytoskeleton includes microfilaments, intermediate filaments, and _____.

Answer: microtubules

Page Ref: 78

18) There is no net movement of water molecules across a membrane separating solutions that are _____ to each other.

Answer: isotonic

Page Ref: 69

19) The two subunits of ribosomes are produced in the _____.

Answer: nucleolus

Page Ref: 86

20) A type of passive transport across a plasma membrane that requires special transporters is _____.

Answer: facilitated diffusion

Page Ref: 69

21) Rough ER is called "rough" because its outer surface is studded with _____.

Answer: ribosomes

Page Ref: 79

22) Export of substances from the cell in which vesicles fuse with the plasma membrane and release their contents into the extracellular fluid is known as _____.

Answer: exocytosis

Page Ref: 75

23) The bulging edges of the membranous sacs forming the Golgi complex are called _____.

Answer: cisterns

Page Ref: 81

24) The process by which lysosomes destroy the cells they are part of is called _____.

Answer: autolysis

Page Ref: 83

25) The proteins around which DNA wraps in a chromatin fiber are called _____.

Answer: histones

Page Ref: 86

26) A coupled transporter that moves two substances in opposite directions across a membrane is called a(n) _____.

Answer: antiporter

Page Ref: 72

27) The folds of the inner mitochondrial membrane are called _____.

Answer: cristae

Page Ref: 84

28) RNA polymerase attaches to a gene at a special nucleotide sequence called a _____, located near the beginning of a gene.

Answer: promoter

Page Ref: 88

29) Each set of three consecutive nucleotide bases on messenger RNA that specifies one amino acid is called a _____.

Answer: codon

Page Ref: 87

30) Division of a parent cell's cytoplasm and organelles is called _____.

Answer: cytokinesis

Page Ref: 94

31) The triplet of nucleotides on tRNA opposite the end carrying the amino acid is called the _____.

Answer: anticodon

Page Ref: 89

32) Organisms that have been altered by the insertion of genes that code for proteins not normally produced by the organism are called _____.

Answer: recombinants

Page Ref: 89

33) _____ cell division replaces dead or injured cells and adds new ones for tissue growth.

Answer: Somatic

Page Ref: 91

34) The process by which cells are programmed to die at a certain point is called _____.

Answer: apoptosis

Page Ref: 94

35) Pathological cell death is known as _____.

Answer: necrosis

Page Ref: 94

ESSAY. Write your answer in the space provided or on a separate sheet of paper.

1) Describe the various functions of membrane proteins.

Answer: Membrane proteins include
  A) **channels** through which a specific substance passes,
  B) **transporters** which change shape to move a bound substance across the membrane,
  C) **receptors** that recognize and bind specific molecules needed for cellular activity,
  D) **enzymes** that catalyze chemical reactions,
  E) **cell–identity markers** that make the cell recognizable as one of one's own cells (vs. a foreign cell), and
  F) **linkers** , or **anchoring proteins**, that stabilize a cell's position.

Page Ref: 63

2) Define *diffusion* and identify the factors that affect the rate of diffusion of substances across plasma membranes. Describe the effect of each factor on the rate of diffusion.

Answer: Diffusion is the passive movement of particles from an area of higher concentration to an area of lower concentration (i.e., "down" a concentration gradient). Factors affecting the rate of diffusion include
  A) steepness of the concentration gradient (the greater the difference in concentration, the greater the rate of diffusion),
  B) temperature (the higher the temperature, the greater the rate of diffusion),
  C) mass of the diffusing substance (the greater the mass, the slower the rate of diffusion),
  D) surface area of the membrane (the greater the surface area, the greater the rate of diffusion), and
  E) diffusion distance (the greater the distance, the slower the rate of diffusion).

Page Ref: 66–67

3) Discuss the fluid mosaic model of plasma membrane structure.

Answer: Proteins "float" among phospholipids; phospholipid bilayer, with hydrophobic ends facing each other and hydrophilic ends facing either ECF or ICF; phospholipids can move sideways within layer; glycolipids (cellular identity markers) face ECF; cholesterol molecules (for stability) among phospholipids of both layers of the bilayer; integral proteins (channels, transporters, etc.) extend across phospholipid bilayer; peripheral proteins (enzymes, cytoskeleton anchors, etc.) loosely attached to either the inner or outer surface of the membrane

Page Ref: 62–64

4) Name and describe the four phases of mitosis in sequence.

Answer: 1. Prophase—chromatin fibers shorten and coil into chromosomes; nucleoli and nuclear envelope disappear; centrosomes with centrioles move to opposite poles of cell; mitotic spindle appears
2. Metaphase—centromeres of chromatid pairs line up on metaphase plate of cell
3. Anaphase—centromeres divide; identical sets of chromosomes move to opposite poles of cell
4. Telophase—nuclear envelope reappears to enclose chromosomes; chromosomes revert to chromatin; nucleoli reappear; mitotic spindle disappears

Page Ref: 92–94

5) In the disease *emphysema* respiratory membranes become thickened, and the tiny air sacs known as alveoli merge into larger units. Using your knowledge of the factors affecting the rate of diffusion across a membrane, predict what will happen to the rate of diffusion of respiratory gases across the membrane between the alveoli and the blood. Explain your answer.

Answer: Thickened membranes increase the diffusion distance and lower the rate of diffusion. Fusion of alveoli reduces the surface area, thus further reducing rate of diffusion. Very clever students may also predict altered concentration gradients, which will also lower the rate of diffusion.

Page Ref: 67

6) Name the three types of RNA and describe the role of each in protein synthesis.

Answer: 1. messenger RNA—produced from sense strand of DNA via transcription; carries code for making a particular protein from the nucleus to the ribosome
2. ribosomal RNA—makes up the ribosome; moves along the mRNA strand to "read" directions for making protein
3. transfer RNA—transports specific amino acids from the cytoplasm to the growing peptide chain; places amino acids in proper sequence by matching its anticodon with an appropriate codon on the mRNA strand

Page Ref: 87–88

7) Compare and contrast primary and secondary active transport.

Answer: Both are mediated, energy-requiring processes moving substances against their concentration gradients. Energy obtained from hydrolysis of ATP drives primary active transport, while energy stored in an ionic concentration gradient drives secondary active transport.

Page Ref: 70–72

8) Compare and contrast simple diffusion and osmosis.

Answer: Both are passive types of movements. Simple diffusion involves the net movement of solute molecules from an area of higher solute concentration to an area of lower solute concentration. Osmosis involves the movement of water (solvent) across a semipermeable membrane from an area of higher water concentration to an area of lower water concentration. Both may occur through the lipid bilayer or through special channels.

Page Ref: 66–68

9) Describe the process of receptor–mediated endocytosis.

Answer: The ligand binds to a specific receptor on the outer side of the membrane. An interaction between the receptor–ligand complex and the peripheral protein, clathrin, triggers an invagination of the membrane to form a clathrin–coated vesicle around the receptor–ligand complex. The clathrin coat is lost and several vesicles fuse to form an endosome. Receptors and ligands separate, and the receptors get recycled via carrier vesicles. Ligands may be degraded in lysosomes or may be transported across cells for exocytosis from the opposite side of the cell.

Page Ref: 73

10) Describe the process of transcription.

Answer: Transcription occurs in the nucleus, and is catalyzed by RNA polymerase. The RNA polymerase binds to the promoter nucleotide sequence, and the sense strand of DNA is exposed. Complementary RNA nucleotides bind to the exposed DNA nucleotides (adenine to thymine, uracil to adenine, cytosine to guanine, and guanine to cytosine). The transcription process ceases at the terminator nucleotide sequence, as the RNA polymerase detaches from the DNA and transcribed RNA molecule.

Page Ref: 87–89

CHAPTER 4   The Tissue Level of Organization

MULTIPLE CHOICE. Choose the one alternative that best completes the statement or answers the question.

   1) Which of the following tissues has the **least** amount of matrix?
     A) stratified squamous epithelium
     B) areolar connective tissue
     C) osseous tissue
     D) dense irregular connective tissue
     E) blood

    Answer: A
    Page Ref: 106

   2) Microvilli and goblet cells are typical modifications of:
     A) skeletal muscle tissue.
     B) simple columnar epithelium.
     C) osseous tissue.
     D) hyaline cartilage.
     E) nervous tissue.

    Answer: B
    Page Ref: 109

   3) The tissue that forms glands is:
     A) epithelial tissue.
     B) connective tissue.
     C) nervous tissue.
     D) muscle tissue.
     E) mesenchyme.

    Answer: A
    Page Ref: 104

   4) Mesoderm is the source of:
     A) some epithelial tissue.
     B) most muscle tissue.
     C) all connective tissue.
     D) most nervous tissue.
     E) A, B, and C are all correct.

    Answer: E
    Page Ref: 104

5) Nervous tissue develops from which germ layer?

   A) ectoderm only

   B) endoderm only

   C) mesoderm only

   D) both ectoderm and endoderm

   E) all three germ layers

   Answer: A
   Page Ref: 104

6) Fibroblasts are the typical cells of:

   A) simple squamous epithelium.

   B) dense connective tissue.

   C) cardiac muscle tissue.

   D) skeletal muscle tissue.

   E) nervous tissue.

   Answer: B
   Page Ref: 118

7) The type of cell junction that prevents the contents of the stomach or urinary bladder from leaking into surrounding tissues is the:

   A) adherens junction.

   B) gap junction.

   C) hemidesmosome.

   D) desmosome.

   E) tight junction.

   Answer: E
   Page Ref: 105

8) A dense layer of proteins, called plaque, forms:

   A) gap junctions.

   B) the glycocalyx.

   C) adherens junctions.

   D) microvilli.

   E) the striations of skeletal muscle.

   Answer: C
   Page Ref: 105

9) Intermediate filaments are important components of:
    A) adherens junctions.
    B) gap junctions.
    C) tight junctions.
    D) desmosomes.
    E) Both B and D are correct.

Answer: D
Page Ref: 105

10) Connexons are:
    A) the typical cells of connective tissue.
    B) fibers that provide nutrient waste and gas exchange for epithelial cells.
    C) proteins found in muscle fibers.
    D) the route by which osteocytes in osseous tissue receive nutrients.
    E) proteins in gap junctions that form the channels that provide a means of ion exchange between cells at gap junctions.

Answer: E
Page Ref: 105

11) Which of the following is typical of an endocrine gland?
    A) It releases hormones.
    B) It is made of epithelial tissue.
    C) It releases its products into ducts that empty onto epithelial surfaces.
    D) Both A and B are correct.
    E) Both B and C are correct.

Answer: D
Page Ref: 116

12) Ions and small molecules can travel between cells via:
    A) tight junctions.
    B) adherens junctions.
    C) gap junctions.
    D) desmosomes.
    E) Both A and C are correct.

Answer: C
Page Ref: 105

13) Which of the following tissues is avascular?

    A) adipose tissue

    B) areolar connective tissue

    C) cardiac muscle tissue

    D) skeletal muscle tissue

    E) stratified squamous epithelium

Answer: E
Page Ref: 106

14) **ALL** of the following are **TRUE** for epithelial tissues **EXCEPT**:

    A) they attach to connective tissues via a basement membrane.

    B) they have a rich blood supply.

    C) they have a high rate of cell division.

    D) they have a nerve supply.

    E) there is little extracellular space between adjacent plasma membranes.

Answer: B
Page Ref: 106

15) Which of the following connective tissue cells secrete antibodies?

    A) adipocytes

    B) fibroblasts

    C) macrophages

    D) mast cells

    E) plasma cells

Answer: E
Page Ref: 118

16) Hyaline cartilage is found in **ALL** of the following locations **EXCEPT** the:

    A) embryonic skeleton.

    B) trachea.

    C) bronchial tubes.

    D) intervertebral discs.

    E) nose.

Answer: D
Page Ref: 125

17) Which of the following tissues provides the greatest protection from mechanical injury?
    A) stratified squamous epithelium
    B) dense regular connective tissue
    C) smooth muscle
    D) simple cuboidal epithelium
    E) elastic cartilage

Answer: A
Page Ref: 110

18) Endothelium forms:
    A) endocrine glands.
    B) exocrine glands.
    C) the lining of the heart and blood vessels.
    D) the inner layer of the skin.
    E) Both A and B are correct.

Answer: C
Page Ref: 107

19) The function of the basement membrane is to:
    A) provide a blood supply to epithelial tissue.
    B) hold cartilage onto bone.
    C) house the reproducing cells of stratified squamous epithelium.
    D) anchor epithelial tissues onto underlying connective tissue.
    E) secrete matrix.

Answer: D
Page Ref: 106

20) Mucus is produced by:
    A) goblet cells.
    B) endocrine glands.
    C) exocrine glands.
    D) microvilli.
    E) Both A and C are correct.

Answer: E
Page Ref: 115

21) Gap junctions are seen in tissues which:

  A) fluid leakage between cells is a particular risk.

  B) cells may be damaged by friction or stretching.

  C) move from one location to another.

  D) electrical or chemical signals must pass between cells.

  E) adjacent cells are many millimeters apart.

  Answer: D
  Page Ref: 105

22) Secretion and absorption are important functions of:

  A) adipose tissue.

  B) smooth muscle.

  C) stratified squamous epithelium.

  D) simple cuboidal epithelium.

  E) Both C and D are correct.

  Answer: D
  Page Ref: 107

23) Microvilli and goblet cells are characteristic of:

  A) areolar connective tissue.

  B) simple squamous epithelium.

  C) simple columnar epithelium.

  D) skeletal muscle tissue.

  E) All of these could have microvilli and goblet cells.

  Answer: C
  Page Ref: 115

24) Cilia are commonly seen on cells in tissues that:

  A) line the blood vessels.

  B) line the respiratory tract.

  C) form the skin.

  D) move from one place to another.

  E) All of these are correct.

  Answer: B
  Page Ref: 115

25) Keratin is seen in tissues that:

    A) resist friction.

    B) move throughout the body.

    C) engulf bacteria.

    D) are important for diffusion and absorption.

    E) transmit nerve impulses.

Answer: A
Page Ref: 115

26) The type of epithelium seen in the **urinary bladder** is:

    A) simple squamous epithelium.

    B) simple cuboidal epithelium.

    C) pseudostratified columnar epithelium.

    D) stratified squamous epithelium.

    E) transitional epithelium.

Answer: E
Page Ref: 115

27) Mesothelium is seen in:

    A) kidney tubules.

    B) serous membranes.

    C) the urinary bladder.

    D) the lining of the heart and blood vessels.

    E) skin.

Answer: B
Page Ref: 107

28) Most of the upper respiratory tract is lined with:

    A) hyaline cartilage.

    B) keratinized stratified squamous epithelium.

    C) ciliated pseudostratified columnar epithelium.

    D) transitional epithelium.

    E) skeletal muscle.

Answer: C
Page Ref: 115

29) Which of the following is considered a unicellular exocrine gland?

A) mast cell

B) plasma cell

C) fibroblast

D) adipocyte

E) goblet cell

Answer: E
Page Ref: 116

30) The surface area for diffusion across the membranes of cells in simple columnar epithelium is increased by the presence of:

A) goblet cells.

B) microvilli.

C) cilia.

D) desmosomes.

E) All of the above increase surface area.

Answer: B
Page Ref: 115

31) An exocrine gland in which a cell filled with a secretory product dies and becomes the secretory product is called a(n):

A) acinar gland.

B) apocrine gland.

C) holocrine gland.

D) merocrine gland.

E) simple gland.

Answer: C
Page Ref: 117

32) One might expect to see microvilli on epithelial tissues whose principal function is:

A) protection.

B) movement.

C) absorption.

D) mineral storage.

E) transmission of electrical impulses.

Answer: C
Page Ref: 115

33) Stratified squamous epithelium can be made waterproof and friction resistant by intracellular deposits of:

A) collagen

B) hyaluronidase.

C) chondroitin sulfate.

D) mucus.

E) keratin.

Answer: E
Page Ref: 115

34) Most exocrine glands in the human body are classified as:

A) acinar glands.

B) apocrine glands.

C) holocrine glands.

D) merocrine glands.

E) endocrine glands.

Answer: D
Page Ref: 117

35) Most exocrine glands in the human body release their products by:

A) pinching them off into the apical surface of the cell.

B) active transport through specific ion channels.

C) death and subsequent rupture of the secretory cell.

D) simple diffusion.

E) exocytosis.

Answer: E
Page Ref: 117

36) The matrix of a connective tissue consists of:

A) ground substance and fibers.

B) all the of the functioning cells of a tissue.

C) microfilaments and microtubules.

D) an embryonic form of the connective tissue.

E) mesoderm and endoderm.

Answer: A
Page Ref: 118

37) The most abundant tissue in the body is:

    A) epithelium tissue.

    B) connective tissue.

    C) muscle tissue.

    D) nervous tissue.

    E) All tissues are equally abundant when the body is in homeostasis.

Answer: B
Page Ref: 118

38) The basic tissue type whose function is particularly related to the form of its matrix (solid, semisolid, or liquid) is:

    A) epithelium tissue.

    B) connective tissue.

    C) muscle tissue.

    D) nervous tissue.

    E) the structure of the matrix is unrelated to the functioning of tissues

Answer: B
Page Ref: 118

39) The suffix *–blast* in a cell name indicates a(n):

    A) cell that has ruptured.

    B) mature cell with reduced capacity for cell division.

    C) cell that is part of an exocrine gland.

    D) immature cell that can still divide.

    E) cell that is part of the stroma of an organ.

Answer: D
Page Ref: 118

40) The embryonic connective tissue from which all other connective tissues arise is:

    A) areolar connective tissue.

    B) mucous connective tissue.

    C) hyaline cartilage.

    D) neuroglia.

    E) mesenchyme.

Answer: E
Page Ref: 120

41) The diffusion of injected drugs can be enhanced by the action of hyaluronidase because it:
   A) increases the rate of ATP synthesis.
   B) raises the local temperature by causing inflammation, so molecules move faster.
   C) lowers the viscosity of the matrix of areolar connective tissue.
   D) forms new, tighter junctions between the cells of connective tissue.
   E) increases the rate of matrix secretion by fibroblasts.

   Answer: C
   Page Ref: 119

42) Histiocytes are:
   A) macrophages in areolar connective tissue.
   B) cells that produce histamine.
   C) cells that produce antibodies.
   D) cells that secrete the matrix of connective tissue.
   E) stem cells that form skeletal muscle cells.

   Answer: A
   Page Ref: 118

43) The principal adhesion protein of connective tissue is:
   A) fibrillin.
   B) chondroitin sulfate.
   C) collagen.
   D) fibronectin.
   E) hyaluronic acid.

   Answer: D
   Page Ref: 119

44) **ALL** of the following are functions of adipose tissue **EXCEPT**:
   A) support.
   B) protection.
   C) formation of certain glands.
   D) insulation.
   E) energy reserve.

   Answer: C
   Page Ref: 122

45) *Nonstriated* and *involuntary* are terms used to describe:

   A) skeletal muscle tissue.

   B) smooth muscle tissue.

   C) cardiac muscle tissue.

   D) hyaline cartilage.

   E) Both B and C are correct.

   Answer: B
   Page Ref: 130

46) Nutrient and waste exchange between osteocytes and blood vessels in the central canals of osteons occurs via structures called:

   A) lacunae.

   B) lamellae.

   C) canaliculi.

   D) trabeculae.

   E) connexons.

   Answer: C
   Page Ref: 129

47) The space between the parietal and visceral layers of a membrane, such as the pericardium, is normally filled with:

   A) air.

   B) blood.

   C) serous fluid.

   D) synovial fluid.

   E) adipose tissue.

   Answer: C
   Page Ref: 130

48) Both desmosomes and gap junctions are found in the intercalated discs connecting cells of:

   A) adipose tissue.

   B) osseous tissue.

   C) skeletal muscle tissue.

   D) cardiac muscle tissue.

   E) simple squamous epithelium.

   Answer: D
   Page Ref: 130

49) If fibrosis occurs during tissue repair, then:
   A) a perfect reconstruction of the injured tissue occurs.
   B) rapid replication of parenchymal cells has occurred.
   C) the function of the repaired tissue is impaired.
   D) only connective tissue was involved in the injury.
   E) Both B and C are correct.

   Answer: C
   Page Ref: 133

50) The scab over a wound to the skin is formed primarily by:
   A) keratin in the epidermis.
   B) calcium salts.
   C) serous fluid as it evaporates.
   D) fibrin in blood clots.
   E) collagen in torn connective tissue.

   Answer: D
   Page Ref: 134

MATCHING. Choose the item in column 2 that best matches each item in column 1.

Choose the item from column 2 that best matches each item in column 1.

1) Column 1: produce mucus
   Column 2: goblet cells
   Answer: goblet cells
   Page Ref: 115

2) Column 1: may contain keratin
   Column 2: stratified squamous epithelial
            cells
      Foil: simple squamous epithelial
            cells
   Answer: stratified squamous epithelial cells
   Page Ref: 115

3) Column 1: secrete collagen
   Column 2: fibroblasts
   Answer: fibroblasts
   Page Ref: 118

4) Column 1: develop from white blood cells
           called monocytes
   Column 2: macrophages
   Answer: macrophages
   Page Ref: 118

5) Column 1: develop from white blood cells
           called B lymphocytes
   Column 2: plasma cells
      Foil: platelets
   Answer: plasma cells
   Page Ref: 118

6) Column 1: produce histamine
   Column 2: mast cells
   Answer: mast cells
   Page Ref: 118

7) Column 1: fat storage cells
   Column 2: adipocytes
   Answer: adipocytes
   Page Ref: 122

8) Column 1: bone cells
   Column 2: osteocytes
   Answer: osteocytes
   Page Ref: 129

9) Column 1: cells described as being
           striated and voluntary
   Column 2: skeletal muscle cells
      Foil: neurons
   Answer: skeletal muscle cells
   Page Ref: 130

10) Column 1: attached to each other via
            intercalated discs
    Column 2: cardiac muscle cells
       Foil: smooth muscle cells
    Answer: cardiac muscle cells
    Page Ref: 130

MATCHING. Choose the item in column 2 that best matches each item in column 1.

Choose the item from column 2 that best matches each item in column 1.

1) Column 1: connective tissue specialized
   for fat storage
   Column 2: adipose tissue
   Answer: adipose tissue
   Page Ref: 122

2) Column 1: embryonic connective tissue
   from which all other
   connective tissues are derived
   Column 2: mesenchyme
   Foil: mucous connective tissue
   Answer: mesenchyme
   Page Ref: 120

3) Column 1: very tough connective tissue
   containing many parallel
   collagen fibers
   Column 2: dense regular connective
   tissue
   Answer: dense regular connective tissue
   Page Ref: 127

4) Column 1: an especially smooth type of
   simple squamous epithelium
   that lines the heart and blood
   vessels
   Column 2: endothelium
   Answer: endothelium
   Page Ref: 107

5) Column 1: multiple layers of flat cells
   designed for protection
   Column 2: stratified squamous
   epithelium
   Answer: stratified squamous epithelium
   Page Ref: 115

6) Column 1: cells may have microvilli
   and/or cilia
   Column 2: simple columnar epithelium
   Answer: simple columnar epithelium
   Page Ref: 115

7) Column 1: found in serous membranes
             and produces serous fluid
   Column 2: mesothelium

   Answer: mesothelium
   Page Ref: 107

8) Column 1: most widely distributed tissue
             in body; located under skin
             and around all organs and
             vessels
   Column 2: areolar connective tissue

   Answer: areolar connective tissue
   Page Ref: 121

9) Column 1: found only in the wall of the
             heart; contains intercalated
             discs
   Column 2: cardiac muscle tissue

   Answer: cardiac muscle tissue
   Page Ref: 130

10) Column 1: covers ends of bones at joints;
             forms much of embryonic
             skeleton
    Column 2: hyaline cartilage
        Foil: fibrocartilage

    Answer: hyaline cartilage
    Page Ref: 128

TRUE/FALSE. Write 'T' if the statement is true and 'F' if the statement is false.

1) Epithelial cells do not have a direct nerve supply.

   Answer: FALSE
   Page Ref: 106

2) There is synovial fluid between the layers of a serous membrane.

   Answer: FALSE
   Page Ref: 130

3) Connective tissues do not occur on free surfaces, such as the external surface of the body.

   Answer: TRUE
   Page Ref: 118

4) The lamina propria is the areolar connective tissue supporting the epithelial layer of a mucous membrane.

Answer: TRUE
Page Ref: 129

5) Both skeletal and cardiac muscle cells are striated.

Answer: TRUE
Page Ref: 130

6) Dendrites and axons are extensions of neuroglia.

Answer: FALSE
Page Ref: 132

7) Of the four main tissue types, nervous tissue has the poorest capacity for renewal.

Answer: TRUE
Page Ref: 133

8) Epithelial tissues derive only from ectoderm.

Answer: FALSE
Page Ref: 104

9) Gap junctions allow communication between cells in a tissue.

Answer: TRUE
Page Ref: 105

10) The cardinal factor in the restoration of normal function during tissue repair is the capacity of the parenchymal cells to replicate quickly.

Answer: TRUE
Page Ref: 133

11) The apical surface of an epithelial cell adheres to adjacent connective tissue.

Answer: FALSE
Page Ref: 106

12) The pleura and the pericardium each have both parietal and visceral layers.

Answer: TRUE
Page Ref: 130

13) Macrophages may travel from one tissue to another.

Answer: TRUE
Page Ref: 118

14) Mesenchyme is the embryonic connective tissue from which all other connective tissues arise.

Answer: TRUE
Page Ref: 120

15) Epithelial tissues contain a large amount of intercellular substance.

Answer: FALSE
Page Ref: 106

SHORT ANSWER. Write the word or phrase that best completes each statement or answers the question.

1) The primary function of stratified squamous epithelium is _____.

Answer: protection
Page Ref: 115

2) Simple squamous epithelium that lines the heart, blood vessels, and lymphatic vessels, and forms the walls of the capillaries is _____.

Answer: endothelium
Page Ref: 107

3) _____ glands secrete their products into ducts.

Answer: Exocrine
Page Ref: 116

4) Antibodies are produced by connective tissue cells known as _____.

Answer: plasma cells
Page Ref: 118

5) The principal adhesion protein of connective tissue is _____.

Answer: fibronectin
Page Ref: 119

6) The stroma of soft organs is formed by _____ fibers.

Answer: reticular
Page Ref: 123

7) The cells of mature cartilage are called _____.

Answer: chondrocytes
Page Ref: 128

8) The connective tissue from which all other connective tissues eventually arise is _____.

Answer: mesenchyme
Page Ref: 120

9) Spaces in the matrix of cartilage or bone in which cells are located are called _____.
Answer: lacunae
Page Ref: 129

10) The type of cartilage that always lacks a perichondrium is _____.
Answer: fibrocartilage
Page Ref: 128

11) The type of membrane that lines a body cavity that does not open to the exterior is a _____.
Answer: serous membrane
Page Ref: 130

12) The connections between cardiac muscle cells are called _____.
Answer: intercalated discs
Page Ref: 130

13) The type of cartilage growth in which new matrix is added on to the surface of existing cartilage is called _____ growth.
Answer: appositional
Page Ref: 128

14) Columns of bone forming spongy bone are called _____.
Answer: trabeculae
Page Ref: 129

15) The surface area of the apical surfaces of epithelial cell membranes is increased by the presence of _____.
Answer: microvilli
Page Ref: 115

16) Goblet cells produce _____.
Answer: mucus
Page Ref: 115

17) The liquid matrix of blood tissue is called _____.
Answer: plasma
Page Ref: 129

18) Membranes lining joints are called _____ membranes.
Answer: synovial
Page Ref: 130

19) The type of cell in areolar connective tissue that produces histamine is the _____.
Answer: mast cell
Page Ref: 118

20) The portion of a serous membrane attached to the cavity wall is called the _____ layer.
Answer: parietal
Page Ref: 130

21) The part of a neuron that contains the nucleus is the _____.
Answer: cell body
Page Ref: 132

22) Cells in nervous tissue that do not generate or conduct nerve impulses are called _____.
Answer: neuroglia
Page Ref: 132

23) Cells that constitute a tissue's or an organ's functioning part are called the _____.
Answer: parenchyma
Page Ref: 133

24) The immature cells of each major type of connective tissue have names that end in the suffix
_____.
Answer: –blast
Page Ref: 118

25) The three types of fibers seen in connective tissue are _____ fibers, _____ fibers, and _____
fibers.
Answer: collagen, elastic, reticular
Page Ref: 119–120

26) The reticular connective tissue that forms the supporting framework for many soft organs is
known as the _____.
Answer: stroma
Page Ref: 123

27) The basic unit of compact bone is the _____.
Answer: osteon (Haversian system)
Page Ref: 128

28) The type of tissue that is described as being striated and voluntary is _____ tissue.
Answer: skeletal muscle
Page Ref: 130

29) The process of scar formation is known as _____.
   Answer: fibrosis
   Page Ref: 133

30) The actively growing connective tissue that provides a framework that supports epithelial cells is known as _____.
   Answer: granulation tissue
   Page Ref: 134

31) _____ are scar tissues that form abnormal joining of tissues.
   Answer: Adhesions
   Page Ref: 134

32) A decrease in the size of cells is called _____.
   Answer: atrophy
   Page Ref: 135

33) Hormones are secreted by _____ glands.
   Answer: endocrine
   Page Ref: 116

34) Reducing heat loss and serving as an energy reserve are important functions of _____ tissue.
   Answer: adipose
   Page Ref: 122

35) Tendons and most ligaments are made of _____ connective tissue.
   Answer: dense regular
   Page Ref: 123

ESSAY. Write your answer in the space provided or on a separate sheet of paper.

1) Name the four principal types of human tissues, and briefly describe the function of each.
   Answer: 1. Epithelial tissue —covers body surfaces; lines hollow organs, body cavities and ducts; forms glands
   2. Connective tissue —protects and supports the body and its organs; binds organs together; stores energy reserves as fat; provides immunity
   3. Muscle tissue —responsible for movement and generation of force
   4. Nervous tissue —initiates and transmits action potentials (nerve impulses) that help coordinate body activities
   Page Ref: 104

2) Name and describe the structures of the various types of cell junctions.

Answer: 1. Tight junctions —outer surfaces of adjacent plasma membranes fused by weblike strip of proteins
2. Adherens junctions —made of dense layer of proteins (plaque) on inside of plasma membrane; microfilaments extend from plaque into cytoplasm; transmembrane glycoproteins anchored in plaque join adjacent cells
3. Desmosomes—made of plaque; link adjacent cell membranes via transmembrane glycoproteins; intermediate filaments extend across cytoplasm from desmosome to desmosome in same cell
4. Hemidesmosomes—structurally like half a desmosome, but proteins link different tissue types
5. Gap junctions —fluid-filled gap between cells bridged by transmembrane channels (connexons)

Page Ref: 105

3) Name and briefly describe the functions of the various types of cell junctions.

Answer: 1. Tight junctions —prevent passage of substances between cells
2. Adherens junctions —help epithelial surfaces resist separation
3. Desmosomes—attach cells to each other; structure provides tissue with greater stability
4. Hemidesmosomes—anchor one kind of tissue to another
5. Gap junctions —allow communication between cells

Page Ref: 105

4) Describe the basic structural characteristics of epithelial tissue.

Answer: Epithelial cells are arranged in continuous sheets, either single or multiple. Cells are packed very close together and have numerous cell junctions. There is very little extracellular material. Apical surfaces of cells are exposed to a body cavity, the lumen of a tube or organ, or the exterior of the body. The basal surfaces are attached to connective tissue via a basement membrane. Epithelial tissues are avascular, but do have a nerve supply.

Page Ref: 106

5) Identify and state the functions of the types of cells commonly seen in areolar connective tissue.

Answer: 1. Fibroblasts —secrete fibers and ground substance of matrix
2. Macrophages —provide protection by engulfing bacteria and cellular debris via phagocytosis
3. Plasma cells —provide protection via secretion of antibodies
4. Mast cells —produce histamine, which promotes inflammation
5. Adipocytes—specialized to store triglycerides
6. White blood cells—provide protection during infections and allergic responses

Page Ref: 118

6) Give an example using connective tissue that illustrates the concept of **differentiation**.

Answer: There are many correct answers here. All should begin with mesenchyme cells. An example would be to continue on to fibroblasts, then to chondroblasts, then to chondrocytes.

Page Ref: 118–128

7) Name and describe the locations of the various types of cartilage.

Answer: 1. Hyaline cartilage —covers ends of long bones; forms epiphyseal plate, most of embryonic skeleton, and parts of most respiratory tubing
2. Fibrocartilage—joins pubic bones at pubic symphysis; forms intervertebral discs and menisci in knee
3. Elastic cartilage —forms external ear, auditory (Eustachian) tubes, and epiglottis

Page Ref: 128

8) Describe the factors influencing successful tissue repair.

Answer: Predominance of parenchymal or stromal cell activity determines regeneration (perfect reconstruction) or fibrosis (scar formation and loss of function). Other factors include nutrition (raw materials), blood flow (ability to deliver helpful substances/cells and remove wastes), and age (changes in collagen and elastin characteristics with age; lower cellular metabolic and reproduction rates with age).

Page Ref: 133–134

9) How does the arrangement of collagen fibers affect the nature of support and strength a connective tissue provides? Give examples to support your answer.

Answer: Collagen fibers that are arranged in parallel bundles, such would be found in the dense regular connective tissue of tendons, provide strength and support in one particular direction. When collagen fibers are arranged randomly, such as in areolar connective tissue, greater flexibility is allowed, and strength and support are distributed more equally in all directions.

Page Ref: 127–128

10) Many bacteria produce the enzyme *hyaluronidase*. What advantage does this provide to bacteria that invade the human body?

Answer: The enzyme breaks down hyaluronic acid, an important component of the interstitial substance of many tissues. Any bacteria that produce this enzymes can more easily make their way between human cells, and spread their infection more quickly.

Page Ref: 119

CHAPTER 5   The Integumentary System

MULTIPLE CHOICE. Choose the one alternative that best completes the statement or answers the question.

1) Keratinocytes are the predominant cells in the:

A) epidermis.

B) papillary region of the dermis.

C) reticular region of the dermis.

D) subcutaneous layer.

E) All of the above are correct.

Answer: A
Page Ref: 140

2) Nourishment to cells in the epidermis is provided by:

A) blood vessels running through the stratum basale.

B) keratinocytes.

C) blood vessels in the dermal papillae.

D) bacteria that live in sebaceous glands.

E) Both A and C are correct.

Answer: C
Page Ref: 144

3) Absorption of damaging light rays is the primary function of:

A) keratin.

B) sebum.

C) cerumen.

D) melanin.

E) keratohyalin.

Answer: D
Page Ref: 140

4) Cells in the epidermis that arise from red bone marrow are the:

A) keratinocytes.

B) Merkel cells.

C) Langerhans cells.

D) melanocytes.

E) arrector pili.

Answer: C
Page Ref: 141

5) The function of keratin is to:

   A) make bone hard.

   B) make skin tough and waterproof.

   C) protect skin from ultraviolet light.

   D) provided added pigment to the skin of Asian races.

   E) provide nourishment to the epidermal cells.

Answer: B
Page Ref: 140

6) In the feedback loop involving the skin that helps control body temperature, the effectors are the:

   A) receptors in the dermis.

   B) melanocytes.

   C) sebaceous glands.

   D) sudoriferous glands.

   E) keratinocytes.

Answer: D
Page Ref: 148

7) The stratum basale contains:

   A) stem cells of keratinocytes.

   B) many blood vessels.

   C) eccrine sweat glands.

   D) hair follicles.

   E) Both A and B are correct.

Answer: A
Page Ref: 142

8) Which of the following is most superficial?

   A) stratum basale

   B) papillary region of the dermis

   C) hypodermis

   D) stratum granulosum

   E) stratum corneum

Answer: E
Page Ref: 143

9) The epidermis is made up of:

   A) dense irregular connective tissue.

   B) stratified squamous epithelium.

   C) areolar connective tissue.

   D) smooth muscle.

   E) All of the above are correct.

Answer: B
Page Ref: 140

10) "Goosebumps" occur due to:

   A) over-stimulation of secretion from sudoriferous glands.

   B) over-stimulation of secretion from sebaceous glands.

   C) separation of the epidermis from the dermis.

   D) vasodilation of blood vessels in the skin.

   E) the action of arrector pili muscles as they raise hairs to an upright position.

Answer: E
Page Ref: 147

11) Keratinocytes are bound to the basement membrane via:

   A) hemidesmosomes.

   B) tight junctions.

   C) gap junctions.

   D) keratohyalin.

   E) the lipid substance in lamellar granules.

Answer: A
Page Ref: 142

12) Sweat is produced by:

   A) keratinocytes.

   B) melanocytes.

   C) ceruminous glands.

   D) sudoriferous glands.

   E) sebaceous glands.

Answer: D
Page Ref: 148

13) Which of the following is present in thick skin but not in thin skin?
   A) stratum germinativum
   B) stratum lucidum
   C) stratum corneum
   D) stratum granulosum
   E) dermal papillae

   Answer: B
   Page Ref: 150

14) An isograft is a skin graft taken from:
   A) another part of one's own body.
   B) another animal species.
   C) cells grown in the laboratory.
   D) an unrelated human.
   E) an identical twin.

   Answer: E
   Page Ref: 142

15) Keratohyalin is a distinctive feature of cells in the:
   A) sudoriferous glands.
   B) stratum granulosum.
   C) stratum basale.
   D) hypodermis.
   E) dermal papillae.

   Answer: B
   Page Ref: 143

16) The stratum corneum is:
   A) the innermost layer of the epidermis.
   B) highly vascular.
   C) made up of dead cells.
   D) seen only in the palms and soles.
   E) the layer in which keratin begins to form.

   Answer: C
   Page Ref: 143

17) The function of lamellar granules is to produce:

   A) keratin.

   B) melanin.

   C) a lipid–rich water–repellent sealant.

   D) apocrine sweat.

   E) breast milk.

   Answer: C
   Page Ref: 143

18) Which of the following statements is **TRUE** regarding the epidermis?

   A) It is keratinized.

   B) Blood vessels travel from the dermis to the outer layers through special channels.

   C) All of the cells in the epidermis reproduce rapidly.

   D) It is made mostly of areolar connective tissue.

   E) Both A and C are correct.

   Answer: A
   Page Ref: 140

19) The "ABCD" signs are used to assess:

   A) the seriousness of decubitus ulcers.

   B) whether sufficient oxygen is being transported by blood.

   C) the percentage of surface area lost to a burn.

   D) a person's total risk of developing skin cancer.

   E) a skin lesion suspected of being a malignant melanoma.

   Answer: E
   Page Ref: 155

20) The average length of time for a cell to be produced by the stratum basale, rise to the surface, become keratinized, and slough off is about how long?

   A) 24–48 hours

   B) two weeks

   C) one month

   D) one year

   E) Once cells are keratinized, they never slough off.

   Answer: C
   Page Ref: 144

21) A skin condition in which abnormal keratin is produced and keratinocytes are shed prematurely is:

   A) psoriasis.

   B) malignant melanoma.

   C) albinism.

   D) alopecia.

   E) impetigo.

   Answer: A
   Page Ref: 144

22) Corpuscles of touch (Meissner's corpuscles) are located in the:

   A) stratum basale.

   B) stratum corneum.

   C) apocrine sweat glands.

   D) dermal papillae.

   E) hair follicles.

   Answer: D
   Page Ref: 144

23) Just beneath the stratum basale of the epidermis is the:

   A) stratum corneum of the epidermis.

   B) hypodermis.

   C) reticular layer of the dermis.

   D) papillary regions of the dermis.

   E) skeletal muscle.

   Answer: D
   Page Ref: 144

24) In the negative feedback loop involving the integumentary system that helps maintain homeostasis by reducing elevated body temperature, the effectors achieve a reduction in body temperature by:

   A) raising body hairs to let more heat escape from the body.

   B) producing oil to coat and insulate skin.

   C) sending messages to your brain to generate mental images of cool environments.

   D) causing constriction of blood vessels in the epidermis.

   E) producing sweat, which evaporates, thus taking heat from the skin surface.

   Answer: E
   Page Ref: 148

25) The papillary region of the dermis consists mostly of:

A) areolar connective tissue.

B) adipose tissue.

C) smooth muscle.

D) stratified squamous epithelium.

E) dense irregular connective tissue.

Answer: A
Page Ref: 144

26) The reticular layer of the dermis consists mostly of:

A) areolar connective tissue.

B) adipose tissue.

C) smooth muscle.

D) stratified squamous epithelium.

E) dense irregular connective tissue.

Answer: E
Page Ref: 144

27) *Striae* are:

A) free nerve endings sensing touch.

B) the epidermal ridges that form fingerprints.

C) stretch marks resulting from tears in the dermis.

D) intermediate filaments connecting desmosomes.

E) areas of fat storage.

Answer: C
Page Ref: 144

28) Fat storage is an important function of the:

A) epidermis.

B) papillary region of the dermis.

C) reticular region of the dermis.

D) subcutaneous layer.

E) All of the above except the epidermis.

Answer: D
Page Ref: 140

29) Tyrosinase is required for the production of:

   A) keratin.

   B) melanin.

   C) cerumen.

   D) sebum.

   E) apocrine sweat.

   Answer: B
   Page Ref: 145

30) Synthesis of vitamin D begins with the activation of a precursor molecule in the skin by:

   A) melanin.

   B) keratin.

   C) sebum.

   D) UV light.

   E) temperatures above 60°F in the external environment.

   Answer: D
   Page Ref: 151

31) Enzymatic activity within melanosomes is increased by:

   A) apoptosis of epidermal cells.

   B) environmental temperatures above normal body temperature.

   C) increased activity of sweat glands.

   D) tension on desmosomes.

   E) exposure to UV light.

   Answer: E
   Page Ref: 145

32) Albinism results from:

   A) liver disease.

   B) low oxygen levels in the blood.

   C) lack of the enzyme tyrosinase

   D) too little exposure to sunlight.

   E) viral infection.

   Answer: C
   Page Ref: 145

33) The substance in skin that is a precursor to the substance needed for synthesis of visual pigments is:

A) keratohyalin.

B) melanin.

C) carotene.

D) vitamin D.

E) calcitriol.

Answer: C
Page Ref: 145

34) Jaundice is indicative of:

A) excessive carotene production.

B) liver disease.

C) too much sun exposure.

D) insufficient oxygen in blood.

E) Both A and B are correct.

Answer: B
Page Ref: 145

35) Cyanosis is indicative of:

A) lack of tyrosinase.

B) liver disease.

C) inflammation.

D) insufficient oxygen in blood.

E) patchy loss of melanocytes.

Answer: D
Page Ref: 145

36) The blood vessels nourishing a hair follicle are located in the:

A) arrector pili.

B) cortex of the hair.

C) cuticle of the hair.

D) matrix cells.

E) papilla of the hair.

Answer: E
Page Ref: 147

37) Production of new hairs is the responsibility of the:

A) arrector pili.

B) cortex of the hair.

C) cuticle of the hair.

D) matrix cells.

E) papilla of the hair.

Answer: D
Page Ref: 147

38) Sebaceous glands usually secrete their products into the:

A) blood.

B) necks of hair follicles.

C) peaks of epidermal ridges.

D) melanosomes.

E) external auditory canal.

Answer: B
Page Ref: 148

39) Fats, cholesterol, and pheromones are important components of:

A) keratin.

B) melanin.

C) sebum.

D) eccrine sweat

E) hair and nails.

Answer: C
Page Ref: 148

40) **ALL** of the following are **TRUE EXCEPT:**

A) apocrine sweat glands are found mainly in the axilla and groin.

B) sebaceous glands are present in all areas of the skin except palms and soles.

C) apocrine sweat is important in the regulation of body temperature.

D) apocrine sweat glands vary in size with changes in a woman's hormone balance.

E) eccrine sweat plays a role in waste elimination.

Answer: C
Page Ref: 148

41) **ALL** of the following are **TRUE EXCEPT**:

A) thick skin covers palms and soles.

B) thick skin has more sudoriferous glands than thin skin.

C) thick skin has more numerous dermal papillae than thin skin.

D) thick skin has more numerous hair follicles than thin skin.

E) thick skin has more densely clustered sensory receptors than thin skin.

Answer: D
Page Ref: 150

42) The term *contact inhibition* refers to the:

A) tendency to avoid touching things that are too hot.

B) inability of blood to flow into the epidermis.

C) social effect of the unpleasant aroma of sweat.

D) end of migration of epidermal cells once touching like cells on all sides.

E) extreme sensitivity of exposed dermis.

Answer: D
Page Ref: 152

43) **ALL** of the following events occur during deep wound healing **EXCEPT**:

A) vasodilation of blood vessels.

B) suspension of the rules of contact inhibition.

C) formation of a blood clot.

D) synthesis of scar tissue by fibroblasts.

E) increased permeability of blood vessels.

Answer: B
Page Ref: 152

44) Granulation tissue is the tissue that forms:

A) from the debris of phagocytosis during deep wound healing.

B) basal cell carcinomas.

C) a greater than normal amount of melanin.

D) during the migratory phase of deep wound healing.

E) hemangiomas.

Answer: D
Page Ref: 152

45) The process of fibrosis results in:
    A) some form of skin cancer.
    B) scar formation.
    C) excessive production of skin pigment.
    D) excessive production of hair and nails.
    E) premature wrinkling of skin.

    Answer: B
    Page Ref: 152

46) Blisters form in second–degree burns because:
    A) the epidermis and dermis separate, and tissue fluid accumulates between the layers.
    B) the dermal papillae extend through the damaged epidermis, and are exposed to the external environment.
    C) damaged nerve endings swell.
    D) accumulated tissue fluid is necessary for scar formation.
    E) the cells of the stratum basale are reproducing at such a rapid rate.

    Answer: A
    Page Ref: 155

47) The most common forms of skin cancer are all caused, at least in part, by:
    A) chronic dryness of skin.
    B) over–secretion by sudoriferous glands.
    C) chronic exposure to sunlight.
    D) over–production of keratin.
    E) chronically reduced blood flow in the dermis.

    Answer: C
    Page Ref: 155

48) Which of the following would you expect to happen if the external temperature is 39 °C?
    A) vasoconstriction of blood vessels in the skin
    B) vasodilation of blood vessels in the skin.
    C) contraction of arrector pili muscles.
    D) Both A and C are correct.
    E) None of these, because the body is already in homeostasis.

    Answer: B
    Page Ref: 151

49) Differences in skin color among human races is due primarily to the:

   A) total number of melanocytes.

   B) total number of keratinocytes.

   C) amount of melanin produced by melanocytes.

   D) amount of keratin produced by keratinocytes.

   E) amount of iron in hemoglobin molecules.

   Answer: C
   Page Ref: 145

50) During deep wound healing, mesenchyme cells that migrate to the site of injury during the inflammatory phase will develop into:

   A) keratinocytes.

   B) melanocytes.

   C) fibroblasts.

   D) phagocytes.

   E) collagen fibers.

   Answer: C
   Page Ref: 152

MATCHING. Choose the item in column 2 that best matches each item in column 1.

Choose the item from column 2 that best matches each item in column 1.

   1) Column 1: provides protection from UV
                    light
      Column 2: melanin

      Answer: melanin

      Page Ref: 140

   2) Column 1: fibrous protein providing
                    mechanical protection in the
                    epidermis
      Column 2: keratin

      Answer: keratin

      Page Ref: 140

   3) Column 1: prevents hair from drying out
                    and prevents excessive water
                    evaporation
      Column 2: sebum

      Answer: sebum

      Page Ref: 148

4) Column 1: darkly staining granules of the stratum granulosum
   Column 2: keratohyalin
   Answer: keratohyalin
   Page Ref: 143

5) Column 1: a precursor to vitamin A; needed for formation of visual pigments
   Column 2: carotene
   Answer: carotene
   Page Ref: 145

6) Column 1: pigment responsible for pinkish red color of "white" skin
   Column 2: hemoglobin
   Answer: hemoglobin
   Page Ref: 145

7) Column 1: forms sticky barrier in external auditory canal
   Column 2: cerumen
   Answer: cerumen
   Page Ref: 149

8) Column 1: helps regulate body temperature
   Column 2: eccrine sweat
   Answer: eccrine sweat
   Page Ref: 148

9) Column 1: secreted during emotional stress and sexual excitement
   Column 2: apocrine sweat
   Answer: apocrine sweat
   Page Ref: 148

10) Column 1: UV light activates a precursor
of this compound, which is
important for absorption of
calcium

Column 2: vitamin D

Answer: vitamin D

Page Ref: 151

MATCHING. Choose the item in column 2 that best matches each item in column 1.

Choose the item from column 2 that best matches each item in column 1.

1) Column 1: produce a substance that
helps protect the body from
UV light

Column 2: melanocytes

Answer: melanocytes

Page Ref: 140

2) Column 1: produce a protein that
provides protection from
mechanical injury and
bacterial invasion

Column 2: keratinocytes

Answer: keratinocytes

Page Ref: 140

3) Column 1: work with helper T cells to
provide immunity

Column 2: Langerhans cells

Answer: Langerhans cells

Page Ref: 141

4) Column 1: produce a product that helps
regulate body temperature

Column 2: sudoriferous glands

Answer: sudoriferous glands

Page Ref: 148

5) Column 1: produce a product that helps
prevent excessive evaporation
of water from the skin and
keeps skin soft and pliable

Column 2: sebaceous glands

Answer: sebaceous glands

Page Ref: 148

6) Column 1: function in sensation of touch
   Column 2: Merkel cells
   Answer: Merkel cells
   Page Ref: 141

7) Column 1: function in sensations of pressure
   Column 2: lamellate (Pacinian) corpuscles
   Answer: lamellate (Pacinian) corpuscles
   Page Ref: 158

8) Column 1: raises hair to vertical position
   Column 2: arrector pili
   Answer: arrector pili
   Page Ref: 147

9) Column 1: provide increased surface area for nutrient, waste, and gas exchange with cells of the stratum basale
   Column 2: dermal papillae
   Answer: dermal papillae
   Page Ref: 144

10) Column 1: produce earwax
    Column 2: ceruminous glands
    Answer: ceruminous glands
    Page Ref: 149

TRUE/FALSE. Write 'T' if the statement is true and 'F' if the statement is false.

1) The skin is the largest organ of the body in surface area and weight.

   Answer: TRUE
   Page Ref: 140

2) The dermis is deep to the epidermis.

   Answer: TRUE
   Page Ref: 140

3) The function of keratin is to provide protection from UV light.

   Answer: FALSE
   Page Ref: 140

4) The number of melanocytes is approximately the same for all races.

Answer: TRUE
Page Ref: 145

5) *Stratum basale* and *stratum germinativum* are terms referring to the same layer of the epidermis.

Answer: TRUE
Page Ref: 142

6) A skin graft taken from the same individual is called an isograft.

Answer: FALSE
Page Ref: 142

7) The stratum granulosum is present only in the skin of the palms and soles.

Answer: FALSE
Page Ref: 143

8) The function of dermal papillae is to provide resistance to friction damage.

Answer: FALSE
Page Ref: 144

9) The dermis is composed of stratified squamous epithelium.

Answer: FALSE
Page Ref: 144

10) The subcutaneous layer of skin consists of areolar and adipose tissues.

Answer: TRUE
Page Ref: 140

11) The cells of the stratum basale are all dead.

Answer: FALSE
Page Ref: 142

12) The epidermis is highly vascular.

Answer: FALSE
Page Ref: 140

13) Carotene is a yellow–orange pigment that is the precursor to vitamin A.

Answer: TRUE
Page Ref: 145

14) The receptors in the negative feedback loop that helps regulate body temperature are the sudoriferous glands.

Answer: FALSE
Page Ref: 148

15) Vasoconstriction of blood vessels in the skin reduces heat loss from radiation.

Answer: TRUE
Page Ref: 151

SHORT ANSWER. Write the word or phrase that best completes each statement or answers the question.

1) Individuals who do not get enough exposure to sunlight or who do not consume enough fortified milk may develop a deficiency of vitamin _____.

Answer: D
Page Ref: 151

2) The red/brown/black pigment in skin that absorbs UV light is _____.

Answer: melanin
Page Ref: 145

3) The pinkish red color of the skin of white people is due to the pigment _____ in red blood cells.

Answer: hemoglobin
Page Ref: 145

4) The outermost layer of a hair is called the _____.

Answer: cuticle
Page Ref: 147

5) Contraction of smooth muscle called _____ pulls a hair shaft perpendicular to the skin surface.

Answer: arrector pili
Page Ref: 147

6) The more common type of sweat gland is the _____ gland.

Answer: eccrine
Page Ref: 148

7) The single layer of continually reproducing cells in the epidermis is called the _____.

Answer: stratum basale
Page Ref: 142

8) The most superficial layer of cells in the epidermis is called the _____.
Answer: stratum corneum
Page Ref: 143

9) The protein in the outer layer of the epidermis that provides protection against mechanical injury and bacterial invasion is _____.
Answer: keratin
Page Ref: 140

10) The main function of eccrine gland sweat is to _____.
Answer: regulate body temperature
Page Ref: 148

11) The layer of the epidermis seen in thick skin that is NOT seen in thin skin is the _____.
Answer: stratum lucidum
Page Ref: 143

12) The most common skin cancers are the _____.
Answer: basal cell carcinomas
Page Ref: 155

13) The branch of medicine that specializes in diagnosing and treating skin disorders is _____.
Answer: dermatology
Page Ref: 140

14) A yellowed appearance of skin and the whites of the eyes due to buildup of bilirubin resulting from liver disease is called _____.
Answer: jaundice
Page Ref: 145

15) Redness of the skin due to increased blood flow is known as _____.
Answer: erythema
Page Ref: 145

16) The most common of the cell types in the epidermis is the _____.
Answer: keratinocyte
Page Ref: 140

17) Cells that arise from the red bone marrow and migrate to the epidermis where they participate in immune responses are the _____.
Answer: Langerhans cells
Page Ref: 141

18) Cells in the epidermis that function in the sensation of touch are the _____.

Answer: Merkel cells

Page Ref: 141

19) The stem cells of the epidermis are located in the stratum _____.

Answer: basale (germinativum)

Page Ref: 142

20) Keratohyalin is a protein distinctive of the stratum _____.

Answer: granulosum

Page Ref: 143

21) A lipid-rich, water-repellent secretion is produced by structures known as _____ within the keratinocytes of the stratum granulosum.

Answer: lamellar granules

Page Ref: 143

22) The characteristic of epidermal cells that causes them to stop migrating during wound healing once they are touching other epidermal cells on all sides is called _____.

Answer: contact inhibition

Page Ref: 152

23) The process of scar tissue formation is called _____.

Answer: fibrosis

Page Ref: 152

24) When body temperature begins to fall, to prevent further heat loss blood vessels in the skin will _____.

Answer: constrict

Page Ref: 151

25) In the negative feedback loop in which the integumentary system helps regulate body temperature, the effectors are the _____ and the _____.

Answer: sudoriferous glands; blood vessels in the skin

Page Ref: 151

26) The deeper portion of the dermis is called the _____ region.

Answer: reticular

Page Ref: 144

27) Nerve endings in the subcutaneous layer that are sensitive to pressure are called _____.
   Answer: lamellated (Pacinian) corpuscles
   Page Ref: 158

28) The medical term for itching is _____.
   Answer: pruritus
   Page Ref: 156

29) Pressure sores (or bedsores) are also known as _____.
   Answer: decubitus ulcers
   Page Ref: 156

30) The type of tissue that forms the epidermis is _____.
   Answer: stratified squamous epithelium
   Page Ref: 140

ESSAY. Write your answer in the space provided or on a separate sheet of paper.

1) List and briefly discuss the functions of skin.
   Answer: 1. regulation of body temperature via sweat production and changes in blood flow
   2. protection from mechanical injury, bacterial invasion (via keratin), dehydration (via product of lamellar granules), and UV light (via melanin)
   3. sensory reception via receptors for temperature, touch, pressure, pain
   4. excretion via sweat
   5. immunity via Langerhans cells
   6. blood reservoir for 8–10% of total blood flow
   7. synthesis of vitamin D from precursors in skin activated by UV light
   Page Ref: 150–151

2) Describe the structural characteristics of the epidermis that relate to its protection function.
   Answer: Multiple layers of cells in stratified squamous epithelium help resist friction. Keratin of intermediate filaments provides strength to tissue by binding cells tightly together and to underlying tissue, and by producing a barrier to microbes. Lamellar granules of keratinocytes produce lipid-rich, water-repellent sealant to protect from dehydration and entry of foreign materials. Melanin, produced by melanocytes, protects underlying tissue from UV light. Sebum secreted onto the surface helps protect from dehydration and microbial invasion. Langerhans cells participate in immune reponse to microbial invasion.
   Page Ref: 151

3) John has just been brought into the emergency room following a fiery explosion at a chemical plant. He is diagnosed with third degree burns over the anterior surfaces of his arms and trunk. What specific structural damage has occurred to his skin? What risks to John's life have resulted from this damage?

Answer: John has lost approximately 36% of his skin's surface area (according to the Rule of Nines), which leads to severe systemic effects. The epidermis, dermis and associated structures have been destroyed. Sensory function is lost. Loss of epidermis (and so, lost keratin and Langerhans cells) leaves John open to microbial invasion. Loss of keratinized structures and lamellar granules allows for extreme water loss, leading to dehydration, reduced blood volume and circulation, and decreased urine output.

Page Ref: 155

4) Describe the process of deep wound healing.

Answer: 1. Inflammatory phase—blood clot forms to loosely unite wound edges; blood vessels dilate and become more permeable; phagocytes and mesenchyme cells migrate to site of injury
2. Migratory phase—clot becomes scab; epithelial cells migrate beneath scab; fibroblasts synthesize scar tissue; begin repair of damaged blood vessels; granulation tissue fills wound
3. Proliferative phase—extensive growth of epithelium beneath scab; fibroblasts deposit collagen fibers in random patterns; further vessel repair
4. Maturation phase—scab falls off; collagen fibers become organized; fibroblasts decrease in number; blood vessels repaired

Page Ref: 152

5) Compare and contrast the locations and structure of thin and thick skin.

Answer: Thick skin is found on palms and palmar surfaces of digits and soles, while thin skin is found in all other areas but not these. Thick skin is 4 −5X thicker than thin skin. The stratum lucidum is present in thick skin but not thin, and strata spinosum and corneum are thicker. Thick skin exhibits epidermal ridges, more sweat glands and denser sensory receptors. Thin skin has hair follicles and sebaceous glands, while thick skin does not.

Page Ref: 150

6) Describe the changes that occur in the skin during the aging process.

Answer: After age 40: collagen fibers decrease in number, become tangled; elastic fibers lose elasticity and fray; wrinkles form; fibroblasts and Langerhans cells decrease in number; macrophages less efficient; hair and nails grow more slowly; sebaceous glands decrease in number and may enlarge, causing blotching of skin; blood vessels in dermis thicker-walled and less permeable; less subcutaneous fat; skin becomes thinner; slower migration of epidermal cells to surface.

Page Ref: 154

7) Describe in detail the negative feedback mechanisms involving the skin that help relieve the stress of elevated body temperature.

Answer: 1. Controlled condition = constant body temperature

2. Stress = elevation of body temperature

3. Receptors = thermoreceptors in skin and hypothalamus, which detect elevated temperature

4. Control center = brain, which receives input from thermoreceptors and notifies effectors of appropriate response

5. Effectors = eccrine sweat glands, which increase secretion of sweat, which evaporates, causing heat loss; blood vessels in dermis, which dilate, causing heat loss by radiation

6. Output = decreased body temperature, returning to homeostasis

Page Ref: 148, 151

8) Name and describe the three common forms of skin cancer.

Answer: Most are basal cell carcinomas arising in the stratum basale. These rarely metastasize. Next most common and with variable tendencies to metastasize are the squamous cell carcinomas, which arise from pre-existing lesions in the epidermis of sun-damaged skin. Most deadly, but least common, are the malignant melanomas that arise in melanocytes damaged by UV light.

Page Ref: 155

9) What are the "ABCD" warning signs of malignant melanoma?

Answer: A = asymmetry of lesions (i.e., irregular shapes)

B = irregular borders of lesions

C = color, which is uneven and varied within the lesion

D = diameter, which is often large compared with ordinary moles

Page Ref: 155

10) Design a questionnaire you could use to assess a person's risk of developing skin cancer.

Answer: Questions should cover the following risk factors: light colored skin that never tans, but always burns; total amount of sun exposure (higher exposure = higher risk); family history of skin cancer; age (older = greater risk); immune status (immunosuppressed people have higher incidence of skin cancer).

Page Ref: 155

CHAPTER 6   Bone Tissue

MULTIPLE CHOICE. Choose the one alternative that best completes the statement or answers the question.

1) The process of hemopoiesis occurs in:
   A) osteons.
   B) the periosteum.
   C) yellow bone marrow.
   D) red bone marrow.
   E) Both C and D are correct.

   Answer: D
   Page Ref: 160

2) The primary function of yellow bone marrow is:
   A) triglyceride storage.
   B) hemopoiesis.
   C) collagen production.
   D) to prevent collapse of trabeculae.
   E) to provide a blood supply to osteocytes in lacunae.

   Answer: A
   Page Ref: 160

3) Hydroxyapatite is the:
   A) combination of calcium compounds in bone matrix.
   B) collagen portion of bone matrix.
   C) concentric ring structure seen in compact bone.
   D) central canal of an osteon.
   E) hormone that stimulates breakdown of bone matrix.

   Answer: A
   Page Ref: 163

4) During endochondral bone formation, the primary center of ossification forms in the:
   A) proximal epiphysis.
   B) distal epiphysis.
   C) epiphyseal plate.
   D) diaphysis.
   E) metaphysis.

   Answer: D
   Page Ref: 168

5) In endochondral bone formation the original pattern for the bone is made of:

   A) osseous tissue.

   B) keratin.

   C) dense irregular connective tissue.

   D) elastic cartilage.

   E) hyaline cartilage.

   Answer: E
   Page Ref: 167

6) The function of the epiphyseal plate is to:

   A) allow more flexibility in a long bone.

   B) allow a means by which the bone can increase in diameter.

   C) allow a means by which the bone can increase in length.

   D) provide nourishment to isolated osteocytes.

   E) Both B and C are correct.

   Answer: C
   Page Ref: 169

7) The shaft of a long bone is the:

   A) osteon.

   B) Haversian canal.

   C) metaphysis.

   D) diaphysis.

   E) epiphysis.

   Answer: D
   Page Ref: 161

8) The function of osteoblasts is to:

   A) break down bone.

   B) produce blood cells.

   C) produce new collagen for bone matrix.

   D) add new tissue to the periosteum.

   E) provide nourishment to the cells of the articular cartilage.

   Answer: C
   Page Ref: 162

9) Osteons are typical of the structure of:
   A) compact bone.
   B) epiphyseal plates.
   C) spongy bone.
   D) the endosteum.
   E) All of these contain osteons.

   Answer: A
   Page Ref: 163

10) The epiphyseal plate is located in the:
    A) trabeculae.
    B) metaphysis.
    C) periosteum.
    D) diaphysis.
    E) epiphysis.

    Answer: B
    Page Ref: 162

11) The distal and proximal extremities of a bone are the:
    A) lacunae.
    B) trabeculae.
    C) metaphyses.
    D) diaphyses.
    E) epiphyses.

    Answer: E
    Page Ref: 161

12) Lamellae are the:
    A) plates of bone in spongy bone.
    B) spaces in osteons in which osteocytes are located.
    C) channels that contain cytoplasmic extensions of osteocytes in compact bone.
    D) layers of bone in an osteon.
    E) active cells in the epiphyseal plate.

    Answer: D
    Page Ref: 163

13) Friction reduction and shock absorption are functions of what part of a long bone?

A) the articular cartilage

B) the periosteum

C) the epiphyseal plate

D) the bone marrow

E) the endosteum

Answer: A
Page Ref: 162

14) Nutrients are provided to osteocytes in compact bone by:

A) transport through canaliculi from blood in vessels in the central canals.

B) blood in the marrow cavity.

C) blood seeping through the matrix of interstitial lamellae.

D) dissolving the matrix around them via enzymes in the lacunae.

E) blood in yellow bone marrow.

Answer: A
Page Ref: 163

15) The endosteum is the:

A) covering of a long bone.

B) marrow in spongy bone.

C) layer of active chondrocytes in the epiphyseal plate.

D) end of a long bone.

E) lining of the medullary cavity.

Answer: E
Page Ref: 162

16) Which of the following cells is the most mature (i.e., the most differentiated)?

A) osteocyte

B) mesenchyme cell

C) osteoblast

D) osteogenic cells

E) All of these are equally differentiated.

Answer: A
Page Ref: 162

17) The tiny channels connecting osteocytes with the central canal of an osteon are called:
    A) Haversian canals.
    B) lamellae.
    C) canaliculi.
    D) lacunae.
    E) perforating (Volkmann's) canals.

    Answer: C
    Page Ref: 163

18) The hormone produced by the thyroid gland that lowers serum calcium levels is:
    A) IGF.
    B) PTH.
    C) calcitonin
    D) growth hormone.
    E) T$_3$

    Answer: C
    Page Ref: 175

19) Inhibition of osteoclast activity is a primary function of:
    A) IGF.
    B) PTH.
    C) calcitonin
    D) growth hormone.
    E) estrogen.

    Answer: C
    Page Ref: 175

20) **ALL** of the following occur during the formation of the parietal bone **EXCEPT**:
    A) mesenchyme cells will migrate into the area where ossification will occur.
    B) osteoblasts will produce collagen.
    C) some osteogenic cells will become chondroblasts.
    D) trabeculae of spongy bone will form.
    E) outer layers of bone will be remodeled.

    Answer: C
    Page Ref: 167

21) During endochondral ossification, calcification of cartilage matrix causes the death of chondrocytes. This leads to:

A) death of the developing bone.

B) hemopoiesis.

C) closing of the epiphyseal plates.

D) erosion o articular cartilage.

E) development of the marrow cavity.

Answer: E
Page Ref: 169

22) Osteogenic cells are located in:

A) the inner portion of the periosteum.

B) lacunae at the edge of lamellae in osteons.

C) the epiphyseal plate.

D) the articular cartilage.

E) All of these are correct.

Answer: A
Page Ref: 162

23) Collagen is secreted by:

A) mesenchyme cells.

B) osteoblasts.

C) osteoclasts.

D) hydroxyapatites.

E) Both B and C are correct.

Answer: B
Page Ref: 162

24) **ALL** of the following are **TRUE** about bone composition **EXCEPT:**

A) immature bone contains more cells than mature bone.

B) bone matrix, unlike other connective tissues, contains abundant mineral salts.

C) mature bone is generally considered to be completely solid.

D) the diaphysis of a long bone is primarily compact bone.

E) the organic part of bone matrix is primarily collagen.

Answer: C
Page Ref: 163

25) **ALL** of the following are normal sites of hemopoiesis **EXCEPT**:
   A) clavicle (collarbone).
   B) hip bone.
   C) rib.
   D) sternum.
   E) vertebral bodies.

   Answer: A
   Page Ref: 165

26) Osteoclasts are located primarily in the:
   A) lining of the central canal.
   B) lacunae at the edges of lamellae.
   C) epiphyses.
   D) endosteum.
   E) epiphyseal plate.

   Answer: D
   Page Ref: 163

27) Hydroxyapatite consists mostly of:
   A) calcium phosphate.
   B) collagen.
   C) magnesium hydroxide.
   D) dense irregular connective tissue.
   E) hyaline cartilage.

   Answer: A
   Page Ref: 163

28) **ALL** of the following are **TRUE** about bone homeostasis **EXCEPT**:
   A) bone formation begins before birth.
   B) bone constantly remodels and redistributes its matrix along lines of mechanical stress.
   C) spongy bone is formed from compact bone.
   D) remodeling allows bone to serve as the body's reservoir for calcium.
   E) even after bones have reached their adult shapes and sizes, old bone matrix is destroyed and replaced by new bone matrix.

   Answer: C
   Page Ref: 167

29) The tensile strength of bone is provided by:

A) the periosteum.

B) mineral salts.

C) collagen fibers.

D) hyaline cartilage.

E) extensions of osteocytes into canaliculi.

Answer: C
Page Ref: 163

30) Which of the following best describes a compound (open) fracture?

A) The bone is broken in more than one place.

B) The broken ends of the bone protrude through the skin.

C) The bone is usually twisted apart.

D) The fracture is at right angles to the long axis of the bone.

E) One bone fragment is driven into the other.

Answer: B
Page Ref: 172

31) Blood vessels, lymphatic vessels, and nerves from the periosteum penetrate compact bone via:

A) central (Haversian) canals.

B) perforating (Volkmann's) canals.

C) canaliculi.

D) nutrient foramina.

E) circumferential lamellae.

Answer: B
Page Ref: 163

32) The function of the nutrient foramina of a long bone is to provide a passageway for:

A) blood vessels through the center of osteons.

B) ionized calcium ions to leave the bone matrix.

C) hormones to enter the bone matrix.

D) osteoblasts to reach the sites of new bone growth.

E) blood vessels into the medullary cavity.

Answer: E
Page Ref: 165

33) As bones increase in length, new bone is added as osteoblasts and capillaries from the diaphysis invade the:

A) zone of resting cartilage.

B) zone of proliferating cartilage.

C) zone of hypertrophic cartilage.

D) zone of calcified cartilage.

E) articular cartilage.

Answer: D
Page Ref: 169

34) **ALL** of the following are **TRUE** regarding epiphyseal plates **EXCEPT**:

A) They "close" between the ages of 18 and 20.

B) They are avascular.

C) They get thinner and thinner as a child ages.

D) Cartilage is replaced by bone on the diaphyseal side of the plate.

E) They consist of hyaline cartilage in four zones.

Answer: C
Page Ref: 170

35) Bone grow in diameter by:

A) appositional growth on the periosteal side of the bone.

B) interstitial growth.

C) activity at the epiphyseal plate.

D) activity of the hemopoietic tissue.

E) A, B, and C are all correct.

Answer: A
Page Ref: 170

36) **ALL** of the following bones would be produced via endochondral ossification **EXCEPT** the:

A) tibia.

B) femur.

C) frontal.

D) humerus.

E) radius.

Answer: C
Page Ref: 167

37) The role of Vitamin C in bone growth is that it:

    A) promotes absorption of calcium from the intestinal tract.

    B) is required for collagen synthesis.

    C) stimulates osteoclast activity.

    D) promotes secretion of calcitonin.

    E) acts as an insulin–like growth factor.

Answer: B
Page Ref: 171

38) The role of human growth hormone in bone growth is that it:

    A) stimulates production of osteoclasts in the endosteum.

    B) trigger calcification of matrix at the epiphyseal plate.

    C) promotes formation of calcitriol.

    D) stimulates production of IGFs.

    E) inhibits osteoclast activity.

Answer: D
Page Ref: 171

39) Growth at the epiphyseal plates is shut down by:

    A) Vitamin A.

    B) human growth hormone.

    C) calcitonin.

    D) PTH.

    E) estrogens.

Answer: E
Page Ref: 172

40) Giantism results from childhood oversecretion of:

    A) hGH.

    B) PTH.

    C) calcitonin.

    D) T_3.

    E) oversecretion of any of these results in giantism.

Answer: A
Page Ref: 172

41) In both intramembranous and endochondral ossification, the first stage of development of bone is:

   A) penetration of the diaphysis by a nutrient artery.

   B) migration of mesenchyme cells to the area of bone formation.

   C) formation of a cartilage model of the bone.

   D) fusion of trabeculae.

   E) development of a periosteal bud.

   Answer: B
   Page Ref: 167

42) The cells responsible for maintaining the daily cellular activities of bone tissue, such as exchange of nutrients and wastes with the blood, are the:

   A) osteogenic cells.

   B) osteoblasts.

   C) osteoclasts.

   D) osteocytes.

   E) chondroblasts.

   Answer: D
   Page Ref: 162

43) The crystallization of mineral salts in bone occurs only in the presence of:

   A) collagen.

   B) PTH.

   C) osteoclasts.

   D) hyaline cartilage.

   E) yellow bone marrow.

   Answer: A
   Page Ref: 163

44) Promotion of apoptosis of osteoclasts is an effect of:

   A) PTH.

   B) hGH.

   C) Vitamin C.

   D) hydroxyapatite.

   E) estrogens.

   Answer: E
   Page Ref: 172

45) Bone constantly remodels and redistributes its matrix along lines of:

A) blood flow.

B) nervous stimulation.

C) canaliculi.

D) mechanical stress.

E) overlying muscles.

Answer: D
Page Ref: 172

46) A bedridden person loses bone mass because of:

A) decreased calcitonin activity due to immobility.

B) lack of sufficient mechanical stress on bones.

C) increased conversion of monocytes to osteoclasts.

D) pressure on the kidney that leads to reduced calcitriol production.

E) insufficient blood flow to bones.

Answer: B
Page Ref: 176

47) **ALL** of the following are effects of parathyroid hormone **EXCEPT**:

A) increased protein synthesis.

B) increased numbers and activity of osteoclasts.

C) reabsorption of calcium ions by the kidney.

D) elimination of phosphate ions by the kidney.

E) promotion of calcitriol production by the kidney.

Answer: A
Page Ref: 175

48) Cells produced by the fusion of monocytes are:

A) mesenchyme cells.

B) osteoblasts.

C) chondroblasts.

D) osteoclasts.

E) parafollicular cells.

Answer: D
Page Ref: 162

49) The "growth spurt" of teenage years is due to an increase in the level of:
   A) hGH.
   B) T$_3$.
   C) sex steroids.
   D) PTH.
   E) calcitonin.

   Answer: C
   Page Ref: 172

50) Bones are more brittle in the elderly because:
   A) levels of calcitonin are higher in the elderly.
   B) there is less collagen relative to the amount of mineral salts.
   C) low levels of growth hormone prevent deposition of calcium in bone.
   D) the calcium salts in the bone matrix are of a different type than those in younger people.
   E) too much collagen takes up space that should be occupied by hydroxyapatites.

   Answer: B
   Page Ref: 178

MATCHING. Choose the item in column 2 that best matches each item in column 1.

Choose the item from column 2 that best matches each item in column 1.

1) Column 1: mesenchyme cells
   Column 2: stem cells from which more
             differentiated bone and
             cartilage cells arise

   Answer: stem cells from which more differentiated bone and cartilage cells arise
   Page Ref: 162

2) Column 1: osteogenic cells
   Column 2: develop into osteoblasts;
             found in periosteum and
             endosteum

   Answer: develop into osteoblasts; found in periosteum and endosteum
   Page Ref: 162

3) Column 1: osteoblasts
   Column 2: do not undergo mitosis;
             secrete collagen

   Answer: do not undergo mitosis; secrete collagen
   Page Ref: 162

4) Column 1: osteocytes

Column 2: sit in lacunae in bone matrix;
maintain daily cellular
activities of bone

Answer: sit in lacunae in bone matrix; maintain daily cellular activities of bone

Page Ref: 162

5) Column 1: osteoclasts

Column 2: located on bone surfaces;
function in bone resorption

Answer: located on bone surfaces; function in bone resorption

Page Ref: 162

6) Column 1: hydroxyapatites

Column 2: the mineral portion of bone
matrix

Answer: the mineral portion of bone matrix

Page Ref: 163

7) Column 1: osteons

Column 2: units of concentric lamellae in
compact bone

Answer: units of concentric lamellae in compact bone

Page Ref: 163

8) Column 1: trabeculae

Column 2: thin plates of bone in spongy
bone

Answer: thin plates of bone in spongy bone

Page Ref: 163

9) Column 1: canaliculi

Column 2: tiny channels that allow
communication between
osteocytes and blood vessels
in central canals

Answer: tiny channels that allow communication between osteocytes and blood vessels in
central canals

Page Ref: 163

10) Column 1: chondroblasts

Column 2: form the matrix of cartilage

Answer: form the matrix of cartilage

Page Ref: 169

MATCHING. Choose the item in column 2 that best matches each item in column 1.

Choose the item from column 2 that best matches each item in column 1.

1) Column 1: osteoarthritis

Column 2: degeneration of articular
cartilage due to overuse or
aging

Answer: degeneration of articular cartilage due to overuse or aging

Page Ref: 179

2) Column 1: osteogenic sarcoma

Column 2: bone cancer primarily
affecting osteoblasts

Answer: bone cancer primarily affecting osteoblasts

Page Ref: 179

3) Column 1: osteomyelitis

Column 2: an infection of bone often
caused by *Staphylococcus
aureus*

Answer: an infection of bone often caused by *Staphylococcus aureus*

Page Ref: 179

4) Column 1: osteoporosis

Column 2: condition in which bone
resorption outpaces bone
deposition

Answer: condition in which bone resorption outpaces bone deposition

Page Ref: 178

5) Column 1: stress fracture

Column 2: microscopic fissures resulting
from repeated, strenuous
activities

Answer: microscopic fissures resulting from repeated, strenuous activities

Page Ref: 173

6) Column 1: Pott's fracture

   Column 2: fracture of the distal end of
   the fibula

   Answer: fracture of the distal end of the fibula

   Page Ref: 172

7) Column 1: open (compound) fracture

   Column 2: broken ends of bone protrude
   through skin

   Answer: broken ends of bone protrude through skin

   Page Ref: 172

8) Column 1: comminuted fracture

   Column 2: bone has splintered at the site
   of impact

   Answer: bone has splintered at the site of impact

   Page Ref: 172

9) Column 1: Colles' fracture

   Column 2: fracture of the distal end of
   the radius

   Answer: fracture of the distal end of the radius

   Page Ref: 173

10) Column 1: rickets

   Column 2: condition in children in which
   bones fail to calcify, resulting
   in bone deformities

   Answer: condition in children in which bones fail to calcify, resulting in bone deformities

   Page Ref: 179

TRUE/FALSE. Write 'T' if the statement is true and 'F' if the statement is false.

1) Osteoblasts break down bone matrix.

   Answer: FALSE
   Page Ref: 162

2) The tensile strength of bone matrix is provided by mineral salts.

   Answer: FALSE
   Page Ref: 163

3) Compact bone tissue forms the external layer of all bones.

Answer: TRUE
Page Ref: 163

4) The activity of the epiphyseal plate is the only means by which the diaphysis can increase in length.

Answer: TRUE
Page Ref: 169

5) Osteocytes are contained in lacunae between the lamellae of compact bone.

Answer: TRUE
Page Ref: 163

6) Injuries to cartilage heal more slowly than those to bone because the blood vessels that serve cartilage do not extend into the cartilage matrix as they do in bone.

Answer: TRUE
Page Ref: 174

7) Yellow bone marrow is a hemopoietic tissue.

Answer: FALSE
Page Ref: 160

8) In intramembranous ossification, bones form directly from mesenchyme without first going through a cartilage stage.

Answer: TRUE
Page Ref: 167

9) Endochondral ossification is formation of bone within hyaline cartilage.

Answer: TRUE
Page Ref: 167

10) Osseous tissue is an avascular tissue.

Answer: FALSE
Page Ref: 165

11) Osteons (Haversian systems) are commonly seen in spongy bone.

Answer: FALSE
Page Ref: 163

12) The last bone to stop growing is the clavicle.

Answer: TRUE
Page Ref: 170

13) Trabeculae are the spaces between plates of bone in spongy bone.

Answer: FALSE
Page Ref: 163

14) Bone can grow in diameter only by appositional growth.

Answer: TRUE
Page Ref: 170

15) Calcitonin stimulates the activity of osteoclasts.

Answer: FALSE
Page Ref: 175

SHORT ANSWER. Write the word or phrase that best completes each statement or answers the question.

1) Destruction of matrix by osteoclasts is called bone _____.
Answer: resorption
Page Ref: 172

2) A partial fracture in which one side of the bone is broken and the other side bends is known as a(n) _____ fracture.
Answer: greenstick
Page Ref: 172

3) The membrane that lines the medullary cavity of a long bone is called the _____.
Answer: endosteum
Page Ref: 162

4) Mature bone cells that are completely surrounded by matrix are called _____.
Answer: osteocytes
Page Ref: 162

5) A fracture of the distal end of the radius in which the distal fragment is displaced posteriorly is called a(n) _____ fracture.
Answer: Colles'
Page Ref: 173

6) The channels in osteons that connect lacunae with central canals are called _____.
Answer: canaliculi
Page Ref: 163

7) The granulation tissue of a healing bone fracture is called a(n) _____.
Answer: procallus
Page Ref: 173

8) In intramembranous ossification, the highly vascularized mesenchyme on the outside of the new bone develops into the _____.

Answer: periosteum

Page Ref: 167

9) A series of microscopic fissures in bone that results from repeated, strenuous activities is known as a(n) _____ fracture.

Answer: stress

Page Ref: 173

10) The part of a long bone that is not covered by periosteum is covered by _____.

Answer: articular cartilage (hyaline cartilage)

Page Ref: 162

11) Cells whose primary function is bone resorption are the _____.

Answer: osteoclasts

Page Ref: 162

12) The process by which the fractured ends of a bone are brought into alignment is called _____.

Answer: reduction

Page Ref: 175

13) Bone is the major reservoir for the minerals _____ and _____.

Answer: calcium; phosphorus

Page Ref: 160

14) The two most important hormones involved in the regulation of calcium ion levels in the blood are _____ and _____.

Answer: parathyroid hormone; calcitonin

Page Ref: 175

15) Increasing the activity of osteoclasts is one of the major effects of the hormone _____.

Answer: parathyroid hormone

Page Ref: 175

16) Blood vessels run longitudinally through compact bone in spaces known as _____.

Answer: central (Haversian) canals

Page Ref: 163

17) Thin plates of bone in spongy bone are called _____.

Answer: trabeculae

Page Ref: 163

18) The flat bones of the skull form by _____ ossification.
   Answer: intramembranous
   Page Ref: 167

19) The flexible rod of mesoderm that defines the midline of the embryo and gives it some rigidity is the _____.
   Answer: notochord
   Page Ref: 178

20) The process by which blood cells are produced in red bone marrow is called _____.
   Answer: hemopoiesis
   Page Ref: 160

21) The main function of yellow bone marrow is _____.
   Answer: triglyceride storage
   Page Ref: 160

22) The shaft of a long bone is called the _____.
   Answer: diaphysis
   Page Ref: 161

23) Bone constantly remodels and redistributes matrix along lines of _____.
   Answer: mechanical stress
   Page Ref: 172

24) The dense irregular connective tissue that surrounds bone surfaces not covered by articular cartilage is the _____.
   Answer: periosteum
   Page Ref: 162

25) Levels of calcium ions in the blood are decreased by the effects of the hormone _____.
   Answer: calcitonin
   Page Ref: 175

26) The blood clot that forms in and around the site of a bone fracture is called a _____.
   Answer: fracture hematoma
   Page Ref: 173

27) The region in a mature bone where the diaphysis joins an epiphysis is the _____.
   Answer: metaphysis
   Page Ref: 162

28) Osteogenic cells are unspecialized stem cells derived from ____.

Answer: mesenchyme

Page Ref: 162

29) The inorganic mineral salts providing the hardness of bone matrix are collectively called

____.

Answer: hydroxyapatite

Page Ref: 163

30) The process of bone formation is called ossification or ____.

Answer: osteogenesis

Page Ref: 166

ESSAY. Write your answer in the space provided or on a separate sheet of paper.

1) List and briefly discuss the functions of the skeletal system.

Answer: 1. Support—point of attachment for skeletal muscles; supports soft organs
2. Protection—bones surround major organs
3. Assists in movement —skeletal muscles attached to bones provide leverage
4. Mineral homeostasis —exchange of minerals (especially Ca and P) between bone and blood
5. Hemopoiesis—red bone marrow produces blood cells
6. Energy storage—yellow bone marrow is triglyceride storage site

Page Ref: 160

2) Describe the structure of a typical long bone.

Answer: The diaphysis is the shaft of the bone, and the epiphyses are the proximal and distal extremities. Metaphyses are the junctions of the diaphysis with the epiphyses and include the epiphyseal plate. Articular cartilage is hyaline cartilage covering the epiphyses where they form an articulation. The remainder of the bone surface is covered with dense irregular connective tissue called the periosteum. The medullary (marrow) cavity is the space within the diaphysis that contains bone marrow. The medullary cavity is lined by the endosteum.

Page Ref: 161

3) Describe the process of intramembranous ossification.

Answer: Mesenchymal cells in the fibrous connective tissue membrane cluster and differentiate into osteogenic cells, then into osteoblasts at a center of ossification. Osteoblasts secrete the organic part of bone matrix until completely surrounded, at which point they become osteocytes. Osteocytes extend cytoplasmic processes into canaliculi. The matrix becomes calcified, forming a trabecula. Many trabeculae merge to form spongy bone. The remaining mesenchyme condenses to form the periosteum, and the outermost layers of spongy bone are remodeled into compact bone. Blood vessels grow into spaces between trabeculae and eventually differentiate into red bone marrow.

Page Ref: 167

4) Compare and contrast the structure of compact vs. spongy bone.

Answer: Compact bone is arranged in osteons. Concentric lamellae of matrix surround a central canal containing blood vessels and nerves. Osteocytes are isolated in lacunae at the edges of the lamellae and communicate with the central canal via canaliculi. Interstitial lamellae are those between osteons. Spongy bone has no osteons. Thin plates of bone called trabeculae surround spaces containing red bone marrow. Osteocytes in lacunae get nutrients directly from blood in marrow.

Page Ref: 163

5) List the various mechanisms by which parathyroid hormone raises serum calcium ion levels.

Answer: 1. increased number and activity of osteoclasts to break down bone matrix and release calcium and phosphate ions into the blood
2. reabsorption of calcium ions by the kidney (at the expense of phosphate ions)
3. formation of calcitriol which promotes absorption of calcium from intestines

Page Ref: 175

6) Describe the effects of aging on the skeletal system.

Answer: The primary effects are demineralization and reduced collagen production. The former results especially from decreased levels of sex steroids, particularly in women. The latter results from a decreased rate of protein synthesis, partly due to decreased levels of hGH, which reduces the amount of collagen in matrix. If the proportion of mineral to collagen increases in matrix, the bones become more brittle.

Page Ref: 178

7) Patient X has a tumor of the parathyroid glands that causes a hypersecretion from these glands. Predict the effect on the skeletal system and on the secretion of calcitonin.

Answer: High levels of PTH would cause high levels of osteoclast activity, thus removing calcium from bones. Bones would become weak and soft. Excess phosphate would be lost from the kidneys. High levels of calcium ions in blood may disrupt nerve and muscle function. Calcitonin levels would probably be high, trying to restore homeostasis by increasing deposition of calcium into bone.

Page Ref: 175

8) Describe the signs and symptoms of osteoporosis and describe the risk factors for developing osteoporosis.

Answer: In osteoporosis, bone resorption outpaces bone deposition so that bone mass is depleted, sometimes to the point of spontaneous fracture. Pain and height loss may occur as vertebrae shrink. Postmenopausal women are especially at risk due to lower initial bone mass than men due to dramatically reduced estrogen levels. Family history may play a role, as does ethnicity (white and Asian women have a higher rate of disease), inactivity, cigarette smoking, excessive alcohol consumption, and a diet low in calcium and vitamin D.

Page Ref: 178

9) Archaeologists have unearthed the upper arm bones of some ancient humans. They note with interest that these bones have greatly enlarged deltoid tuberosities, which are the points where the deltoid (shoulder) muscles attach to the lateral surfaces of these bones. What might they infer from this finding about the life and activities of these people, and why?

Answer: Possibly some activity that required the repeated use of this muscle (such as archery or rowing), that causes continual mechanical stress on this point of muscle attachment, thus inducing remodeling via addition of bone.

Page Ref: 172

10) Describe the process by which bone increases in length and diameter.

Answer: The only means by which bone can increase in length is by activity at the epiphyseal plate. Until full height is reached, the plate consists of layers of chondrocytes which generate matrix which is then calcified and replaced by bone matrix secreted by osteoblasts on the diaphyseal side of the plate. Around ages 18 −20 the cartilage is replaced completely by bone and no more lengthwise growth can occur. Bone increases in diameter via appositional growth as new bone matrix is laid down by osteoblasts in the periosteum.

Page Ref: 169–170

CHAPTER 7   The Skeletal System: The Axial Skeleton

MULTIPLE CHOICE. Choose the one alternative that best completes the statement or answers the question.

1) The auditory ossicles are located in the
   A) sella turcica of the sphenoid bone.
   B) middle ear.
   C) external auditory meatus.
   D) internal auditory meatus.
   E) mastoid processes of the temporal bone.

   Answer: B
   Page Ref: 183

2) Which of the following best defines a short bone?
   A) a bone with greater length than width
   B) a bone consisting of two parallel plates of compact bone
   C) a bone whose length and width are nearly equal
   D) a bone in a suture
   E) a bone measuring not more than five centimeters in length

   Answer: C
   Page Ref: 185

3) Which of the following best defines a flat bone?
   A) any bone in the skull
   B) a bone consisting of two parallel plates of compact bone
   C) a bone whose length and width are nearly equal
   D) a bone that has no curves in its structure
   E) a bone in a suture

   Answer: B
   Page Ref: 185

4) The carpals and tarsal are classified as:
   A) flat bones.
   B) irregular bones.
   C) Wormian bones.
   D) short bones.
   E) long bones.

   Answer: D
   Page Ref: 185

5) The scapula is an example of a(n):
   A) flat bone.
   B) irregular bone.
   C) Wormian bone.
   D) short bone.
   E) long bone.

   Answer: A
   Page Ref: 185

6) The patellae are examples of:
   A) flat bones.
   B) irregular bones.
   C) Wormian bones.
   D) short bones.
   E) sesamoid bones.

   Answer: E
   Page Ref: 185

7) **ALL** of the following are part of the axial skeleton **EXCEPT** the:
   A) occipital bone.
   B) hyoid bone.
   C) vertebrae.
   D) coxal bones.
   E) sternum.

   Answer: D
   Page Ref: 184

8) Which of the following bones is considered to be part of the axial skeleton?
   A) humerus
   B) coxal
   C) hyoid
   D) patella
   E) talus

   Answer: C
   Page Ref: 185

9) The only movable bone of the skull is the:
   A) temporal.
   B) maxilla.
   C) mandible.
   D) zygomatic.
   E) nasal.

   Answer: C
   Page Ref: 196

10) Which of the following sutures generally does **NOT** persist into adulthood?
   A) frontal
   B) sagittal
   C) coronal
   D) lambdoid
   E) squamous

   Answer: A
   Page Ref: 197

11) The bones forming the greater portions of the sides and roof of the cranial cavity are the:
   A) frontals.
   B) temporals.
   C) sphenoids.
   D) occipitals.
   E) parietals.

   Answer: E
   Page Ref: 188

12) **ALL** of the following terms refer to processes or projections from bones **EXCEPT**:
   A) tubercle.
   B) fossa.
   C) trochanter.
   D) condyle.
   E) spine.

   Answer: B
   Page Ref: 187

13) The zygomatic process is part of the:

   A) sphenoid bone.

   B) frontal bone.

   C) temporal bone.

   D) zygomatic bone.

   E) maxilla.

   Answer: C
   Page Ref: 189

14) The internal auditory meatus is the opening through which:

   A) cranial nerves VII and VIII pass.

   B) sound waves are directed into the ear.

   C) the ossicles vibrate.

   D) air passes to enter the middle ear.

   E) ligaments suspending the hyoid bone pass.

   Answer: A
   Page Ref: 190

15) **ALL** of the following are considered part of the appendicular skeleton **EXCEPT** the:

   A) humerus.

   B) coxal bones.

   C) fibula.

   D) ribs.

   E) calcaneus.

   Answer: D
   Page Ref: 185

16) There are normally **TWO** of **EACH** of the following bones **EXCEPT** the:

   A) vomer.

   B) maxilla.

   C) nasal.

   D) temporal.

   E) zygomatic.

   Answer: A
   Page Ref: 186

17) The carotid artery passes through the carotid foramen in the:

   A) greater wings of the sphenoid.

   B) cribriform plate of the ethmoid.

   C) mastoid process of the temporal bone.

   D) petrous portion of the temporal bone.

   E) occipital condyles.

   Answer: D
   Page Ref: 199

18) The ligamentum nuchae is a fibroelastic ligament extending between the seventh cervical vertebra and the:

   A) external occipital protuberance.

   B) mastoid processes of the temporal bone.

   C) coccyx.

   D) dens of the axis.

   E) crista galli of the ethmoid.

   Answer: A
   Page Ref: 191

19) The superior orbital fissure is located:

   A) in the supraorbital margin.

   B) between the anterior aspects of the greater and lesser wings of the sphenoid bone.

   C) between the petrous portion of the temporal bone and the occipital bone.

   D) in the orbit between the sphenoid and ethmoid bones.

   E) between the lacrimal and nasal bones.

   Answer: B
   Page Ref: 194

20) Some muscles that move the mandible attach to the:

   A) sella turcica of the sphenoid bone.

   B) styloid processes of the temporal bone.

   C) external occipital protuberance.

   D) perpendicular plate of the ethmoid.

   E) pterygoid processes of the sphenoid bone.

   Answer: E
   Page Ref: 194

21) The internal and middle ear are housed by the:

    A) external auditory meatus.

    B) mastoid process of the temporal bone.

    C) sella turcica of the sphenoid bone.

    D) petrous portion of the temporal bone.

    E) greater wings of the sphenoid bone.

Answer: D
Page Ref: 190

22) The mandibular fossa of the temporal bone articulates with what part of the mandible?

    A) condylar process

    B) coronoid process

    C) alveolar process

    D) zygomatic process

    E) mental foramen

Answer: A
Page Ref: 197

23) The temporal bone articulates with **ALL** of the following **EXCEPT** the:

    A) parietal bone.

    B) zygomatic bone.

    C) mandible.

    D) frontal bone.

    E) sphenoid bone.

Answer: D
Page Ref: 189

24) Directly anterior to the sphenoid bone and posterior to the nasal bones is the:

    A) zygomatic bone.

    B) palatine bone.

    C) maxilla.

    D) hyoid.

    E) ethmoid bone.

Answer: E
Page Ref: 194

25) The hyoid bone is suspended from the:
    A) mastoid processes of the temporal bones.
    B) occipital condyles.
    C) superior nasal conchae of the ethmoid bones.
    D) sella turcica of the sphenoid bone.
    E) styloid processes of the temporal bones.

    Answer: E
    Page Ref: 201

26) The superior articular facets of the atlas articulate with the:
    A) occipital condyles.
    B) mastoid processes of the temporal bones.
    C) dens of the axis.
    D) inferior articular facets of the axis.
    E) first ribs.

    Answer: A
    Page Ref: 204

27) Which of the following is located between the greater wing of the sphenoid bone and the maxilla?
    A) optic foramen
    B) infraorbital foramen
    C) supraorbital foramen
    D) superior orbital fissure
    E) inferior orbital fissure

    Answer: E
    Page Ref: 194

28) Cleft palate results from incomplete fusion of the:
    A) vomer and perpendicular plate.
    B) alveolar processes of the maxillae.
    C) palatine processes of the maxillae.
    D) pterygoid processes of the sphenoid.
    E) nasal bones.

    Answer: C
    Page Ref: 194

29) Tears pass into the nasal cavity via the:

A) mental foramen.

B) jugular foramen.

C) carotid foramen.

D) infraorbital foramen.

E) lacrimal fossa.

Answer: E
Page Ref: 196

30) The pituitary gland is located in the:

A) sella turcica of the sphenoid bone.

B) petrous portion of the temporal bone.

C) mastoid process of the temporal bone.

D) hypoglossal canal of the occipital bone.

E) crista galli of the ethmoid bone.

Answer: A
Page Ref: 194

31) Which of the following are **NOT** part of the ethmoid bone?

A) superior nasal conchae

B) middle nasal conchae

C) inferior nasal conchae

D) lateral masses

E) olfactory foramina

Answer: C
Page Ref: 194

32) The bone whose superior border articulates with the perpendicular plate of the ethmoid to form the nasal septum is the:

A) lacrimal.

B) nasal.

C) palatine.

D) sphenoid.

E) vomer.

Answer: E
Page Ref: 196

33) Which of the following has both an alveolar process and a coronoid process?

A) mandible

B) maxilla

C) zygomatic

D) vomer

E) palatine

Answer: A
Page Ref: 197

34) The function of the nasal conchae is to:

A) provide a surface for muscle attachment.

B) create turbulence in inspired air for cleansing purposes.

C) provide extensive surface area for gas exchange.

D) act as an anchor for periodontal ligaments.

E) protect olfactory nerves as they travel to the brain.

Answer: B
Page Ref: 196

35) Paranasal sinuses are found in **ALL** of the following bones **EXCEPT** the:

A) frontal.

B) sphenoid.

C) zygomatic.

D) ethmoid.

E) maxilla.

Answer: C
Page Ref: 197

36) **ALL** of the following form part of the orbit **EXCEPT** the:

A) zygomatic.

B) maxilla.

C) sphenoid.

D) vomer.

E) lacrimal.

Answer: D
Page Ref: 198

37) The nasal septum is formed by cartilage and the:

   A) pterygoid processes and perpendicular plate of the sphenoid.

   B) horizontal plate of the palatine and the perpendicular plate of the ethmoid.

   C) vomer and perpendicular plate of the ethmoid.

   D) vomer and perpendicular plate of the sphenoid.

   E) nasal bones.

   Answer: C
   Page Ref: 195

38) The tongue is supported by the:

   A) hyoid.

   B) maxilla.

   C) zygomatic.

   D) vomer.

   E) palatines.

   Answer: A
   Page Ref: 201

39) The spinal cord passes through the:

   A) intervertebral foramen.

   B) transverse foramen.

   C) vertebral foramen.

   D) centrum.

   E) Both C and D are correct.

   Answer: C
   Page Ref: 204

40) When whiplash injuries result in death, the usual cause is damage to the medulla oblongata of the brain by the:

   A) rupturing of intervertebral discs.

   B) dens of the axis.

   C) spinous processes of the cervical vertebrae.

   D) vertebra prominens.

   E) lateral masses of the atlas.

   Answer: B
   Page Ref: 205

41) The meninges that cover the brain attach anteriorly to the:

    A) sella turcica of the sphenoid bone.

    B) styloid processes of the temporal bones.

    C) external occipital protuberance.

    D) perpendicular plate of the ethmoid.

    E) crista galli of the ethmoid bone.

Answer: E
Page Ref: 194

42) The laminae of a vertebra are the parts:

    A) through which spinal nerves pass.

    B) that form the posterior portion of the vertebral arch.

    C) that form the transverse processes.

    D) to which the ribs attach.

    E) to which the intervertebral discs attach.

Answer: B
Page Ref: 203

43) Transverse foramina are seen in:

    A) cervical vertebrae.

    B) thoracic vertebrae

    C) lumbar vertebrae

    D) sacral vertebrae

    E) Both A and B are correct.

Answer: A
Page Ref: 204

44) **ALL** of the following foramina are in the sphenoid bone **EXCEPT** the:

    A) foramen rotundum.

    B) superior orbital fissure.

    C) foramen ovale.

    D) optic foramen.

    E) jugular foramen.

Answer: E
Page Ref: 194

45) Anesthetic agents used in caudal anesthesia are sometimes injected into the:
   A) lumbosacral joint.
   B) sacral hiatus.
   C) coccygeal cornua.
   D) nucleus pulposus.
   E) sacral ala.

   Answer: B
   Page Ref: 210

46) The xiphoid process is part of the:
   A) atlas.
   B) axis.
   C) sternum.
   D) sacrum.
   E) coccyx.

   Answer: C
   Page Ref: 211

47) Herniated discs occur most often in which vertebral region?
   A) cervical
   B) thoracic
   C) lumbar
   D) sacral
   E) coccygeal

   Answer: C
   Page Ref: 213

48) Which of the following lists the regions of the vertebral column in the correct order from superior to inferior?
   A) cervical, lumbar, thoracic, coccygeal, sacral
   B) coccygeal, sacral, lumbar, thoracic, cervical
   C) coccygeal, lumbar, sacral, thoracic, cervical
   D) cervical, thoracic, lumbar, sacral, coccygeal
   E) thoracic, cervical lumbar, sacral, coccygeal

   Answer: D
   Page Ref: 202

49) The lumbar curve of the vertebral column develops:

   A) only if the intervertebral discs are damaged.

   B) when an infant begins to hold its head erect.

   C) when a child begins to sit, stand, and walk.

   D) during the third month of fetal development.

   E) just prior to birth.

   Answer: C
   Page Ref: 203

50) The glossopharyngeal, vagus, and accessory nerves pass through the:

   A) foramen rotundum.

   B) foramen lacerum

   C) carotid foramen.

   D) hypoglossal canal.

   E) jugular foramen.

   Answer: E
   Page Ref: 199

MATCHING. Choose the item in column 2 that best matches each item in column 1.

Choose the item from column 2 that best matches each item is column 1.

   1) Column 1: sella turcica
      Column 2: sphenoid
      Answer: sphenoid
      Page Ref: 194

   2) Column 1: horizontal plate
      Column 2: palatine
      Answer: palatine
      Page Ref: 196

   3) Column 1: palatine process
      Column 2: maxilla
      Answer: maxilla
      Page Ref: 194

   4) Column 1: condylar process
      Column 2: mandible
      Answer: mandible
      Page Ref: 197

5) Column 1: supraorbital margin
   Column 2: frontal
   Answer: frontal
   Page Ref: 188

6) Column 1: temporal process
   Column 2: zygomatic
   Answer: zygomatic
   Page Ref: 196

7) Column 1: styloid process
   Column 2: temporal
   Answer: temporal
   Page Ref: 190

8) Column 1: crista galli
   Column 2: ethmoid
   Answer: ethmoid
   Page Ref: 194

9) Column 1: superior nuchal line
   Column 2: occipital
   Answer: occipital
   Page Ref: 191

10) Column 1: manubrium
    Column 2: sternum
    Answer: sternum
    Page Ref: 211

MATCHING. Choose the item in column 2 that best matches each item in column 1.

Choose the item from column 2 that best matches each item is column 1.

1) Column 1: foramen
   Column 2: an opening through which
           blood vessels, nerves, or
           ligaments pass
   Answer: an opening through which blood vessels, nerves, or ligaments pass
   Page Ref: 187

2) Column 1: fossa

   Column 2: a depression in or on a bone

   Answer: a depression in or on a bone

   Page Ref: 187

3) Column 1: sulcus

   Column 2: a groove that accommodates a
   soft structure

   Answer: a groove that accommodates a soft structure

   Page Ref: 187

4) Column 1: meatus

   Column 2: a tubelike passageway
   running within a bone

   Answer: a tubelike passageway running within a bone

   Page Ref: 187

5) Column 1: fissure

   Column 2: a narrow, cleftlike opening
   between adjacent parts of
   bones

   Answer: a narrow, cleftlike opening between adjacent parts of bones

   Page Ref: 187

6) Column 1: facet

   Column 2: a smooth, flat surface

   Answer: a smooth, flat surface

   Page Ref: 187

7) Column 1: crest

   Column 2: a prominent border or ridge

   Answer: a prominent border or ridge

   Page Ref: 187

8) Column 1: tubercle

   Column 2: a small, rounded process

   Answer: a small, rounded process

   Page Ref: 187

9) Column 1: tuberosity

Column 2: a large, rounded, roughened process

Answer: a large, rounded, roughened process

Page Ref: 187

10) Column 1: ramus

Column 2: part of a bone that forms an angle with the main body of a bone

Answer: part of a bone that forms an angle with the main body of a bone

Page Ref: 196

TRUE/FALSE. Write 'T' if the statement is true and 'F' if the statement is false.

1) Flat bones are generally composed of two plates of spongy bone enclosing a layer of compact bone.

Answer: FALSE
Page Ref: 185

2) The sphenoid articulates with all other cranial bones.

Answer: TRUE
Page Ref: 192

3) A trochanter is a large projection seen only on the femur.

Answer: TRUE
Page Ref: 187

4) A tubercle is a small, rounded process on a bone.

Answer: TRUE
Page Ref: 187

5) The olfactory foramina pass through the perpendicular plate.

Answer: FALSE
Page Ref: 194

6) The coronal suture joins the parietal bones to each other.

Answer: FALSE
Page Ref: 197

7) The posterior portion of the hard palate is formed by the horizontal plates of the palatine bones.

Answer: TRUE
Page Ref: 196

8) Thoracic vertebrae have bifid spinous processes.

Answer: FALSE
Page Ref: 205

9) The optic nerve passes through the optic foramen.

Answer: TRUE
Page Ref: 194

10) The alveoli of the maxillae are air–filled spaces.

Answer: FALSE
Page Ref: 194

11) There is a paranasal sinus within the sphenoid bone.

Answer: TRUE
Page Ref: 197

12) The hyoid bone is suspended from the mastoid processes.

Answer: FALSE
Page Ref: 201

13) The foramen ovale passes through the sphenoid bone.

Answer: TRUE
Page Ref: 194

14) Women normally have only one pair of floating ribs.

Answer: FALSE
Page Ref: 211

15) Cranial nerve VIII (vestibulocochlear) passes through the external auditory meatus.

Answer: FALSE
Page Ref: 189

SHORT ANSWER. Write the word or phrase that best completes each statement or answers the question.

1) The suture between the frontal and parietal bones is the _____ suture.
Answer: coronal
Page Ref: 197

2) The superior portion of the sternum is called the _____.
Answer: manubrium
Page Ref: 211

3) There are _____ bones in the axial division of the skeletal system, and _____ bones in the appendicular division.
Answer: 80, 126
Page Ref: 183

4) The clavicular notches are seen on the _____.
Answer: sternum
Page Ref: 211

5) There are _____ pairs of vertebrosternal ribs.
Answer: seven
Page Ref: 211

6) The spaces between the ribs are called _____ spaces.
Answer: intercostal
Page Ref: 213

7) An exaggeration of the thoracic curve of the vertebral column commonly seen in women with advanced osteoporosis is called _____.
Answer: kyphosis
Page Ref: 214

8) The first cervical vertebra is called the _____.
Answer: atlas
Page Ref: 204

9) Spinal nerves pass through openings between the vertebrae called _____.
Answer: intervertebral foramina
Page Ref: 201

10) Bones located in tendons are referred to as _____ bones.
Answer: sesamoid
Page Ref: 185

11) The passageway through the temporal bone that directs sound waves into the ear is the _____.
Answer: external auditory meatus
Page Ref: 189

12) The suture located between the parietal bones and the occipital bone is the _____ suture.
    Answer: lambdoid
    Page Ref: 197

13) The hyoid bone is suspended by ligaments from the _____ of the temporal bones.
    Answer: styloid processes
    Page Ref: 201

14) Ribs that attach anteriorly to the cartilage of other ribs are referred to as false ribs or _____ ribs.
    Answer: vertebrochondral
    Page Ref: 211

15) The internal and middle ear are housed within the _____ of the temporal bone.
    Answer: petrous portion
    Page Ref: 190

16) When an infant begins to hold its head up, its vertebral column begins to develop a _____ curve.
    Answer: cervical
    Page Ref: 203

17) The occipital condyles articulate with the _____.
    Answer: atlas
    Page Ref: 191

18) The foramen magnum is a large hole in the _____ bone.
    Answer: occipital
    Page Ref: 191

19) The major supporting structure of the nasal cavity is the _____ bone.
    Answer: ethmoid
    Page Ref: 194

20) The olfactory foramina are located in the _____ of the ethmoid bone.
    Answer: cribriform plate
    Page Ref: 194

21) The nasal septum is formed by the _____ and the _____.
    Answer: perpendicular plate of the ethmoid; vomer
    Page Ref: 194, 196

22) The triangular point of the ethmoid that serves as a point of attachment for the meninges is the _____.
Answer: crista galli
Page Ref: 194

23) Two foramina in the mandible that serve as important sites for injection of dental anesthetics are the mandibular foramen and the _____ foramen.
Answer: mental
Page Ref: 197

24) The superior and middle conchae are part of the _____ bone.
Answer: ethmoid
Page Ref: 194

25) The adult vertebral column consists of _____ cervical vertebrae, _____ thoracic vertebrae, _____ lumbar vertebrae, _____ sacral vertebrae fused into one bone, and _____ coccygeal vertebrae fused into one or two bones.
Answer: 7; 12; 5; 5; 4
Page Ref: 201

26) The hard palate is formed by the _____ of the _____ , and the _____ of the _____.
Answer: palatine processes; maxillae; horizontal plates; palatine bones
Page Ref: 194, 196

27) The prominences of the cheeks are formed by the _____ bones.
Answer: zygomatic
Page Ref: 196

28) The tiny bones just posterior and lateral to the nasal bones are the _____.
Answer: lacrimal bones
Page Ref: 196

29) The condylar process of the mandible articulates with the mandibular fossa of the _____.
Answer: temporal bone
Page Ref: 197

30) The suture between the parietal and temporal bones is the _____ suture.
Answer: squamous
Page Ref: 197

31) An opening in a bone through which blood vessels, nerves, or ligaments pass is called a(n) _____.

Answer: foramen

Page Ref: 187

32) A shallow depression in a bone is called a(n) _____.

Answer: fossa

Page Ref: 187

33) Cranial nerve II passes through the _____ foramen.

Answer: optic

Page Ref: 199

34) Branches of the trigeminal nerve pass through two foramina —the foramen _____ and the foramen _____.

Answer: ovale; rotundum

Page Ref: 199

35) The bony structure that protects the pituitary gland is the _____.

Answer: sella turcica of the sphenoid

Page Ref: 194

ESSAY. Write your answer in the space provided or on a separate sheet of paper.

1) Describe the location and anatomical features of the sphenoid bone.

Answer: The bat–shaped sphenoid bone forms much of the cranial floor and articulates anteriorly with the frontal, laterally with the temporal, and posteriorly with the occipital. The body, containing the sphenoidal sinus, is centrally located between the ethmoid and the occipital. The sella turcica, which protects the pituitary, sits atop the body. The greater wings form the anterolateral cranial floor and part of the lateral wall of the skull. The lesser wings, anterior and superior to the greater wings, form the posterior part of the orbit. Foramina include the optic foramen, forman ovale, foramen rotundum, and superior and inferior orbital fissures. The pterygoid processes project inferiorly from the junction of the body and the greater wings.

Page Ref: 192–194

2) Where are the turbinates located and what is their function?

Answer: Superior and middle nasal conchae (turbinates) project like scrolls from the lateral masses of the ethmoid. The inferior turbinates are separate bones. All form the lateral walls of the nasal cavity. The scrolled structure forms a mucus–coated surface area that traps inhaled particles and warms and moistens air.

Page Ref: 194, 196

3) Describe the function of the orbit, and give the names and locations of the bones of the orbit.

Answer: The function is protection of the eyeball and associated structures. The roof is formed by the frontal and sphenoid, the lateral wall by the sphenoid and the zygomatic, the floor by the maxilla, zygomatic and palatine, and the medial wall by the maxilla, lacrimal, ethmoid, and sphenoid.

Page Ref: 198

4) Where is the hyoid bone located? What is its function? What is the significance of finding a broken hyoid on autopsy?

Answer: The hyoid bone is suspended by ligaments and muscles from the styloid processes of the temporal bones. It is located in the anterior neck between the mandible and the larynx. It supports the tongue, providing attachment sites for some tongue muscles and for muscles of the neck and pharynx. Crushing injury to the neck, such as would occur in strangulation, is indicated by a broken hyoid.

Page Ref: 201

5) Define the term *fontanel* and describe the functions of fontanels.

Answer: A fontanel is a membrane–filled space between the cranial bones of a newborn. Fontanels enable the fetal skull to modify its size and shape as it passes through the birth canal, permit rapid brain growth in infancy, help determine the degree of brain development by their state of closure, and act as landmarks for blood drawing.

Page Ref: 197

6) Describe the classification of ribs based on their articulations with other bones.

Answer: True ribs (vertebrosternal) are pairs 1–7, and attach directly to the sternum via costal cartilages. False ribs (vertebrochondral) are pairs 8 –10, and attach directly to each other's cartilage then to the cartilage of pair 7. False ribs (vertebral) also include pairs 11 –12, which have no anterior attachment.

Page Ref: 211

7) Describe the functions of the cranial and facial bones.

Answer: Cranial bones protect the brain and provide an attachment point for the meninges and the muscles moving the head. The facial bones form the framework of the face, protect and provide support for the entrances to the digestive and respiratory tracts, and provide attachment points for the muscles of facial expression. Both support organs of special senses.

Page Ref: 187

8) Archaeologists have unearthed several vertebrae. Vertebrae A and B are extremely tiny, and appear to be fused. Vertebrae C–F have transverse foramina and bifid spinous processes. Vertebra G has a spinous process that projects straight posteriorly, and has superior articular facets that project medially. How should the vertebrae be arranged to put them in the most realistic order? Why?

Answer: The features described suggest the following order: Vertebrae C–F most superior (cervical); Vertebra G (lumbar); Vertebrae A and B (coccygeal).

Page Ref: 204–209

9) Describe the structure and function of intervertebral discs. Describe what happens when a disc "slips." Why is this such a painful condition?

Answer: An intervertebral disc consists of a fibrocartilage ring (annulus fibrosus) surrounding an inner soft, pulpy, elastic substance (nucleus pulposus). Damaged or weakened ligaments associated with the discs may allow such pressure to develop that the fibrocartilage ruptures, allowing the nucleus pulposus to protrude posteriorly to put pressure on spinal nerves. This causes acute pain.

Page Ref: 213

10) Name and describe the abnormal curvatures of the spine. How does each commonly develop?

Answer: 1. Scoliosis —abnormal lateral bending on the thoracic region; congenital, malformed vertebrae, chronic sciatica, one-sided paralysis, poor posture, one leg shorter than the other
2. Kyphosis—exaggerated thoracic curvature; TB of spine or osteoporosis leading to collapse of vertebral bodies; also rickets, poor posture, geriatric disc degeneration
3. Lordosis—exaggerated lumbar curvature; increased abdominal weight, poor posture, rickets, TB of spine

Page Ref: 214

CHAPTER 8   The Skeletal System: The Appendicular Skeleton

MULTIPLE CHOICE. Choose the one alternative that best completes the statement or answers the question.

1) **ALL** of the following are part of the appendicular skeleton **EXCEPT** the:

   A) scapula.

   B) coxal bones.

   C) sternum.

   D) fibula.

   E) radius.

   Answer: C
   Page Ref: 184, 218

2) Most of the structural differences between the male and female skeletons are related to adaptation for:

   A) problems associated with height differences.

   B) problems associated with weight differences.

   C) hunting vs. gathering.

   D) pregnancy and childbirth.

   E) roles in sexual activity.

   Answer: C
   Page Ref: 231

3) **ALL** of the following are typical of a female pelvis **EXCEPT**:

   A) oval obturator foramen.

   B) acetabulum faces anteriorly.

   C) less movable coccyx.

   D) wider greater sciatic notch.

   E) shorter, wider sacrum.

   Answer: C
   Page Ref: 230

4) The coronoid and olecranon fossae are depressions found on the:
   A) ulna.
   B) radius.
   C) scapula.
   D) humerus.
   E) femur.

   Answer: D
   Page Ref: 222

5) Most of the muscles of the forearm attach to the:
   A) greater and lesser tubercles of the humerus.
   B) coronoid and olecranon fossae of the humerus.
   C) deltoid tuberosity of humerus.
   D) acromion and coracoid processes of the scapula.
   E) medial and lateral epicondyles of the humerus.

   Answer: E
   Page Ref: 222

6) The proximal end of the femur articulates with the:
   A) acetabulum.
   B) patella.
   C) obturator foramen.
   D) condyles of the tibia.
   E) Both B and D are correct.

   Answer: A
   Page Ref: 231

7) Which of the following is part of the elbow joint?
   A) trochlear notch of the ulna
   B) ulnar notch of the radius
   C) glenoid fossa of the humerus
   D) styloid process of the radius
   E) head of the ulna

   Answer: A
   Page Ref: 224

8) **ALL** of the following are in the proximal row of carpal bones **EXCEPT** the:

   A) hamate.

   B) lunate.

   C) scaphoid.

   D) pisiform.

   E) triquetrum.

   Answer: A
   Page Ref: 225

9) **ALL** of the following are in the distal row of carpal bones **EXCEPT** the:

   A) trapezium.

   B) trapezoid.

   C) triquetrum.

   D) hamate.

   E) capitate.

   Answer: C
   Page Ref: 225

10) Which of the following is on the anterior side of the femur?

   A) gluteal tuberosity

   B) linea aspera

   C) intertrochanteric line

   D) intertrochanteric crest

   E) Both B and C are correct.

   Answer: D
   Page Ref: 232

11) *Genu varum* is:

   A) a landmark of the pelvic brim.

   B) the medical term for bowleggedness.

   C) a part of the carpal tunnel.

   D) the junction between the tibia and talus.

   E) the imaginary line the baby's head follows through the pelvis.

   Answer: B
   Page Ref: 237

12) The tibial tuberosity is the attachment point for the:
   A) interosseous membrane.
   B) biceps brachii.
   C) patellar ligament.
   D) deltoid.
   E) flexor retinaculum.

   Answer: C
   Page Ref: 234

13) The bone that is considered a sesamoid bone is the:
   A) clavicle.
   B) scaphoid.
   C) cuboid.
   D) patella.
   E) All are sesamoid bones except A.

   Answer: D
   Page Ref: 232

14) The base of the patella is the:
   A) superior end.
   B) inferior end.
   C) anterior surface.
   D) posterior surface.
   E) lateral edge.

   Answer: A
   Page Ref: 234

15) The articular facets of the patella articulate with the:
   A) medial and lateral epicondyles of the femur.
   B) medial and lateral condyles of the femur.
   C) medial and lateral epicondyles of the tibia.
   D) tibial tuberosity.
   E) head of the fibula.

   Answer: B
   Page Ref: 232

16) The "shinbone" is the:

   A) femur.

   B) fibula.

   C) pubis.

   D) radius.

   E) tibia.

   Answer: E
   Page Ref: 234

17) The part of the tibia that articulates with the head of the fibula is the:

   A) tibial tuberosity.

   B) medial malleolus.

   C) medial condyle.

   D) lateral condyle.

   E) None of these—the tibia does not articulate with the head of the femur.

   Answer: D
   Page Ref: 234

18) When someone says an elderly person "broke her hip," it is most likely the fracture occurred in the:

   A) sacroiliac joint.

   B) pubic symphysis.

   C) neck of the femur.

   D) acetabulum.

   E) ilium.

   Answer: C
   Page Ref: 238

19) The prominence that can be felt on the medial surface of the ankle is part of the:

   A) tibia.

   B) fibula.

   C) talus.

   D) calcaneus.

   E) navicular.

   Answer: A
   Page Ref: 234

20) The greater and lesser trochanters are projections seen on the:
   A) humerus.
   B) scapula.
   C) tibia.
   D) femur.
   E) ischium.

   Answer: D
   Page Ref: 232

21) The distal end of the fibula articulates with the:
   A) lateral condyle of the tibia.
   B) lateral condyle of the femur.
   C) fibular notch of the tibia.
   D) medial malleolus of the tibia.
   E) calcaneus.

   Answer: C
   Page Ref: 234

22) The lateral malleolus is part of the:
   A) tibia.
   B) fibula.
   C) femur.
   D) humerus.
   E) ulna.

   Answer: B
   Page Ref: 234

23) During walking, the talus transmits about half of the weight of the body to the:
   A) navicular.
   B) cuboid.
   C) calcaneus.
   D) metatarsals.
   E) phalanges.

   Answer: C
   Page Ref: 234

24) The head of metatarsal I articulates with the:

   A) base of the proximal phalanx of the hallux.

   B) first cuneiform

   C) cuboid.

   D) base of metatarsal II.

   E) hamate.

   Answer: A
   Page Ref: 234

25) The acromion process of the scapula articulates with the:

   A) greater tubercle of the humerus.

   B) head of the humerus.

   C) lateral end of the clavicle.

   D) medial end of the clavicle.

   E) vertebral column.

   Answer: C
   Page Ref: 221

26) Which of the following is located on the ventral surface of the scapula?

   A) acromion process

   B) spine

   C) supraspinous fossa

   D) subscapular fossa

   E) All of these are correct.

   Answer: D
   Page Ref: 221

27) The medial part of the longitudinal arch includes **ALL** of the following **EXCEPT** the:

   A) cuboid.

   B) cuneiforms.

   C) talus.

   D) navicular.

   E) heads of the three metatarsals I, II and III.

   Answer: A
   Page Ref: 236

28) The roughened area on the middle portion of the shaft of the humerus is the:

   A) deltoid tuberosity.

   B) anatomical neck.

   C) capitulum.

   D) trochlea.

   E) lesser tubercle.

   Answer: A
   Page Ref: 222

29) A lateral deviation of the proximal phalanx of the great toe and medial displacement of metatarsal I describes:

   A) clawfoot.

   B) flatfoot.

   C) clubfoot.

   D) bunion.

   E) genu valgus.

   Answer: D
   Page Ref: 237

30) The prominence of the elbow is formed by the:

   A) coronoid process of the ulna.

   B) olecranon process of the ulna.

   C) head of the radius.

   D) head of the humerus.

   E) ulnar tuberosity.

   Answer: B
   Page Ref: 223

31) The main function of the appendicular skeleton is to:

   A) facilitate movement.

   B) protect internal organs.

   C) produce hormones for regulation of calcium balance.

   D) store iron for blood cell production.

   E) help regulate body temperature.

   Answer: A
   Page Ref: 218

32) Which of the following lists the proximal row of carpal bones in the correct order from lateral to medial?

A) scaphoid, pisiform, lunate, triquetrum

B) pisiform, triquetrum, lunate, scaphoid

C) scaphoid, lunate, triquetrum, pisiform

D) scaphoid, triquetrum, lunate, pisiform

E) None of these, because these are the distal carpal bones.

Answer: C
Page Ref: 225

33) Which of the following lists the distal row of carpal bones in the correct order from lateral to medial?

A) hamate, capitate, trapezoid, trapezium

B) trapezium, trapezoid, capitate, hamate

C) capitate, hamate, trapezium, trapezoid

D) trapezoid, trapezium, capitate, hamate

E) None of these, because these are the proximal carpal bones.

Answer: E
Page Ref: 225

34) The costal tuberosity is located on the:

A) lateral midshaft of the humerus.

B) anterior surface of the distal end of the humerus.

C) superior ramus of the pubis.

D) posterior aspect of the femur.

E) inferior surface of the medial end of the clavicle.

Answer: E
Page Ref: 218

35) ALL of the following are TRUE for the scapula EXCEPT the:

A) scapular notch is in the superior border.

B) acromion is the high point of the shoulder.

C) glenoid cavity opens toward the lateral side of the body.

D) medial border articulates with the vertebral column.

E) spine is on the posterior surface.

Answer: D
Page Ref: 221

36) The bones making up the palm of the hand are the:

A) metatarsals.

B) metacarpals.

C) carpals.

D) tarsals.

E) phalanges.

Answer: B
Page Ref: 225

37) The trochlea is located:

A) between the greater and lesser tubercles of the humerus.

B) between the coronoid process and the olecranon of the ulna.

C) on the lateral midshaft of the humerus.

D) lateral to the capitulum of the humerus.

E) medial to the capitulum of the humerus.

Answer: E
Page Ref: 222

38) Which metacarpal is proximal to the little finger?

A) number I

B) number II

C) number III

D) number IV

E) number V

Answer: E
Page Ref: 225

39) When the forearm is flexed, which of the following is TRUE?

A) The olecranon moves into the olecranon fossa.

B) The coronoid process moves into the coronoid fossa.

C) The radial head moves into the radial fossa.

D) The radial head moves into the glenoid fossa.

E) Both B and C are correct.

Answer: B
Page Ref: 225

40) When you sit on a stool, which part of the coxal bones touch the stool first?

A) ischial spines

B) ischial tuberosities

C) iliac crests

D) pubic symphysis

E) inferior pubic rami

Answer: B
Page Ref: 227

41) The interosseous membrane joins the:

A) radius and ulna.

B) bones of the metacarpals.

C) femur and tibia.

D) two scapulae.

E) medial malleolus and lateral malleolus.

Answer: A
Page Ref: 223

42) The radius articulates with the:

A) lateral metacarpals.

B) trapezoid.

C) capitate.

D) lunate.

E) medial metacarpals.

Answer: D
Page Ref: 225

43) The superior border of the most superior of the subdivisions of the hipbone is the:

A) ischial tuberosity.

B) superior ramus of the pubis.

C) pubic crest.

D) ischial spine.

E) iliac crest.

Answer: E
Page Ref: 226

44) The head of the capitate articulates with the:
   A) radius.
   B) head of metacarpal III.
   C) scaphoid.
   D) pisiform.
   E) hamate.

   Answer: E
   Page Ref: 225

45) The large hole in the coxal bone through which blood vessels and nerves pass is the:
   A) acetabulum.
   B) pubic symphysis.
   C) obturator foramen.
   D) iliac fossa.
   E) glenoid cavity.

   Answer: C
   Page Ref: 227

46) The lesser sciatic notch is a feature of the:
   A) ilium.
   B) ischium.
   C) pubis.
   D) femur.
   E) sacrum.

   Answer: B
   Page Ref: 227

47) The posterior landmark of the pelvic brim is the:
   A) sacral promontory.
   B) posterior superior iliac spines.
   C) posterior inferior iliac spines.
   D) ischial tuberosities.
   E) tip of the coccyx.

   Answer: A
   Page Ref: 227

48) **ALL** of the following are **TRUE** for the true pelvis **EXCEPT**:

    A) it surrounds the pelvic cavity.

    B) its inferior opening is the pelvic outlet.

    C) it is bounded anteriorly by the abdominal wall.

    D) it is bounded posteriorly by the sacrum and coccyx.

    E) it is the part of the bony pelvic below the pelvic brim.

Answer: C
Page Ref: 228

49) Which of the following is **TRUE** for the false pelvis?

    A) It does not normally contain pelvic organs.

    B) It is bounded posteriorly by the sacrum and coccyx.

    C) Its superior opening is the pelvic inlet.

    D) Its inferior opening is the pelvic outlet.

    E) It is bordered anteriorly by the pubic symphysis.

Answer: A
Page Ref: 228

50) A pair of coxal bones unearthed from an unmarked grave have oval–shaped obturator foramina and a pubic arch of greater than 90 degrees. What can you tell from this information?

    A) The person was probably very old because the bones have spread apart from the original position.

    B) The bones are probably those of a male because the pubic angle would be less in a female.

    C) The bones are probably those of a female because the pubic angle would be less in a male.

    D) The bones are probably from someone who suffered from a vitamin D deficiency, which caused abnormal flexibility in the bones.

    E) The bones are probably from a very young person because the obturator foramen is round in adults.

Answer: C
Page Ref: 230

MATCHING. Choose the item in column 2 that best matches each item in column 1.

Choose the item from column 2 that best matches each item in column 1.

1) Column 1: head of femur

    Column 2: acetabulum of coxal bone

    Answer: acetabulum of coxal bone

    Page Ref: 227

2) Column 1: head of humerus
   Column 2: glenoid cavity of humerus
   Answer: glenoid cavity of humerus
   Page Ref: 221

3) Column 1: lateral extremity of clavicle
   Column 2: acromion of scapula
   Foil: coracoid process of scapula
   Answer: acromion of scapula
   Page Ref: 221

4) Column 1: medial extremity of clavicle
   Column 2: sternum
   Answer: sternum
   Page Ref: 218

5) Column 1: head of radius
   Column 2: capitulum of humerus
   Foil: trochlea of humerus
   Answer: capitulum of humerus
   Page Ref: 225

6) Column 1: distal end of radius
   Column 2: scaphoid
   Foil: hamate
   Answer: scaphoid
   Page Ref: 225

7) Column 1: medial condyle of tibia
   Column 2: medial condyle of femur
   Answer: medial condyle of femur
   Page Ref: 234

8) Column 1: lateral condyle of tibia
   Column 2: head of fibula
   Answer: head of fibula
   Page Ref: 234

9) Column 1: lateral malleolus of fibula
Column 2: talus
Foil: calcaneus
Answer: talus
Page Ref: 234

10) Column 1: metatarsals
Column 2: cuneiforms
Answer: cuneiforms
Page Ref: 234

MATCHING. Choose the item in column 2 that best matches each item in column 1.

Choose the item from column 2 that best matches each item in column 1.

1) Column 1: trochlear notch
Column 2: ulna
Answer: ulna
Page Ref: 223

2) Column 1: ulnar notch
Column 2: radius
Answer: radius
Page Ref: 225

3) Column 1: greater sciatic notch
Column 2: ilium
Answer: ilium
Page Ref: 226

4) Column 1: lesser sciatic notch
Column 2: ischium
Answer: ischium
Page Ref: 227

5) Column 1: coronoid fossa
Column 2: humerus
Answer: humerus
Page Ref: 222

6) Column 1: glenoid cavity
   Column 2: scapula
   Answer: scapula
   Page Ref: 221

7) Column 1: gluteal tuberosity
   Column 2: femur
   Answer: femur
   Page Ref: 232

8) Column 1: fibular notch
   Column 2: tibia
   Answer: tibia
   Page Ref: 234

9) Column 1: lateral malleolus
   Column 2: fibula
   Answer: fibula
   Page Ref: 234

10) Column 1: conoid tubercle
    Column 2: clavicle
    Answer: clavicle
    Page Ref: 218

TRUE/FALSE. Write 'T' if the statement is true and 'F' if the statement is false.

1) The pectoral girdle consists of the clavicle and the scapula.

   Answer: TRUE
   Page Ref: 218

2) The head of the ulna is on its distal end, while the head of the radius is on its proximal end.

   Answer: TRUE
   Page Ref: 225

3) The medial end of the clavicle articulates with the scapula.

   Answer: FALSE
   Page Ref: 218

4) The spine of the scapula is on the anterior surface.

Answer: FALSE
Page Ref: 221

5) The coracoid process is part of the ulna.

Answer: FALSE
Page Ref: 221

6) The distal end of the femur articulates with both the tibia and the fibula.

Answer: FALSE
Page Ref: 234

7) The ulnar nerve lies on the posterior surface of the medial epicondyle of the humerus.

Answer: TRUE
Page Ref: 222

8) The scaphoid is in the proximal row of carpal bones.

Answer: TRUE
Page Ref: 225

9) The anatomical neck is the site of most fractures of the humerus.

Answer: FALSE
Page Ref: 221

10) The coronoid fossa is a depression on the anterior surface of the distal end of the humerus.

Answer: TRUE
Page Ref: 222

11) The heads of the phalanges articulate with the bases of the metacarpals.

Answer: FALSE
Page Ref: 225

12) The scapular notch articulates with the head of the humerus.

Answer: FALSE
Page Ref: 221

13) During a fall on an outstretched arm, force is transmitted from the upper limb to the trunk by the clavicle.

Answer: TRUE
Page Ref: 218

14) The distal end of the radius articulates with the capitate and hamate.

Answer: FALSE
Page Ref: 225

15) The inferior end of the patella is the base.

Answer: FALSE
Page Ref: 232

SHORT ANSWER. Write the word or phrase that best completes each statement or answers the question.

1) The scapula articulates with the clavicle and the _____.
Answer: humerus
Page Ref: 221

2) The former site of the epiphyseal plate on the proximal end of the humerus is the _____.
Answer: anatomical neck
Page Ref: 221

3) The fossa that is formed by the union of the ilium, ischium, and pubis, and that receives the head of the femur is the _____.
Answer: acetabulum
Page Ref: 227

4) The medial end of the clavicle is the _____ extremity.
Answer: sternal
Page Ref: 218

5) At the lateral end of the superior border of the scapula is a projection of the anterior surface called the _____ process.
Answer: coracoid
Page Ref: 221

6) The only foot bone that articulates with the tibia and fibula is the _____.
Answer: talus
Page Ref: 234

7) The head of the humerus articulates with the _____ of the _____.
Answer: glenoid cavity; scapula
Page Ref: 221

8) The lateral end of the clavicle articulates with the _____ of the _____.
Answer: acromion; scapula
Page Ref: 221

9) The spool–shaped surface at the distal end of the humerus that articulates with the ulna is the _____.
Answer: trochlea
Page Ref: 222

10) The proximal end of the fibula is called the _____.
Answer: head
Page Ref: 234

11) The distal end of the humerus has two indentations that receive parts of the ulna during flexion and extension of the forearm; these are the _____ fossa on the anterior surface and the _____ fossa on the posterior surface.
Answer: coronoid; olecranon
Page Ref: 222

12) The ulna and radius are connected by a broad, flat fibrous connective tissue called the _____.
Answer: interosseous membrane
Page Ref: 223

13) The pointed projection on the posterior side of the distal end of the ulna is the _____.
Answer: styloid process
Page Ref: 225

14) The radial notch of the ulna and the capitulum of the humerus both articulate with the _____ of the _____.
Answer: head; radius
Page Ref: 225

15) The head of the ulna articulates with the ulnar notch of the _____.
Answer: radius
Page Ref: 225

16) The force of a fall on an outstretched hand is transmitted from the capitate to the radius through the _____.
Answer: scaphoid
Page Ref: 225

17) The distal end of each metacarpal bone is its _____.
Answer: head
Page Ref: 225

18) The most medial bone of the distal row of carpals in the _____.
Answer: hamate
Page Ref: 225

19) The hip bones are also called _____ bones.
Answer: coxal
Page Ref: 225

20) The three bones making up a single hip bone are the _____ , the _____ , and the _____.
Answer: ilium; ischium; pubis
Page Ref: 226

21) The most laterally palpable bony landmark of the shoulder region is the _____ of the _____.
Answer: greater tubercle; humerus
Page Ref: 221

22) The roughened, V-shaped area in the middle portion of the shaft of the humerus is the _____.
Answer: deltoid tuberosity
Page Ref: 222

23) The sciatic nerve passes through a large indentation in the posterior part of the ilium called the _____.
Answer: greater sciatic notch
Page Ref: 226

24) The anterior, posterior, and inferior gluteal lines are all on the lateral surface of the _____.
Answer: ilium
Page Ref: 227

25) The beginning of the iliopectineal line is a projection called the _____.
Answer: pubic tubercle
Page Ref: 227

26) The edge of the scapula near the vertebral column is called the _____.
Answer: medial border
Page Ref: 218

27) The portion of the bony pelvis above the pelvic brim is the _____.
Answer: false (greater) pelvis
Page Ref: 228

28) The projection on the inferior surface of the lateral end of the clavicle is the _____.

Answer: conoid tubercle

Page Ref: 218

29) The auricular surface of the ilium articulates with the _____.

Answer: sacrum

Page Ref: 226

30) The larger projection on the proximal end of the femur that is lateral to the head of the femur is the _____.

Answer: greater trochanter

Page Ref: 232

ESSAY. Write your answer in the space provided or on a separate sheet of paper.

1) Describe the differences between the male pelvis and the female pelvis.

Answer: The female pelvis is specialized for childbirth in the following ways: false pelvis is shallower; pelvic brim is larger and more oval (vs. heart-shaped in male); pubic arch is greater than 90 degrees (male less than 90 degrees); ilium less vertical; iliac fossa shallower; iliac crest less curved; acetabulum smaller; obturator foramen oval (vs. rounded in male).

Page Ref: 230

2) On her way to her car after class, Louise slipped on the ice and fell on her outstretched hand. She cried out, "I think I've broken something!" What are the weak points in the upper extremity and shoulder girdle that might be broken? Why are these places so vulnerable?

Answer: Weak points include: midregion of clavicle, distal end of radius, and scaphoid. These are the regions through which the mechanical force of the landing will be transmitted.

Page Ref: 225

3) Describe the points of articulation among the proximal ends of the ulna and radius and the distal end of the humerus.

Answer: The following articulations are seen: trochlea of humerus fits into trochlear notch of ulna; head of radius articulates with capitulum and radial fossa of humerus; coronoid process of ulna fits into coronoid fossa of humerus during flexion of forearm; olecranon of ulna fits into olecranon fossa of humerus during extension of forearm; head of radius articulates with radial notch of ulna.

Page Ref: 222–225

4) Carolyn has had a long career as a dental hygienist. After 15 years of making small, repetitive wrist and finger movements, she has been diagnosed with carpal tunnel syndrome. What is the "carpal tunnel?"

Answer: The carpal tunnel is a concavity formed by the pisiform, hamate, scaphoid, and trapezium, plus the flexor retinaculum, through which the flexor tendons of the digits and thumb and median nerve pass.

Page Ref: 225

5) Describe/define the pelvic brim.

   Answer: The pelvic brim is the boundary between the true and false pelves, and is the circumference of an oblique plane formed as follows: begin posteriorly at sacral promontory, trace laterally and inferiorly along arcuate lines of pubis, anteriorly to superior portion of pubic symphysis.

   Page Ref: 227

6) Contrast the structures of the true and false pelves.

   Answer: The true pelvis is the portion below the pelvic brim. It is bounded by the sacrum and coccyx, laterally by the ilium and ischium, and anteriorly by the pubic bone. It surrounds the pelvic cavity. The superior opening is the pelvic brim (pelvic inlet). The inferior opening is the pelvic outlet. The pelvic axis is an imaginary line followed by the baby's head during birth. The false pelvis is the portion above the pelvic brim. It is bounded posteriorly by the lumbar vertebrae, laterally by the upper hip bones, and anteriorly by the abdominal wall. It is part of the abdomen, and does not contain pelvic organs unless the bladder is full or the uterus is pregnant.

   Page Ref: 228

7) Chuck is an aging, yet avid, basketball and baseball player who has dislocated his shoulder several times, but never dislocated a hip in any of his many falls. Why is the shoulder more easily dislocated than the hip?

   Answer: The pectoral girdle is designed for mobility over strength. The glenoid fossae are much shallower than the acetabulum. The neck of the humerus is much shorter and less angled than the neck of the femur. The pelvic girdle is attached to the vertebral column, thus making it more stable than the pectoral girdle, which is not attached to the vertebral column.

   Page Ref: 218–222

8) You are confronted with a disarticulated femur. How will you determine whether this is a left femur or a right one?

   Answer: Look for patellar surface (anterior) and intercondylar fossa (posterior). Also look for gluteal tuberosity and linea aspera (posterior). Once anterior and posterior are determined, aim head medially.

   Page Ref: 232

9) You are confronted with a disarticulated humerus. How will you determine whether this is a left humerus or a right one?

   Answer: Look for lesser tubercle (anterior), sizes of epicondyles (medial is larger), depths of fossae on distal end (olecranon is deeper), and capitulum and trochlea (anterior). Once anterior and posterior have been determined, aim head medially.

   Page Ref: 222

10) You are confronted with a single coxal bone. How will you determine whether this is a left coxal bone or a right one?

   Answer: Look for ischial tuberosity, ischial spine, and sciatic notches, all of which are posterior, and acetabulum on lateral surface. Auricular surface identifies posterior medial surface.

   Page Ref: 225–227

CHAPTER 9   Joints

MULTIPLE CHOICE. Choose the one alternative that best completes the statement or answers the question.

1) A synarthrosis is a(n):
   A) slightly movable joint.
   B) joint in which bones are connected by fibrocartilage.
   C) freely movable joint.
   D) joint with lubricating fluid between articulating bones.
   E) immovable joint.

   Answer: E
   Page Ref: 241

2) Which of the following is a freely movable joint?
   A) amphiarthrosis
   B) synostosis
   C) diarthrosis
   D) synarthrosis
   E) symphysis

   Answer: C
   Page Ref: 241

3) A movement that increases the angle between articulating bones is:
   A) abduction.
   B) adduction.
   C) flexion.
   D) extension.
   E) rotation.

   Answer: D
   Page Ref: 253

4) Which of the following best describes *inversion*?
   A) raising up on balls of feet to stand on toes
   B) rocking back on heels
   C) turning soles of feet away from each other
   D) turning soles of feet to face each other
   E) bending the knee to raise sole of foot toward back

   Answer: D
   Page Ref: 253

5) An amphiarthrosis is a(n):

   A) slightly movable joint.

   B) joint in which bones are connected by fibrocartilage.

   C) freely movable joint.

   D) joint with lubricating fluid between articulating bones.

   E) immovable joint.

   Answer: A
   Page Ref: 241

6) In a symphysis, articulating bones are:

   A) connected by hyaline cartilage.

   B) connected by fibrocartilage.

   C) separated by a joint cavity.

   D) connected by a fibrous membrane.

   E) fused by new bone.

   Answer: B
   Page Ref: 243

7) Sutures and synchondroses are similar in that they both:

   A) are functionally classified as amphiarthroses.

   B) have joint cavities between articulating bones.

   C) become synostoses as bodies age.

   D) are functionally classified as synarthroses.

   E) Both B and C are correct.

   Answer: E
   Page Ref: 242

8) A fibrocartilage disc that extends into a joint cavity describes a(n):

   A) ligament.

   B) bursa.

   C) meniscus.

   D) articular cartilage.

   E) synovial membrane.

   Answer: C
   Page Ref: 244

9) A sac of synovial fluid between bones and overlying tissues describes a(n):

A) ligament.

B) bursa.

C) meniscus.

D) syndesmosis.

E) gomphosis.

Answer: B
Page Ref: 247

10) Dense connective tissue connecting one bone to another bone describes a(n):

A) ligament.

B) bursa.

C) meniscus.

D) tendon.

E) synovial membrane.

Answer: A
Page Ref: 244

11) Hyaline cartilage makes up the:

A) articular discs.

B) connection between bones in sutures.

C) bursae.

D) articular cartilage.

E) All of the above are correct.

Answer: D
Page Ref: 243

12) Synovial fluid is produced by:

A) chondrocytes in the articular cartilage.

B) osteocytes in the articulating bones.

C) cells in the inner layer of the articular capsule.

D) fibroblasts in ligaments surrounding the joint.

E) chondrocytes in menisci.

Answer: C
Page Ref: 244

13) Which of the following is functionally classified as an amphiarthrosis?

   A) suture

   B) ball–and–socket joint

   C) syndesmosis

   D) planar joint

   E) Both A and B are correct.

   Answer: C
   Page Ref: 242

14) Flexion and extension are the principal movements performed at:

   A) planar joints.

   B) pivot joints.

   C) syndesmoses.

   D) symphyses.

   E) hinge joints.

   Answer: E
   Page Ref: 248

15) The greatest range of motion occurs at:

   A) hinge joints.

   B) ellipsoidal joints.

   C) pivot joints.

   D) ball–and–socket joints.

   E) synchondroses.

   Answer: D
   Page Ref: 248

16) The fibrous connective tissue that connects a muscle to a bone is called a(n):

   A) tendon.

   B) meniscus.

   C) ligament.

   D) bursa.

   E) labrum.

   Answer: A
   Page Ref: 247

17) The type of movement normally seen at pivot joints is:

A) abduction and adduction.

B) rotation.

C) flexion and extension.

D) protraction and retraction.

E) inversion and eversion.

Answer: B
Page Ref: 248

18) Which of the following is an example of a symphysis?

A) coxal joint

B) intercarpal joint

C) intervertebral joint

D) joint between frontal and parietal bones

E) Both A and B are correct.

Answer: C
Page Ref: 248

19) Which of the following is an example of a planar joint?

A) coxal joint

B) intercarpal joint

C) intervertebral joint

D) joint between frontal and parietal bones

E) Both A and B are correct.

Answer: B
Page Ref: 248

20) Doing a backbend is an example of:

A) flexion.

B) hyperflexion.

C) hyperextension.

D) rotation.

E) dorsiflexion.

Answer: C
Page Ref: 250

21) Which of the following is an example of a ball-and-socket joint?
   A) tibiofemoral joint
   B) glenohumeral joint
   C) atlanto-axial joint
   D) temporomandibular joint
   E) Both B and D are correct.

   Answer: B
   Page Ref: 248

22) The joint formed by the root of a tooth and its socket is called a:
   A) condyloid joint.
   B) syndesmosis.
   C) synchondrosis.
   D) gomphosis.
   E) synostosis.

   Answer: D
   Page Ref: 242

23) The dense connective tissue joining structure in a gomphosis is called a(n):
   A) articular disc.
   B) bursa.
   C) tendon.
   D) synovial membrane.
   E) periodontal ligament.

   Answer: E
   Page Ref: 242

24) Which of the following is an example of a synchondrosis?
   A) intervertebral joint
   B) epiphyseal plate
   C) intertarsal joint
   D) joint between root of tooth and alveolus
   E) Both A and B are correct.

   Answer: B
   Page Ref: 243

25) Turning the palm posterior or inferiorly is referred to as:

A) dorsiflexion of the hand.

B) abduction of the hand

C) supination of the forearm.

D) pronation of the forearm.

E) rotation of the hand.

Answer: D
Page Ref: 253

26) The mouth is opened when:

A) depression occurs at the temporomandibular joint.

B) elevation occurs at the temporomandibular joint.

C) flexion occurs at the temporomandibular joint.

D) extension occurs at the temporomandibular joint.

E) protraction occurs at the temporomandibular joint.

Answer: A
Page Ref: 253

27) Standing on the toes, such as ballet dancers do, is an example of:

A) inversion.

B) eversion.

C) plantar flexion.

D) dorsiflexion.

E) hyperextension.

Answer: C
Page Ref: 253

28) Making circles with the arms is best described as:

A) abduction.

B) hyperextension.

C) circumduction.

D) elevation.

E) flexion.

Answer: C
Page Ref: 253

29) The transverse humeral ligament extends from the greater tubercle of the humerus to the:

A) anatomical neck of the humerus.

B) coracoid process of the scapula.

C) glenoid labrum.

D) lesser tubercle of the humerus.

E) deltoid tuberosity of the humerus.

Answer: D
Page Ref: 254

30) Fibrocartilage that stabilizes the shoulder joint is the:

A) articular capsule.

B) coracohumeral ligament.

C) glenoid labrum.

D) subscapular bursa.

E) Both A and C are fibrocartilage structures.

Answer: C
Page Ref: 254

31) Spreading the legs apart, as in doing jumping jacks, is an example of:

A) abduction.

B) adduction.

C) flexion.

D) extension.

E) protraction.

Answer: A
Page Ref: 253

32) Articular fat pads are accumulations of adipose tissue in the:

A) articular cartilage.

B) articular discs.

C) synovial membrane.

D) bursae.

E) extracapsular ligaments.

Answer: C
Page Ref: 244

33) The anterior cruciate ligament extends from the lateral condyle of the femur to the:
   A) medial condyle of the femur.
   B) lateral epicondyle of the femur.
   C) medial condyle of the femur.
   D) head of the fibula.
   E) area anterior to the intercondylar eminence of the tibia.

   Answer: E
   Page Ref: 259

34) The patellar ligament extends from the patella to the:
   A) linea aspera of the femur.
   B) tibial tuberosity of the tibia.
   C) head of the fibula.
   D) medial and lateral condyles of the femur.
   E) lesser trochanter of the femur.

   Answer: B
   Page Ref: 259

35) The synovial membrane is made of:
   A) areolar connective tissue.
   B) mesothelium.
   C) hyaline cartilage.
   D) dense irregular connective tissue.
   E) endothelium.

   Answer: A
   Page Ref: 244

36) Synovial fluid consists of interstitial fluid and:
   A) phospholipids.
   B) hydroxyapatite.
   C) collagen.
   D) hyaluronic acid.
   E) elastin.

   Answer: D
   Page Ref: 244

37) Subdivision of the synovial cavity and directing the flow of synovial fluid are functions of:

A) articular cartilage.

B) bursae.

C) menisci.

D) extracapsular ligaments.

E) Both B and C are correct.

Answer: C
Page Ref: 244

38) The type of movement possible at a planar joint is:

A) gliding.

B) flexion.

C) circumduction.

D) abduction.

E) All of the above are possible.

Answer: A
Page Ref: 248

39) Bursae are filled with:

A) venous blood.

B) air.

C) synovial fluid.

D) dense irregular connective tissue.

E) adipose tissue.

Answer: C
Page Ref: 247

40) You can elevate and depress your:

A) forearms.

B) legs.

C) mandible.

D) feet at the ankles.

E) All of these can be elevated and depressed.

Answer: C
Page Ref: 253

41) When your palms are lying flat on the table, you forearms are:
    A) inverted.
    B) everted.
    C) pronated.
    D) supinated.
    E) dorsiflexed.

    Answer: C
    Page Ref: 253

42) You are bent over at the waist touching your toes. **ALL** of the following body parts are
    extended **EXCEPT** your:
    A) fingers.
    B) legs.
    C) arms.
    D) vertebral column.
    E) elbows.

    Answer: D
    Page Ref: 253

43) You are sitting **up straight in a chair** with your fingers curled into your palm on the table in
    front of you. **ALL** of the following body parts are *flexed* **EXCEPT** your
    A) fingers.
    B) forearms.
    C) legs.
    D) knees.
    E) vertebral column.

    Answer: E
    Page Ref: 253

44) **ALL** of the following are normal movements of the shoulder **EXCEPT**:
    A) abduction.
    B) hyperextension.
    C) circumduction.
    D) lateral rotation.
    E) medial rotation.

    Answer: B
    Page Ref: 254

45) The coracohumeral ligament extends from the:

    A) conoid tubercle of the clavicle to the greater tubercle of the humerus.

    B) acromion of the scapula to the greater tubercle of the humerus.

    C) coracoid process of the scapula to the greater tubercle of the humerus.

    D) coracoid process of the scapula to the anatomical neck of the humerus.

    E) coracoid process of the scapula to the lesser tubercle of the humerus.

Answer: C
Page Ref: 254

46) The medial epicondyle of the humerus and the coronoid process of the ulna are attachment points for the:

    A) transverse humeral ligament.

    B) subcoracoid bursa.

    C) radial collateral ligament.

    D) ulnar collateral ligament.

    E) coracohumeral ligament.

Answer: D
Page Ref: 254

47) The acetabular labrum is:

    A) an accessory ligament attaching the fovea capitis of the femur to the acetabulum.

    B) a ring of circular collagen fibers within the articular capsule of the hip that surrounds the neck of the femur.

    C) an accessory ligament running from the acetabulum to the intertrochanteric line of the femur.

    D) the central, deepest point of the acetabulum to which the fovea capitis of the femur connects.

    E) the fibrocartilage rim of the acetabulum the enhances its depth.

Answer: E
Page Ref: 257

48) Abduction and adduction are possible for **ALL** of the following **EXCEPT** the:

    A) coxal joint.

    B) glenohumeral joint.

    C) metacarpophalangeal joint.

    D) radiocarpal joint.

    E) elbow.

Answer: E
Page Ref: 256

49) Rotation is the only movement possible at the:

   A) radioulnar joint.

   B) radiocarpal joint.

   C) vertebrocostal joints.

   D) atlanto–occipital joint.

   E) temporomandibular joint.

Answer: A
Page Ref: 262

50) Which of the following is considered to be an autoimmune disease?

   A) rheumatoid arthritis.

   B) osteoarthritis.

   C) gouty arthritis.

   D) osteosarcoma.

   E) Both A and C are autoimmune diseases.

Answer: A
Page Ref: 264

MATCHING. Choose the item in column 2 that best matches each item in column 1.

Choose the item from column 2 that best matches each item in column 1.

1) Column 1: movement of the sole of the
           foot outward so that the soles
           face toward from each other

   Column 2: eversion

   Answer: eversion

   Page Ref: 253

2) Column 1: movement of the sole of the
           foot outward so that the soles
           face away from each other

   Column 2: eversion

   Answer: eversion

   Page Ref: 253

3) Column 1: bending of the foot in the
           direction of the upper surface

   Column 2: dorsiflexion

   Answer: dorsiflexion

   Page Ref: 253

4) Column 1: bending of the foot in the
   direction of the sole
   Column 2: plantar flexion
   Answer: plantar flexion
   Page Ref: 253

5) Column 1: movement of the mandible
   forward on a plane parallel to
   the ground
   Column 2: protraction
   Answer: protraction
   Page Ref: 253

6) Column 1: movement of the mandible
   backward on a plane parallel
   to the ground
   Column 2: retraction
   Answer: retraction
   Page Ref: 253

7) Column 1: movement of the forearm in
   which the palm is turned
   anteriorly or superiorly
   Column 2: supination
   Answer: supination
   Page Ref: 253

8) Column 1: movement of the forearm in
   which the palm is turned
   posteriorly or inferiorly
   Column 2: pronation
   Answer: pronation
   Page Ref: 253

9) Column 1: movement of the mandible
   upward
   Column 2: elevation
   Answer: elevation
   Page Ref: 253

10) Column 1: movement of the mandible
        downward
   Column 2: depression
   Answer: depression
   Page Ref: 253

MATCHING. Choose the item in column 2 that best matches each item in column 1.

Choose the item from column 2 that best matches each item in column 1.

1) Column 1: suture
   Column 2: joint between frontal and
        parietal bones
   Answer: joint between frontal and parietal bones
   Page Ref: 242

2) Column 1: syndesmosis
   Column 2: distal tibiofibular joint
   Answer: distal tibiofibular joint
   Page Ref: 242

3) Column 1: synchondrosis
   Column 2: epiphyseal plate
   Answer: epiphyseal plate
   Page Ref: 243

4) Column 1: symphysis
   Column 2: intervertebral joint
   Answer: intervertebral joint
   Page Ref: 243

5) Column 1: planar joint
   Column 2: intertarsal joint
   Answer: intertarsal joint
   Page Ref: 248

6) Column 1: hinge joint
   Column 2: interphalangeal joint
   Answer: interphalangeal joint
   Page Ref: 248

7) Column 1: pivot joint
Column 2: atlanto–axial joint
Answer: atlanto–axial joint
Page Ref: 248

8) Column 1: condyloid joint
Column 2: radiocarpal joint
Answer: radiocarpal joint
Page Ref: 248

9) Column 1: ball–and–socket joint
Column 2: glenohumeral joint
Answer: glenohumeral joint
Page Ref: 248

10) Column 1: gomphosis
Column 2: roots of teeth in alveoli
Answer: roots of teeth in alveoli
Page Ref: 242

TRUE/FALSE. Write 'T' if the statement is true and 'F' if the statement is false.

1) A cartilaginous joint has no joint cavity.

Answer: TRUE
Page Ref: 243

2) In a suture, the bones are held together by fibrocartilage.

Answer: FALSE
Page Ref: 242

3) A suture eventually becomes a synostosis.

Answer: TRUE
Page Ref: 242

4) A syndesmosis is classified as an ampiarthrosis.

Answer: TRUE
Page Ref: 242

5) Pads of elastic cartilage between bones in a symphysis make it a slightly movable joint.

Answer: FALSE
Page Ref: 243

6) The articular cartilage covering the ends of bones at synovial joints is fibrocartilage.

Answer: FALSE
Page Ref: 243

7) The epiphyseal plate is a temporary synchondrosis.

Answer: TRUE
Page Ref: 243

8) A bursa is a fat pad located at high friction points in large joints.

Answer: FALSE
Page Ref: 247

9) The fibrous capsule of a synovial joint attaches to the periosteum of the articulating bones.

Answer: TRUE
Page Ref: 244

10) Someone who has a "torn cartilage" in the knee has pulled the articular cartilage from the surface of the tibia or femur.

Answer: FALSE
Page Ref: 244

11) The viscosity of synovial fluid decreases as joint movement increases.

Answer: FALSE
Page Ref: 244

12) A *strain* is a stretched or partially torn muscle that often occurs as a result of a sudden, powerful muscle contraction.

Answer: TRUE
Page Ref: 245

13) The sternoclavicular joint is an example of a planar joint.

Answer: TRUE
Page Ref: 245

14) Circumduction is a movement normally seen at the tibiofemoral joint.

Answer: FALSE
Page Ref: 259

15) Inversion and eversion are special movements that occur only at the wrist.

Answer: FALSE
Page Ref: 253

SHORT ANSWER. Write the word or phrase that best completes each statement or answers the question.

1) The functional classification of joints defined as slightly movable is the _____.
Answer: amphiarthrosis
Page Ref: 241

2) Interphalangeal joints are examples of synovial joints called _____ joints.
Answer: hinge
Page Ref: 248

3) The angle between articulating bones is decreased by a movement called _____.
Answer: flexion
Page Ref: 253

4) A bone moves away from the body's midline during _____.
Answer: abduction
Page Ref: 253

5) The atlanto-axial joint is an example of a freely movable joint called a(n) _____.
Answer: pivot
Page Ref: 248

6) The trapezium and metacarpal I form a freely movable joint called a(n) _____ joint.
Answer: saddle
Page Ref: 248

7) A partial or incomplete dislocation is called a(n) _____.
Answer: subluxation
Page Ref: 264

8) A joint in which more flexible connective tissue has been replaced by bone as the body ages is called a(n) _____.
Answer: synostosis
Page Ref: 242

9) The interosseous membrane between the tibia and fibula is an example of a(n) _____.
Answer: syndesmosis
Page Ref: 242

10) In a symphysis, the articulating bones are joined by _____.
Answer: fibrocartilage
Page Ref: 243

11) The dense connective tissue holding a tooth in its socket is called the _____.
Answer: periodontal ligament
Page Ref: 242

12) All synovial joints are classified functionally as _____.
Answer: diarthroses
Page Ref: 243

13) Fibrous connective tissue that connects one bone to another in a joint capsule is called a(n) _____.
Answer: ligament
Page Ref: 244

14) Nutrients are supplied to the chondrocytes of the articular cartilage by _____.
Answer: synovial fluid
Page Ref: 244

15) Fluid-filled sacs located between bones and overlying tissues that help alleviate pressure are called _____.
Answer: bursae
Page Ref: 247

16) Someone who has a "torn cartilage" in the knee has damaged a(n) _____.
Answer: articular disc (meniscus)
Page Ref: 244

17) Examination of the interior of a joint is known as _____.
Answer: arthroscopy
Page Ref: 244

18) Intercarpal joints are examples of synovial joints known as _____ joints.
Answer: planar
Page Ref: 248

19) Bending the trunk backward at the intervertebral joints is an example of _____.
Answer: hyperextension
Page Ref: 250

20) The combined movements of flexion, extension, abduction, and adduction is called _____.
Answer: circumduction
Page Ref: 253

21) A hormone that increases the flexibility of the fibrocartilage of the pubic symphysis is _____.
Answer: relaxin
Page Ref: 263

22) Pain in a joint is called _____.
Answer: arthralgia
Page Ref: 264

23) The glenohumeral joint and the coxal joint are the only examples of the _____ joint.
Answer: ball–and–socket
Page Ref: 248

24) Movement of the thumb across the palm to touch the fingertips on the same hand is called _____.
Answer: opposition
Page Ref: 253

25) Movement of the trunk in the frontal plane is called _____.
Answer: lateral flexion
Page Ref: 250

26) The parietal and occipital bones are held together by a joint called a(n) _____.
Answer: suture
Page Ref: 242

27) The tendons of the supraspinatus, infraspinatus, teres minor, and subscapularis muscles form a structure called the _____.
Answer: rotator cuff
Page Ref: 254

28) Rising up on your toes is known as _____ of the foot at the ankle joint.
Answer: plantar flexion
Page Ref: 253

29) Shrugging the shoulders at the acromioclavicular joint is called _____ of the scapula.
Answer: elevation
Page Ref: 253

30) The ligament stretched or torn in 70% of all serious knee injuries is the _____.
Answer: anterior cruciate ligament
Page Ref: 259

ESSAY. Write your answer in the space provided or on a separate sheet of paper.

1) Describe the factors affecting the range of motion at synovial joints.

Answer: 1. Structure or shape of articulating bones —i.e., how closely they fit together
2. Strength and tension of ligaments —restricts direction and degree of movement
3. Arrangement and tension of muscles —complements ligaments
4. Apposition of soft parts —i.e., point at which one body surface meets another during a movement
5. Hormones—may affect flexibility of connective tissues
6. Disuse—decreases synovial fluid, connective tissue flexibility and muscle mass
Page Ref: 262

2) Describe the affects of aging on joints.

Answer: Changes include: decreased production of synovial fluid; thinning of articular cartilage; ligaments shorten and lose flexibility; osteoarthritis develops from wear and tear —bone exposed at joints, spurs form and synovial membrane becomes inflamed, all affecting range of motion.
Page Ref: 263

3) Describe the functions of synovial fluid.

Answer: 1. lubrication of joints
2. shock absorption
3. providing nutrients to articular cartilage
4. removal of debris and microbes via phagocyte activity
5. removal of metabolic wastes from articular cartilage
Page Ref: 244

4) Describe the structure of s synovial joint.

Answer: A sleevelike articular capsule surrounds the synovial cavity, uniting articular bones. The capsule has an outer fibrous layer of dense irregular connective tissue, possibly arranged into ligaments. The inner layer is the synovial membrane that secretes synovial fluid, which fills the joint cavity. Accessory ligaments, bursae, and/or menisci may be seen in larger joints.
Page Ref: 244

5) Name and briefly describe the common types of arthritis.

Answer: 1. Rheumatoid arthritis is an autoimmune disease in which the immune system attacks cartilage and joint linings, causing swelling, pain, and loss of function. Bones may fuse, making them immovable.
2. Osteoarthritis results from deterioration of articular cartilage due to wear and tear. Bone spurs form, which restricts movement.
3. Gouty arthritis occurs due to deposition of uric acid crystals in soft tissues of joints, eroding cartilage and causing inflammation.
Page Ref: 264

6) Describe the structure of the hip joint.

Answer: The head of the femur fits into the acetabulum. The cartilage of the acetabular labrum deepens the socket. A very strong articular capsule extends from the rim of the acetabulum to the neck of the femur, and is reinforced by accessory ligaments — the iliofemoral ligament (from anterior inferior iliac spine to intertrochanteric line), pubofemoral ligament (from pubic rim of acetabulum to neck of femur), and ischiofemoral ligament (from ischial wall of acetabulum to the neck of the femur). Other reinforcement includes: the ligament of the head of the femur (from fossa of acetabulum to the fovea capitis of femoral head); transverse ligament of acetabulum (supports labrum and connects ligament of head of femur and articular capsule).

Page Ref: 257

7) Name the six types of diarthroses, and give an example of each.

Answer: 1. planar joint —intercarpal; intertarsal; vertebrocostal; sternoclavicular; acromioclavicular
2. hinge joint —knee; elbow; ankle; interphalangeal
3. pivot—atlanto-axial; proximal ends of radius and ulna
4. condyloid —radiocarpal
5. saddle —trapezium and metacarpal of thumb
6. ball-and-socket —shoulder; hip

Page Ref: 248

8) Roger has spent 20 years pitching fastballs during his childhood and adult career. An unfortunate automobile accident dislocated his shoulder. Although he received immediate medical treatment, he can still feel his shoulder begin to slip out of joint every time he tries to raise his arms to begin his pitching motion. What could be the anatomical problem?

Answer: A torn rotator cuff weakens support that holds the head of the humerus in the glenoid cavity. A torn glenoid labrum makes the glenoid cavity shallower. Both allow the large humeral head to slip more easily out of relatively shallow glenoid cavity.

Page Ref: 254

9) Todd must design a set of calisthenics as warm-ups for his aerobics class. Suggest three possible exercises and describe what specific movements are involved. In terms of joint action, why are these warm-ups useful?

Answer: Many possibilities for answers —e.g., jumping jacks (abduction/adduction of arms and legs plus foot and ankle movements); arm circles (circumduction); bend to touch toes (flexion/extension at hip); raise up on balls of feet (plantar/dorsiflexion of foot), etc. Benefits include loosening of connective tissues, decreased viscosity of synovial fluid, and increased production and secretion of synovial fluid.

Page Ref: 253

10) Describe the locations of the intracapsular ligaments and articular discs associated with the tibiofemoral ligament.

Answer: 1. Anterior cruciate ligament (ACL)—extends posteriorly and laterally from area anterior to intercondylar eminence of tibia to posterior part of medial surface of lateral condyle of femur
2. Posterior cruciate ligament (PCL)—extends anteriorly and medially from depression posterior to intercondylar area of tibia and lateral meniscus to anterior part of medial surface of medial condyle of femur
3. Medial meniscus —C-shaped fibrocartilage attached to anterior intercondylar fossa of tibia and ACL anteriorly and posteriorly to intercondylar fossa of tibia between PCL and lateral meniscus
4. Lateral meniscus —O-shaped fibrocartilage attached anteriorly to area anterior to intercondylar eminence of tibia and lateroposteriorly to ACL; attached posteriorly to area posterior to intercondylar eminence of tibia and anteriorly to posterior end of medial meniscus
(add also transverse ligament and coronary ligament as desired)

Page Ref: 259

CHAPTER 10   Muscle Tissue

MULTIPLE CHOICE. Choose the one alternative that best completes the statement or answers the question.

1) The striations seen in some types of muscle tissue are due to:
   A) variable amounts of myoglobin.
   B) the arrangement of blood vessels in the endomysium.
   C) the arrangement of proteins within the cells.
   D) the types of cell junctions present.
   E) the arrangement of phospholipids in the sarcolemma.

   Answer: C
   Page Ref: 268

2) A type of muscle tissue the is both striated and involuntary is:
   A) skeletal muscle tissue.
   B) smooth muscle tissue.
   C) cardiac muscle tissue.
   D) both cardiac and smooth muscle tissues.
   E) no type of muscle tissue is both striated and involuntary.

   Answer: C
   Page Ref: 268

3) Sphincters are structures that allow muscle tissue to perform which of the following functions?
   A) gross body movements
   B) stabilizing body position
   C) regulating organ volume
   D) producing heat
   E) Both B and D are correct.

   Answer: C
   Page Ref: 269

4) Cylindrical muscle cells that contain multiple nuclei located peripherally within the cell would be:

   A) skeletal muscle cells only.

   B) single unit smooth muscle cells only.

   C) multiunit smooth muscle cells only.

   D) cardiac muscle cells.

   E) both single unit and multiunit smooth muscle cells.

   Answer: A
   Page Ref: 294

5) The ability of a muscle to stretch without being damaged is:

   A) excitability.

   B) contractility.

   C) extensibility.

   D) elasticity.

   E) conductivity.

   Answer: C
   Page Ref: 269

6) Smooth muscle tissue is found:

   A) attached to bones.

   B) lining hollow organs and body tubes.

   C) in the wall of the heart.

   D) lining long bones.

   E) Both B and C are correct.

   Answer: B
   Page Ref: 268

7) Deep fascia is:

   A) the areolar connective tissue of the hypodermis.

   B) dense irregular connective tissue holding muscles with similar functions together.

   C) areolar connective tissue surrounding individual muscle fibers.

   D) dense regular connective tissue attaching muscle to bone.

   E) the site of calcium ion storage in skeletal muscle.

   Answer: B
   Page Ref: 271

8) The endomysium is:

   A) the areolar connective tissue of the hypodermis.

   B) dense irregular connective tissue holding muscles with similar functions together.

   C) areolar connective tissue surrounding individual muscle fibers.

   D) dense regular connective tissue attaching muscle to bone.

   E) the site of calcium ion storage in skeletal muscle.

   Answer: C
   Page Ref: 271

9) The sarcolemma is the:

   A) storage site for calcium ions in myofibers.

   B) plasma membrane of a myofiber.

   C) compound that binds oxygen for use in slow, oxidative muscle cells.

   D) separation between sarcomeres in a myofiber.

   E) structure that produces acetylcholine.

   Answer: B
   Page Ref: 273

10) Myosin is seen in:

   A) thin filaments.

   B) thick filaments.

   C) the sarcoplasmic reticulum.

   D) the sarcolemma.

   E) Both A and B are correct.

   Answer: B
   Page Ref: 273

11) Skeletal muscle fibers are multinucleate because:

   A) the original nucleus reproduced as the cell grew.
   B) when neighboring cells undergo apoptosis, cells that remain absorb their nuclei before
      they degenerate.
   C) the fibers grew so fast they engulfed any cells in their way.
   D) the fibers formed from the fusion of many smaller cells during embryonic development.
   E) All of the above have occurred.

   Answer: D
   Page Ref: 273

12) Satellite cells are cells:

   A) in mature muscle that retain the capacity to regenerate functional muscle fibers.

   B) that produce a neurotransmitter that excites muscle cells.

   C) in the deep fascia that generate matrix.

   D) that protect muscle tissue by phagocytosis.

   E) that provide cardiac muscle tissue with the property of autorhythmicity.

   Answer: A
   Page Ref: 273

13) Glucose is stored in muscle cells as:

   A) actin.

   B) myoglobin.

   C) glycogen.

   D) creatine.

   E) calmodulin.

   Answer: C
   Page Ref: 283

14) The function of calcium ions in skeletal muscle contraction is to:
   A) bind to receptors on the sarcolemma at the neuromuscular junction to stimulate muscle contraction.

   B) cause a pH change in the sarcoplasm to trigger muscle contraction.

   C) bind to the myosin binding sites on actin so that myosin will have something to attach to.
   D) bind to the troponin on the thin filaments so that the myosin binding sites on the actin can be exposed.

   E) bind oxygen to fuel cellular respiration in oxidative fibers.

   Answer: D
   Page Ref: 277

15) Skeletal muscles are stimulated to contract when:

   A) calcium ions bind to the sarcolemma, causing an action potential.

   B) acetylcholine diffuse into the sarcoplasm.

   C) acetylcholine binds to receptors on the sarcolemma, causing an action potential.

   D) ATP is released from the sarcoplasmic reticulum.

   E) oxygen binds to myoglobin.

   Answer: C
   Page Ref: 280

16) Energy released during the complete oxidation of glucose is either used for ATP production or:

    A) given off as heat.

    B) turned into water.

    C) converted to lactic acid.

    D) given off as carbon dioxide.

    E) converted to glycogen.

Answer: A
Page Ref: 285

17) What structures meet at the neuromuscular junction?

    A) T tubules and sarcoplasmic reticulum

    B) the sarcolemma and T tubules

    C) an axon and the sarcoplasmic reticulum

    D) an axon and the sarcolemma

    E) an axon and thick myofilaments

Answer: D
Page Ref: 280

18) The function of myoglobin is to:

    A) bind oxygen for aerobic respiration.

    B) bind actin to shorten myofibrils.

    C) block the myosin binding sites on thin filaments.

    D) store ATP.

    E) separate one sarcomere from another.

Answer: A
Page Ref: 285

19) The purpose of the phosphagen system is to:

    A) bind oxygen for aerobic respiration.

    B) bind actin to shorten myofibrils.

    C) block the myosin binding sites on thin filaments.

    D) store high energy phosphate groups for ATP production.

    E) actively transport acetylcholine into skeletal muscle fibers.

Answer: D
Page Ref: 283

20) The Sliding Filament Theory of muscle contraction says that myofibers shorten when:
   A) actin filaments become shorter when they combine with myosin heads.
   B) thin filaments are pulled toward the center of the sarcomere by swiveling of the myosin heads.
   C) myosin heads rotate when they attach to actin, causing the myosin filaments to fold in the middle.
   D) acetylcholine reduces the friction between thin and thick filaments, so the slide over each other more easily.
   E) a neurotransmitter alters the arrangement of collagen fibers in the endomysium, causing it to shrink more tightly around the myofiber.

   Answer: B
   Page Ref: 276

21) The refractory period is the time:
   A) between stimulation and the start of contraction.
   B) when the muscle is shortening.
   C) when the muscle is lengthening.
   D) following a stimulus during which a muscle cell cannot respond to another stimulus.
   E) it takes for acetylcholine to cross the synaptic cleft.

   Answer: D
   Page Ref: 286

22) Fused tetanus is:
   A) a pathological condition in which stimulation of one muscle triggers contraction of all others in the same motor unit.
   B) a sustained contraction with partial relaxation between stimuli.
   C) a sustained contraction in which individual twitches cannot be discerned.
   D) a brief contraction of all the fibers in a motor unit.
   E) a phenomenon that occurs in only muscle cells without refractory periods.

   Answer: C
   Page Ref: 287

23) Jack is sitting on the floor with his legs outstretched in front of him. He lowers his torso so that he is lying flat on the floor. Which of the following describes the contraction of his rectus abdominus muscle?
   A) concentric isometric contraction
   B) eccentric isometric contraction
   C) eccentric isotonic contraction
   D) concentric isotonic contraction
   E) fasciculation

   Answer: C
   Page Ref: 288

24) A motor unit is:

    A) all the muscles that act as prime movers for a particular action.

    B) the sarcomeres in an individual myofibril.

    C) all of the neurons that stimulate a particular skeletal muscle.

    D) a motor neuron plus all the skeletal muscle fibers it stimulates.

    E) the quantity of neurotransmitter that is sufficient to stimulate muscle contraction.

    Answer: D
    Page Ref: 286

25) Jane's car is stuck in the snow. Sally is pushing it as hard as she can, but it won't budge. Which of the following describes the type of contractions occurring in Sally's arm muscles?

    A) concentric isotonic contractions

    B) eccentric isotonic contractions

    C) isometric contractions

    D) fasciculations

    E) twitches

    Answer: C
    Page Ref: 288

26) The Z disc is the:

    A) separation between sarcomeres.

    B) area of a sarcomere where only thick myofilaments are found.

    C) point where the axon and the sarcolemma meet.

    D) place where two cardiac muscle cells meet.

    E) electrical voltage at which a muscle cell fires an action potential.

    Answer: A
    Page Ref: 273

27) The motor protein in all three types of muscle tissue is:

    A) actin.

    B) myosin.

    C) tropomyosin.

    D) titin.

    E) nebulin.

    Answer: B
    Page Ref: 275

28) The muscle protein whose function is related to its golf club–like shape is:

   A) actin.

   B) troponin.

   C) tropomyosin.

   D) myosin.

   E) titin.

   Answer: D
   Page Ref: 275

29) The protein making up the M line that binds titin and connect thick filaments to each other is:

   A) actin.

   B) troponin.

   C) myomesin.

   D) dystrophin.

   E) nebulin.

   Answer: C
   Page Ref: 276

30) Which of the following conditions exists in a resting myofiber?

   A) Levels of calcium ions are relatively high in the sarcoplasm.

   B) Thin myofilaments extend across the H zone.

   C) ATP is attached to myosin cross bridges.

   D) Levels of acetylcholine are high inside the sarcoplasmic reticulum.

   E) Both A and C are correct.

   Answer: C
   Page Ref: 277

31) The function of dystrophin is to:

   A) bind thick filaments to each other.

   B) hold thin filaments to the Z disc.

   C) form a latticework that supports all other muscle proteins.

   D) block the myosin binding sites on actin.

   E) link thin filaments to integral proteins of the sarcolemma.

   Answer: E
   Page Ref: 276

32) The protein responsible for much of the elasticity and extensibility of myofibrils is:

   A) nebulin.

   B) alpha–actinin.

   C) titin.

   D) troponin.

   E) tropomyosin.

   Answer: C
   Page Ref: 275

33) The protein that helps reinforce the sarcolemma and transmit tension generated by the sarcomeres to the tendons is:

   A) actin.

   B) nebulin.

   C) myomesin.

   D) dystrophin.

   E) troponin.

   Answer: D
   Page Ref: 276

34) The term *power stroke*, when used relative to skeletal muscle contraction, refers to the:

   A) flooding of the sarcoplasm with calcium ions.

   B) release of acetylcholine from the motor neuron via exocytosis.

   C) sudden increase in the sarcolemma's permeability to sodium ions following the binding of acetylcholine.

   D) pulling of the tendon on the bone as a whole muscle contracts.

   E) swiveling of the myosin heads as they combine with actin.

   Answer: E
   Page Ref: 277

35) What is happening during the latent period of a muscle contraction?

   A) nothing.

   B) Calcium ions are being actively transported back into the sarcoplasmic reticulum.

   C) New contractile proteins are being synthesized.

   D) Calcium ions are beginning to enter the sarcoplasm from the sarcoplasmic reticulum.

   E) ATP molecules are attaching to myosin heads.

   Answer: D
   Page Ref: 286

36) The role of acetylcholine in skeletal muscle contractions is to:
   A) diffuse into the sarcoplasm to open calcium ion channels in the sarcoplasmic reticulum.
   B) bind to troponin to expose myosin binding sites.
   C) hydrolyze ATP to release energy.
   D) bind to specific receptors on the sarcolemma to open sodium ion channels.
   E) react with titin molecules to cause relaxation of a muscle fiber.

   Answer: D
   Page Ref: 280

37) Two molecules of pyruvic acid are the products of:
   A) reactions catalyzed by creatine kinase.
   B) the breakdown of glucose via glycolysis.
   C) aerobic cellular respiration.
   D) the binding of actin and myosin.
   E) removal of oxygen from myoglobin.

   Answer: B
   Page Ref: 283

38) The fate of pyruvic acid formed during muscle activity depends on the:
   A) amount of oxygen available.
   B) rate of creatine kinase activity.
   C) relative proportions of actin and myosin present.
   D) number of nuclei per cell.
   E) surface area of the sarcolemma.

   Answer: A
   Page Ref: 283

39) Most of the lactic acid remaining after exercise is:
   A) converted to glycogen and stored.
   B) converted to creatine and stored.
   C) converted to pyruvic acid and used for ATP production.
   D) used as a building block for new contractile proteins.
   E) stored as fat.

   Answer: C
   Page Ref: 284

40) Slow oxidative fibers are said to be "slow" because they:

   A) break down acetylcholine slowly.

   B) conduct action potentials slowly.

   C) manufacture creatine phosphate slowly.

   D) recover from fatigue slowly.

   E) hydrolyze ATP slowly.

   Answer: E
   Page Ref: 289

41) Muscle cells with relatively few mitochondria that generate most of their ATP via glycolysis and that have low resistance to fatigue are most likely:

   A) slow oxidative skeletal muscle fibers.

   B) fast oxidative skeletal muscle fibers.

   C) fast glycolytic skeletal muscle fibers.

   D) cardiac muscle fibers.

   E) smooth muscle fibers.

   Answer: C
   Page Ref: 289

42) **ALL** of the following about training-induced changes in skeletal muscle are **TRUE EXCEPT**:

   A) Endurance–type exercises can cause a gradual transformation of fast glycolytic fibers into fast oxidative fibers.

   B) Exercises requiring great strength for short periods of time increase the synthesis of thin and thick filaments.

   C) Endurance–type exercises are though to greatly increase the total number of skeletal muscle cells.

   D) Anabolic steroids can increase muscle size, but moderate doses probably do not increase either strength or endurance.

   E) Endurance–type exercises increase the efficiency of oxygen delivery to skeletal muscle cells.

   Answer: C
   Page Ref: 288

43) The role of tropomyosin in skeletal muscle is to:

   A) provide an additional source of ATP during periods of high intensity exercise.

   B) bind to myosin cross bridges during the power stroke.

   C) block the myosin binding sites on actin during periods of rest.

   D) actively transport calcium ions back into the sarcoplasmic reticulum following the power stroke.

   E) connect the thick myofilaments to the Z discs.

   Answer: C
   Page Ref: 275

44) The amount of force (tension) developed by a skeletal muscle depends on **ALL** of the following **EXCEPT**:

A) rate of conduction of the muscle action potential along the sarcolemma.

B) number of motor units recruited.

C) length of muscle fiber prior to contraction.

D) frequency of stimulation.

E) size of motor units recruited.

Answer: A
Page Ref: 285–288

45) Cardiac muscle can stay contracted 10 −15 times longer than skeletal muscle because:

A) intercalated discs are stronger than Z discs.

B) there is less acetylcholinesterase available in cardiac muscle.

C) channels allowing calcium ions to enter from the extracellular fluid add to that released from the sarcoplasmic reticulum.

D) the contractile proteins in the sarcomeres are different.

E) the passive tension on the heart is greater.

Answer: C
Page Ref: 290

46) The type of tissue in the iris that causes very precise adjustments in pupil diameter is:

A) visceral smooth muscle.

B) multiunit smooth muscle.

C) cardiac muscle.

D) skeletal muscle.

E) dense regular connective tissue.

Answer: B
Page Ref: 291

47) **ALL** of the following are **TRUE** for smooth muscle cells **EXCEPT**:

A) when they contract they twist in a helix.

B) they contain thin and thick filaments.

C) contraction may be triggered by certain hormones.

D) intermediate filaments pull on dense bodies during contraction.

E) they use troponin as their primary regulatory protein.

Answer: E
Page Ref: 291

48) The stress-relaxation response refers to the:

   A) mechanism by which smooth muscle can undergo great length changes while still retaining the ability to contract effectively.

   B) mechanism by which oxygen is used to restore resting metabolic conditions.

   C) process by which skeletal muscles fatigue.

   D) fact that cardiac muscle that is well-conditioned beats more slowly than cardiac muscle that is in good condition.

   E) fact that titin allows a sarcomere to return to its original shape and size.

   Answer: A
   Page Ref: 293

49) An abundance of fast glycolytic fibers is seen in:

   A) the walls of large arteries because they must stretch.

   B) neck muscles because they must stay contracted for long periods to hold up the head.

   C) arm muscles because they must move quickly and intensely.

   D) leg muscles because they must move constantly.

   E) the wall of the heart because it must maintain autorhythmicity.

   Answer: C
   Page Ref: 289

50) The effect of acetylcholine on skeletal muscle fibers ends when:

   A) an action potential is generated.

   B) myosin attaches to actin.

   C) sodium ions begin diffusing out of the fiber.

   D) it is broken down by acetylcholinesterase.

   E) a phosphate attaches to creatine.

   Answer: D
   Page Ref: 280

MATCHING. Choose the item in column 2 that best matches each item in column 1.

Choose the item from column 2 that best matches each item in column 1.

   1) Column 1: protein in thin myofilaments that binds to myosin heads
   Column 2: actin
   Answer: actin
   Page Ref: 275

   2) Column 1: acts as an ATPase in skeletal and cardiac muscle
   Column 2: myosin
   Answer: myosin
   Page Ref: 275

3) Column 1: protein that anchors thick
   myofilaments to the Z discs
   Column 2: titin
   Answer: titin
   Page Ref: 275

4) Column 1: regulatory protein that binds
   calcium ions in smooth
   muscle tissue
   Column 2: calmodulin
   Answer: calmodulin
   Page Ref: 292

5) Column 1: regulatory protein that binds
   calcium ions in skeletal and
   cardiac muscle
   Column 2: troponin
   Answer: troponin
   Page Ref: 275

6) Column 1: binds oxygen for use in
   aerobic cellular respiration
   Column 2: myoglobin
   Answer: myoglobin
   Page Ref: 285

7) Column 1: released by motor neurons to
   stimulate skeletal muscle
   contraction
   Column 2: acetylcholine
   Answer: acetylcholine
   Page Ref: 280

8) Column 1: binds calcium ions inside the
   sarcoplasmic reticulum
   Column 2: calsequestrin
   Answer: calsequestrin
   Page Ref: 278

9) Column 1: binds a high-energy phosphate group for use in future ATP production
Column 2: creatine

Answer: creatine

Page Ref: 283

10) Column 1: regulatory protein in thin myofilaments that binds neither calcium ions nor thick myofilaments
Column 2: tropomyosin

Answer: tropomyosin

Page Ref: 275

MATCHING. Choose the item in column 2 that best matches each item in column 1.

Choose the item from column 2 that best matches each item in column 1.

1) Column 1: a motor neuron and all the skeletal muscle fibers it stimulates
Column 2: motor unit

Answer: motor unit

Page Ref: 286

2) Column 1: a bundle of muscle fibers
Column 2: fascicle

Answer: fascicle

Page Ref: 271

3) Column 1: dense irregular connective tissue that holds together whole muscles with similar functions
Column 2: deep fascia

Answer: deep fascia

Page Ref: 271

4) Column 1: dense irregular connective tissue that encircles single whole muscles
Column 2: epimysium

Answer: epimysium

Page Ref: 271

5) Column 1: dense irregular connective
    tissue that wraps bundles of
    muscle fibers
   Column 2: perimysium
   Answer: perimysium
   Page Ref: 271

6) Column 1: areolar connective tissue
    separating individual muscle
    fibers
   Column 2: endomysium
   Answer: endomysium
   Page Ref: 271

7) Column 1: structure in smooth muscle
    that links intermediate
    filaments with the
    sarcolemma
   Column 2: dense body
   Answer: dense body
   Page Ref: 292

8) Column 1: areas between cardiac muscle
    cells containing desmosomes
    and gap junctions
   Column 2: intercalated discs
   Answer: intercalated discs
   Page Ref: 290

9) Column 1: the plasma membrane of a
    myofiber
   Column 2: sarcolemma
   Answer: sarcolemma
   Page Ref: 273

10) Column 1: storage site for calcium ions
    within skeletal muscle fibers
   Column 2: sarcoplasmic reticulum
   Answer: sarcoplasmic reticulum
   Page Ref: 273

TRUE/FALSE. Write 'T' if the statement is true and 'F' if the statement is false.

1) To say that muscle tissue exhibits the property of *elasticity* means that muscle can be stretched without damaging the tissue.

Answer: FALSE
Page Ref: 269

2) Skeletal muscle tissue is both striated and voluntary.

Answer: TRUE
Page Ref: 268

3) Acteylcholine stimulates skeletal muscle cells by diffusing into T tubules and binding to the sarcoplasmic reticulum.

Answer: FALSE
Page Ref: 280

4) The sarcolemma of a myofiber is the connective tissue layer that surrounds the cell.

Answer: FALSE
Page Ref: 273

5) The contractile elements of skeletal muscle are called myofibrils.

Answer: TRUE
Page Ref: 273

6) Myosin binding sites are found on troponin.

Answer: FALSE
Page Ref: 275

7) Z discs separate one sarcomere from the next.

Answer: FALSE
Page Ref: 273

8) Myosin is considered a *motor protein* in all three types of muscle tissue.

Answer: TRUE
Page Ref: 275

9) During a power stroke myoglobin binds to actin.

Answer: FALSE
Page Ref: 277

10) In resting skeletal muscle tissue, ATP molecules are bound to myosin heads.

Answer: TRUE
Page Ref: 277

11) Fast glycolytic skeletal muscle fibers contain relatively large amounts of myoglobin.

Answer: FALSE
Page Ref: 291

12) Nebulin stabilizes the position of myosin filaments.

Answer: FALSE
Page Ref: 276

13) Muscle contraction is triggered by release of acetylcholine from the sarcoplasmic reticulum.

Answer: FALSE
Page Ref: 280

14) Calsequestrin is the neurotransmitter that stimulates contraction of smooth muscle.

Answer: FALSE
Page Ref: 278

15) Dystrophin helps transmit the tension generated by sarcomeres to the tendons.

Answer: TRUE
Page Ref: 275

SHORT ANSWER. Write the word or phrase that best completes each statement or answers the question.

1) Muscle tissue that is both nonstriated and involuntary is _____.
Answer: smooth muscle tissue
Page Ref: 268

2) The gap between a motor neuron and a muscle cell is called the _____.
Answer: synaptic cleft
Page Ref: 280

3) The inability of a muscle to contract forcefully after prolonged activity is called _____.
Answer: muscle fatigue
Page Ref: 285

4) The smallest, most fatigue-resistant skeletal muscle fibers are the _____ fibers.
Answer: slow oxidative
Page Ref: 289

5) An oxygen-binding protein in skeletal muscle cells is _____.
Answer: myoglobin
Page Ref: 285

6) The dense irregular connective tissue that carries nerves and blood vessels, fills the spaces between muscles, and separates muscles into functional groups is the _____.

Answer: deep fascia

Page Ref: 271

7) The region of a sarcolemma adjacent to the axon terminals at a neuromuscular junction is called the _____.

Answer: motor end plate

Page Ref: 280

8) The region of the sarcomere that contains only thick myofilaments is the _____.

Answer: H zone

Page Ref: 274

9) The structures in smooth muscle fibers that are functionally analogous to the Z discs of skeletal muscle fibers are the _____.

Answer: dense bodies

Page Ref: 292

10) A regulatory protein that binds calcium ions in the cytosol of smooth muscle fibers is _____.

Answer: calmodulin

Page Ref: 294

11) The stem cells of smooth muscle cells are called _____.

Answer: pericytes

Page Ref: 295

12) During embryonic development mesoderm destined to become skeletal muscle forms columns that undergo segmentation into a series of blocks of cells called _____.

Answer: somites

Page Ref: 273

13) A disease that results from inappropriate production of antibodies that block acetylcholine receptors is _____.

Answer: myasthenia gravis

Page Ref: 296

14) Myosin binding sites on actin are exposed when troponin changes shape as a result of binding _____.

Answer: calcium ions

Page Ref: 278

15) Muscle contraction without muscle shortening is called a(n) _____ contraction.

Answer: isometric

Page Ref: 288

16) The time between the application of a stimulus and the beginning of contraction, when calcium ions are being released from the sarcoplasmic reticulum, is called the _____ period.

Answer: latent

Page Ref: 286

17) The time following a stimulus during which a muscle cell is unable to respond to another stimulus is called the _____ period.

Answer: refractory

Page Ref: 286

18) An inherited myopathy that results in the rupture and death of muscle fibers is _____.

Answer: muscular dystrophy

Page Ref: 296

19) Involuntary inactivation of a small number of motor units causes sustained, small contractions that give relaxed skeletal muscle a firmness known as _____.

Answer: muscle tone

Page Ref: 288

20) The contractile protein in thin myofilaments is _____.

Answer: actin

Page Ref: 275

21) The palest muscle fibers that are not fatigue-resistant and that get their ATP primarily via anaerobic respiration are _____ fibers.

Answer: fast glycolytic

Page Ref: 289

22) Muscle fibers that are branched with a single, central nucleus are _____ muscle fibers.

Answer: cardiac

Page Ref: 294

23) A muscle contraction in which the force developed by the muscle remains almost constant while the muscle shortens is said to be a(n) _____ contraction.

Answer: isotonic

Page Ref: 288

24) An isotonic contraction in which the muscle lengthens to produce movement and to increase the angle at a joint is called a(n) _____ contraction.

Answer: eccentric

Page Ref: 288

25) In the phosphagen system, high-energy phosphate groups can be stored for future ATP production by combining with _____.

Answer: creatine

Page Ref: 283

26) The reactions of cellular respiration occurring in the mitochondria are said to be *aerobic* because they require _____.

Answer: oxygen

Page Ref: 284

27) The electrical signals produced by the sarcolemma in response to appropriate stimuli are called _____.

Answer: action potentials

Page Ref: 273

28) A bundle of muscle fibers surrounded by perimysium is called a(n) _____.

Answer: fascicle

Page Ref: 271

29) Individual skeletal muscle cells are separated from each other by a thin sheath of areolar connective tissue called the _____.

Answer: endomysium

Page Ref: 271

30) Muscle is attached to the periosteum of a bone by a(n) _____.

Answer: tendon

Page Ref: 271

31) During embryonic development, each skeletal muscle fiber forms from the fusion of 100 or more small mesodermal cells called _____.

Answer: myoblasts

Page Ref: 273

32) Myoblasts that persists in mature skeletal muscle are called _____.

Answer: satellite cells

Page Ref: 273

33) The dark middle portion of a sarcomere that extends the entire length of the thick filaments is called the _____.

Answer: A band

Page Ref: 273

34) The filaments inside a myofibril of a skeletal muscle fiber are arranged in compartments called _____.

Answer: sarcomeres

Page Ref: 273

35) The two regulatory proteins seen in thin myofilaments are _____ and _____.

Answer: troponin; tropomyosin

Page Ref: 275

ESSAY. Write your answer in the space provided or on a separate sheet of paper.

1) Describe the functions of muscle tissue.

Answer: Functions include: production of body movements (with bones and joints); stabilizing body positions (posture); regulating organ volume of hollow organs (via sphincters); moving substances within the body (e.g., blood through vessels; food through gastrointestinal tract); heat production.

Page Ref: 269

2) Outline the steps of skeletal muscle contraction.

Answer: 1. stimulus provided by binding of ACh to the sarcolemma;
2. resulting action potential travels along sarcolemma and into T tubules, triggering release of calcium ions from SR;
3. calcium ions bind to troponin; resulting shape change causes myosin binding site to be exposed;
4. myosin heads bind to actin, and swivel (power stroke), pulling Z discs closer together, shortening myofiber.
[add details of ATP use as desired]

Page Ref: 277

3) Eileen lives in Canada and goes out every morning in her slippers and pajamas to pick up her newspaper from the box at the end of the driveway. Do you think her muscle tone as she moves outside is any greater at one time of the year than any other time? Why or why not?

Answer: Probably muscle tone is increased in winter, possibly to the point of shivering, for purposes of heat production. On very hot days, muscle tone might be reduced to generate less heat.

Page Ref: 288

4) Describe the mechanisms by which skeletal muscle tissue obtains ATP to fuel contraction.

Answer: 1. ATP is attached to resting myosin heads.
2. Creatine stores high-energy phosphate groups that can be added to ADP as needed.
3. Anaerobic glycolysis breaks down glucose into two molecules of pyruvic acid, releasing enough energy to net 2 ATP molecules per glucose.
4. Mitochondria oxidize pyruvic acid to carbon dioxide and water via aerobic cellular respiration. Energy released nets about 36 ATP molecules per glucose molecule, plus heat.

Page Ref: 283-285

5) Identify and define the four special properties that enable muscle tissue to carry out its functions.

Answer: 1. Electrical excitability —triggering of action potential in muscle cells by appropriate stimuli
2. Contractility —ability to generate force by pulling on attachment points when stimulated
3. Extensibilty —ability to stretch without being damaged
4. Elasticity —ability to return to original length and shape after contraction or extension

Page Ref: 269

6) Colette's six-year-old son is very inquisitive and notices that a woman in a wheelchair in the grocery store has "the thinnest legs he's ever seen." He wants to know why. What explanation would you give him?

Answer: The woman may have denervation atrophy in which nerve supplies have been cut and muscle replaced by connective tissue (not reversible). She may have been bed-ridden for a long time or in a cast for a long time (disuse atrophy).

Page Ref: 273

7) Compare and contrast the processes by which striated and nonstriated muscle tissues contract.

Answer: Smooth muscle: contraction begins more slowly; lasts longer due to slow influx of calcium ions; regulator protein (calmodulin) binds calcium ions and activates myosin light chain kinase to phosphorylate myosin and trigger attachment to actin; wide variety of stimuli.
Striated muscle: regulator protein (troponin) binds calcium ions, changes shape, and exposes myosin binding sites on actin, causing spontaneous attachment of myosin to actin; acetylcholine stimulates contraction skeletal muscle

Page Ref: 294

8) You need to lift a pail of water and carry it across the room. Describe the types of whole muscle contractions that occur during this activity.

Answer: Concentric isotonic contractions to lift pail; isometric contractions to maintain pail in position; eccentric isotonic contractions to set pail down (include complete tetanus, etc., as desired)

Page Ref: 288

9) Name and describe the functions of the two contractile, two regulatory, and five structural proteins seen in skeletal muscle fibers.

Answer: 1. Contractile—myosin in thick filaments is motor protein; actin in thin filaments binds to myosin
2. Regulatory proteins—troponin blocks myosin-binding sites on actin at rest; tropomyosin holds troponin in place
3. Structural—titin stabilizes position of thick filaments; myomesin binds to titin and holds thick filaments together; nebulin helps maintain alignment of thin filaments; alpha-actinin forms latticework to hold actin, nebulin, and titin in Z disc; dystrophin links thin filaments to integral membrane proteins of sarolemma to help transmit tension generated by sarcomeres to tendons

Page Ref: 275

10) Old Farmer Brown complains that at age 88, "I can't get around like I used to." What changes in his muscle tissue might make this true? What would you recommend to slow the process?

Answer: With age general loss of muscle mass occurs, and there is replacement of muscle by fibrous connective tissue and adipose tissue —possibly due to progressive inactivity. Also, maximal strength of contraction decreases and reflexes are slowed. There is an increase in the number of slow oxidative fibers. One could recommend that he keep moving and lifting around the farm. Possibly creatine supplements could help.

Page Ref: 295-296

CHAPTER 11   The Muscular System

MULTIPLE CHOICE. Choose the one alternative that best completes the statement or answers the question.

1) In a muscle group, the muscle that relaxes during a particular action is the:
   A) prime mover.
   B) antagonist.
   C) fixator.
   D) synergist.
   E) Both B and D are correct.

   Answer: B
   Page Ref: 305

2) The insertion of a skeletal muscle is the:
   A) connection to the bone that remains stationary while the muscle contracts.
   B) connection to the bone that moves while the muscle contracts.
   C) point at which effort is applied in an anatomical lever system.
   D) point at which the tendon attaches to the muscle itself.
   E) Both B and C are correct.

   Answer: E
   Page Ref: 302

3) Which of the following would allow a greater range of motion around a joint?
   A) having the insertion point of the muscle be very close to the joint
   B) having the insertion point of the muscle be as far as possible from the joint
   C) having very short fascicles
   D) Both B and C are correct.
   E) Range of motion is not related to the point of muscle insertion or fascicle length.

   Answer: A
   Page Ref: 304

4) The masseter:
   A) sucks in the cheeks.
   B) protracts the mandible.
   C) elevates the mandible.
   D) depresses the mandible.
   E) Both B and D are correct.

   Answer: E
   Page Ref: 317

5) Thoracic volume is increased during normal breathing by the:

A) internal intercostals.

B) external obliques.

C) diaphragm.

D) trapezius.

E) Both B and C are correct.

Answer: C
Page Ref: 328

6) **ALL** of the following move the mandible **EXCEPT** the:

A) masseter.

B) buccinator.

C) temporalis.

D) digastric.

E) lateral pterygoid.

Answer: B
Page Ref: 317

7) The tongue is protracted by the:

A) masseter.

B) buccinator.

C) platysma.

D) styloglossus.

E) genioglossus.

Answer: E
Page Ref: 319

8) Which of the following elevates the hyoid bone and depresses the mandible?

A) styloglossus

B) genioglossus

C) risorius

D) digastric

E) sternocleidomastoid

Answer: D
Page Ref: 321

9) The neck is divided into anterior and posterior triangles by the:

   A) sternocleidomastoid.

   B) masseter.

   C) trapezius.

   D) splenius capitis.

   E) semispinalis capitis.

   Answer: A
   Page Ref: 323

10) The anterior triangle of the neck contains **ALL** of the following **EXCEPT** the:

   A) parotid salivary gland.

   B) brachial plexus.

   C) vagus nerve.

   D) internal jugular vein.

   E) submandibular lymph nodes.

   Answer: B
   Page Ref: 323

11) Jim has been lifting weights and doing exercises, such as sit–ups, to get that rippled "washboard" abdomen look. What muscle provides those "rippled abs?"

   A) transverse abdominis

   B) quadratus lumborum

   C) rectus abdominis

   D) latissimus dorsi

   E) pectoralis major

   Answer: C
   Page Ref: 327

12) The bone(s) that is (are) the origin of the rectus abdominis is (are) the:

   A) ilium.

   B) ischium.

   C) pubis.

   D) sternum.

   E) last pair of vertebrochondral ribs.

   Answer: C
   Page Ref: 326

13) The bone(s) that is (are) the origin of the internal oblique and transverse abdominis is (are) the:

A) ilium.

B) ischium.

C) pubis.

D) sternum.

E) last pair of vertebrochondral ribs.

Answer: A
Page Ref: 326

14) The phrenic nerve stimulates the:

A) sternocleidomastoid.

B) rectus abdominis.

C) splenius capitis.

D) diaphragm.

E) external intercostals.

Answer: D
Page Ref: 328

15) During inspiration (i.e., breathing in), which of the following happens to increase the size of the thoracic cavity?

A) The abdominal muscles relax.

B) The internal intercostals contract to pull on the ribs.

C) The external intercostals relax to "release" the ribs.

D) The diaphragm contracts to flatten out.

E) All of the above are correct.

Answer: D
Page Ref: 328

16) Which of the following is part of the pelvic diaphragm?

A) iliococcygeus

B) external urethral sphincter

C) bulbospongiosus

D) ischiocavernosus

E) Both A and C are correct.

Answer: A
Page Ref: 330

17) The perineum is:

A) the anterior of the two triangles separated by the sternocleidomastoid.

B) the floor of the thoracic cavity.

C) a band of fibrous tissue extending from the pubis to the sternum.

D) a group of muscles that move the foot.

E) the region of the trunk inferior to the pelvic diaphragm.

Answer: E
Page Ref: 332

18) **ALL** of the following are muscles of the perineum **EXCEPT** the:

A) iliococcygeus

B) external urethral sphincter

C) bulbospongiosus

D) ischiocavernosus

E) Both A and C are correct.

Answer: A
Page Ref: 332

19) The muscle that helps maintain the erection of the penis and clitoris is the:

A) external urethral sphincter.

B) deep transverse perineus.

C) ischiocavernosus.

D) coccygeus.

E) pubococcygeus.

Answer: C
Page Ref: 332

20) **ALL** of the following move the scapula **EXCEPT** the:

A) rhomboideus major.

B) serratus anterior.

C) pectoralis major.

D) trapezius.

E) pectoralis minor.

Answer: C
Page Ref: 335

21) A hole in the linea alba that allows passage of the spermatic cord in males is the:
   A) rotator cuff.
   B) inguinal canal.
   C) extensor retinaculum
   D) levator ani.
   E) carpal tunnel.

   Answer: B
   Page Ref: 325

22) **ALL** of the following are part of the rotator cuff **EXCEPT** the:
   A) teres minor.
   B) infraspinatus.
   C) supraspinatus.
   D) subscapularis.
   E) pectoralis major.

   Answer: E
   Page Ref: 337

23) The group of muscles known as the hamstrings includes the:
   A) rectus femoris, vastus lateralis, and vastus medialis.
   B) sartorius and gracilis.
   C) gluteus maximus, medius, and minimus.
   D) external oblique, internal oblique, and rectus abdominis.
   E) biceps femoris, semitendinosus, and semimembranosus.

   Answer: E
   Page Ref: 363

24) The deltoid performs which of the following actions?
   A) adduction of the arm
   B) abduction of the arm
   C) flexion of the forearm
   D) extension of the forearm
   E) Both B and C are correct.

   Answer: B
   Page Ref: 338

25) The radial tuberosity is the insertion point for the:
   A) triceps brachii.
   B) biceps brachii.
   C) brachialis.
   D) deltoid.
   E) Both A and B are correct.

   Answer: B
   Page Ref: 341

26) Which of the following is part of the flexor compartment of the arm?
   A) anconeus
   B) triceps brachii
   C) brachialis
   D) biceps brachii
   E) Both C and D are correct.

   Answer: E
   Page Ref: 341

27) The olecranon of the ulna is the insertion point for the:
   A) triceps brachii.
   B) biceps brachii.
   C) brachialis.
   D) deltoid.
   E) Both A and B are correct.

   Answer: A
   Page Ref: 342

28) The deep fascia covering the palmar surface of the carpal bones is the:
   A) linea alba.
   B) fascia lata.
   C) galea aponeurotica.
   D) flexor retinaculum.
   E) extensor retinaculum.

   Answer: D
   Page Ref: 347

29) The origin of a muscle refers to the:

A) embryonic derivation from a particular germ layer.

B) attachment to the moving bone.

C) attachment to the stationary bone.

D) point at which the tendon meets the bone.

E) point at which blood vessels and nerves enter the muscle.

Answer: C
Page Ref: 302

30) Which of the following refers to the relative size of a muscle?

A) pectinate

B) biceps

C) vastus

D) rectus

E) quadratus

Answer: C
Page Ref: 308

31) Which of the following terms seen in muscle names means "shortest?"

A) minimus

B) brevis

C) minor

D) piriformis

E) vastus

Answer: B
Page Ref: 308

32) A word in a muscle name that indicates that the muscle decreases the size of an opening is:

A) sphincter.

B) extensor.

C) levator.

D) tensor.

E) rotator.

Answer: A
Page Ref: 308

33) In a third class lever system, the arrangement of the system's components is such that the:

A) fulcrum is between the effort and the resistance.

B) effort is between the fulcrum and the resistance.

C) resistance is between the fulcrum and the effort.

D) effort and the resistance are equidistant from the fulcrum.

E) there is no fulcrum.

Answer: B
Page Ref: 304

34) The extrinsic muscles that move the wrist, hand and digits originate on the:

A) humerus.

B) proximal ends of the radius and ulna.

C) carpals.

D) distal ends of the radius and ulna.

E) metacarpals.

Answer: A
Page Ref: 345

35) The hypothenar muscles act on the:

A) thumb.

B) little finger.

C) big toe.

D) carpals.

E) metatarsals.

Answer: B
Page Ref: 350

36) The nerve that passes through the carpal tunnel is the:

A) sciatic.

B) phrenic.

C) median.

D) vagus.

E) trigeminal.

Answer: C
Page Ref: 350

37) Which of the following originates on the transverse processes of the thoracic vertebrae?
   A) iliocostalis thoracis
   B) longissimus thoracis
   C) interspinales
   D) middle scalene
   E) All of these are correct.

   Answer: B
   Page Ref: 354

38) The head is laterally flexed and rotated by the:
   A) iliocostalis thoracis
   B) longissimus thoracis
   C) interspinales
   D) middle scalene
   E) All of these are correct.

   Answer: D
   Page Ref: 335

39) The superior and inferior rectus muscles are prime movers for:
   A) flexion and extension of the lower leg.
   B) flexion and extension of the thigh.
   C) elevation and depression of the eyelid.
   D) flexion and extension of the vertebral column.
   E) movements of the eyeball.

   Answer: E
   Page Ref: 315

40) Muscles with the combining form –*glossus* in the name cause movements of the:
   A) eyeball.
   B) eyelid.
   C) tongue.
   D) vocal cords.
   E) ossicles in the ear.

   Answer: C
   Page Ref: 308

41) Which of the following muscles is deepest?

    A) rectus abdominis

    B) external oblique

    C) internal oblique

    D) transverse abdominis

    E) pectoralis major

Answer: D
Page Ref: 325

42) Which of the following muscles that move the humerus is designated as an *axial* muscle?

    A) latissmus dorsi

    B) deltoid

    C) teres minor

    D) subscapularis

    E) supraspinatus

Answer: A
Page Ref: 337

43) Which of the following would act as an antagonist to the tibialis anterior?

    A) rectus femoris

    B) biceps femoris

    C) tensor fasciae latae

    D) peroneus longus

    E) gracilis

Answer: D
Page Ref: 368

44) Which of the following acts as an antagonist to the rectus femoris?

    A) vastus lateralis

    B) semimembranosus

    C) gastrocnemius

    D) tibialis anterior

    E) adductor magnus

Answer: B
Page Ref: 364

45) Which of the following acts as an antagonist to the deltoid?
   A) biceps brachii
   B) triceps brachii
   C) pectoralis major
   D) sternocleidomastoid
   E) external intercostals

   Answer: C
   Page Ref: 338

46) Which of the following acts as an antagonist to the platysma?
   A) occipitalis
   B) trapezius
   C) sternocleidomastoid
   D) masseter
   E) orbicularis oculi

   Answer: D
   Page Ref: 312

47) In an anatomical lever system, the effort is the:
   A) bone on which the muscle originates.
   B) joint.
   C) muscular contraction pulling on the insertion point.
   D) weight of the body part to be moved.
   E) brain activity that stimulates movement.

   Answer: C
   Page Ref: 304

48) Two structurally identical muscles cross a joint. Muscle X inserts one inch from the joint. Muscle Y inserts three inches from the joint. Which of the following statements is most likely to be **TRUE**?
   A) Muscle X will produce a stronger movement due to greater leverage.
   B) Muscle Y will produce a stronger movement due to greater leverage.
   C) Muscle Y will produce a stronger movement because the tendon must be longer.
   D) Muscle Y will produce a greater range of motion because the lever is longer.
   E) Muscles X and Y must produce movements of equal strength, regardless of point of insertion, because they are structurally identical.

   Answer: B
   Page Ref: 304

49) The most powerful abductor of the femur at the hip joint is the:

   A) semitendinosus.

   B) quadriceps femoris.

   C) quadratus femoris.

   D) gluteus medius.

   E) gluteus maximus.

   Answer: D
   Page Ref: 358

50) The adductors of the thigh have their origins and insertions on the:

   A) ilium and greater trochanter of the femur.

   B) ischial tuberosities and condyles of the femur.

   C) pubis and linea aspera of the femur.

   D) anterior inferior iliac spines and tibial tuberosities.

   E) pubis and tibial tuberosities.

   Answer: C
   Page Ref: 359

51) The tibial tuberosity is the insertion point for the:

   A) gluteus maximus.

   B) biceps femoris.

   C) gracilis.

   D) vastus lateralis.

   E) All of these are correct.

   Answer: D
   Page Ref: 363

52) Flexing the trunk at the hip, as in sitting up from the supine position, is an action of the:

   A) psoas major.

   B) gluteus maximus.

   C) longissimus muscles.

   D) tensor fasciae latae.

   E) semimembranosus.

   Answer: A
   Page Ref: 359

53) A muscle that both adducts the thigh and flexes the leg at the knee joint is the:

   A) gluteus medius.

   B) rectus femoris.

   C) semitendinosus.

   D) sartorius.

   E) gracilis.

   Answer: E
   Page Ref: 363

54) Plantar flexion of the foot is an action of **ALL** of the following **EXCEPT** the:

   A) peroneus longus.

   B) soleus.

   C) tibialis anterior.

   D) gastrocnemius.

   E) tibialis posterior.

   Answer: C
   Page Ref: 367

55) The gastrocnemius has its origin and insertions on the:

   A) condyles of femur; calcaneus

   B) tibia and fibula; calcaneus

   C) tibial tuberosity; calcaneus

   D) calcaneus; linea aspera of femur

   E) calcaneus; lateral malleolus of fibula

   Answer: A
   Page Ref: 368

MATCHING. Choose the item in column 2 that best matches each item in column 1.

Choose the item from column 2 that best matches each item in column 1.

   1) Column 1: extensor

   Column 2: increases a joint angle

   Answer: increases a joint angle

   Page Ref: 308

   2) Column 1: sphincter

   Column 2: decreases the size of an
             opening

   Answer: decreases the size of an opening

   Page Ref: 308

3) Column 1: orbicularis
   Column 2: circular
   Answer: circular
   Page Ref: 308

4) Column 1: vastus
   Column 2: great
   Answer: great
   Page Ref: 308

5) Column 1: rectus
   Column 2: parallel to midline
   Answer: parallel to midline
   Page Ref: 308

6) Column 1: brevis
   Column 2: shortest
   Answer: shortest
   Page Ref: 308

7) Column 1: pectinate
   Column 2: comblike
   Answer: comblike
   Page Ref: 308

8) Column 1: piriformis
   Column 2: pear-shaped
   Answer: pear-shaped
   Page Ref: 308

9) Column 1: platys
   Column 2: flat
   Answer: flat
   Page Ref: 308

10) Column 1: deltoid
    Column 2: triangular
    Answer: triangular
    Page Ref: 308

MATCHING. Choose the item in column 2 that best matches each item in column 1.

Choose the item from column 2 that best matches each item in column 1.

1) Column 1: semitendinosus
   Column 2: flexes leg

   Answer: flexes leg
   Page Ref: 364

2) Column 1: vastus lateralis
   Column 2: extends leg

   Answer: extends leg
   Page Ref: 364

3) Column 1: tibialis anterior
   Column 2: dorsiflexes foot

   Answer: dorsiflexes foot
   Page Ref: 367

4) Column 1: soleus
   Column 2: plantar flexes foot

   Answer: plantar flexes foot
   Page Ref: 368

5) Column 1: gluteus medius
   Column 2: abducts thigh

   Answer: abducts thigh
   Page Ref: 359

6) Column 1: gracilis
   Column 2: adducts thigh

   Answer: adducts thigh
   Page Ref: 364

7) Column 1: deltoid
   Column 2: abducts arm

   Answer: abducts arm
   Page Ref: 338

8) Column 1: latissimus dorsi
   Column 2: adducts arm
   Answer: adducts arm
   Page Ref: 338

9) Column 1: platysma
   Column 2: depresses mandible
   Answer: depresses mandible
   Page Ref: 312

10) Column 1: masseter
    Column 2: elevates mandible
    Answer: elevates mandible
    Page Ref: 317

TRUE/FALSE. Write 'T' if the statement is true and 'F' if the statement is false.

1) The attachment of a muscle tendon to the movable bone is called the origin.

   Answer: FALSE
   Page Ref: 302

2) The word *serratus* in a muscle name means "saw-toothed."

   Answer: TRUE
   Page Ref: 308

3) A greater range of motion is achieved by placing the insertion further away from the joint.

   Answer: FALSE
   Page Ref: 304

4) Most lever systems in the body are first class levers.

   Answer: FALSE
   Page Ref: 305

5) In an anatomical lever system, the fulcrum is the bone.

   Answer: FALSE
   Page Ref: 304

6) The longer the fibers in a muscle, the greater the range of motion it can produce.

   Answer: TRUE
   Page Ref: 305

7) The superior and inferior rectus muscles insert on the eyeball.

Answer: TRUE
Page Ref: 315

8) Fixators block the action of the prime mover.

Answer: FALSE
Page Ref: 306

9) The masseter elevates the mandible.

Answer: TRUE
Page Ref: 317

10) The hamstrings flex the thigh.

Answer: FALSE
Page Ref: 364

11) The strength of a muscle depends on the total number of fibers it contains.

Answer: TRUE
Page Ref: 305

12) The sternocleidomastoid extends the head.

Answer: FALSE
Page Ref: 323

13) The tibialis anterior and the gastrocnemius are antagonists in the movement of the foot.

Answer: TRUE
Page Ref: 367, 368

14) The internal oblique is the deepest of the muscles that compress the abdomen.

Answer: FALSE
Page Ref: 326

15) The external intercostals assist in forced expiration by decreasing the lateral and anteroposterior dimensions of the thorax.

Answer: FALSE
Page Ref: 328

SHORT ANSWER. Write the word or phrase that best completes each statement or answers the question.

1) The attachment of a muscle to the movable bone is called the _____.
Answer: insertion
Page Ref: 302

2) In a third class lever, the _____ is between the _____ and the _____.

Answer: effort; resistance; fulcrum

Page Ref: 304

3) When the resistance is close to the fulcrum and the effort is applied farther away, the lever operates at a mechanical _____.

Answer: advantage

Page Ref: 304

4) The word used in muscle names that means "diagonal to the midline" is _____.

Answer: oblique

Page Ref: 308

5) In anatomical lever systems, bones act as _____.

Answer: levers

Page Ref: 304

6) In an anatomical lever system, the fulcrum is the _____.

Answer: joint

Page Ref: 304

7) A muscle that causes a particular action is called the _____.

Answer: prime mover

Page Ref: 305

8) When a prime mover contracts, the _____ relaxes.

Answer: antagonist

Page Ref: 305

9) The word in a muscle name that means "produces superior movements" is _____.

Answer: levator

Page Ref: 308

10) Muscles that help stabilize movements and help prime movers work more efficiently are called _____ and _____.

Answer: synergists; fixators

Page Ref: 305

11) The muscle that closes and protrudes the lips is the _____.

Answer: orbicularis oris

Page Ref: 311

12) The upper eyelid is elevated by the _____.
   Answer: levator palpebrae superioris
   Page Ref: 312

13) The masseter originates on the maxilla and zygomatic arch and inserts onto the _____ of the _____.
   Answer: angle and ramus; mandible
   Page Ref: 317

14) When general anesthesia is administered during surgery, a total relaxation of the _____ muscle results, allowing the tongue to fall posteriorly.
   Answer: genioglossus
   Page Ref: 319

15) The sternocleidomastoid has its origins on the sternum and the _____.
   Answer: clavicle
   Page Ref: 323

16) A tough fibrous band that extends from the xiphoid process to the pubic symphysis is the _____.
   Answer: linea alba
   Page Ref: 325

17) The inferior free border of the external oblique aponeurosis forms the _____.
   Answer: inguinal ligament
   Page Ref: 325

18) The floor of the thoracic cavity is formed by the _____.
   Answer: diaphragm
   Page Ref: 328

19) The muscles that move the humerus that originate on the axial skeleton are the latissimus dorsi and the _____.
   Answer: pectoralis major
   Page Ref: 338

20) The pubococcygeus and iliococcygeus muscles make up the _____ muscle.
   Answer: levator ani
   Page Ref: 330

21) The triceps brachii inserts onto the _____ of the _____.
   Answer: olecranon process; ulna
   Page Ref: 342

22) The region of the trunk inferior to the pelvic diaphragm is a diamond-shaped area called the _____.
   Answer: perineum
   Page Ref: 332

23) The hamstrings are the biceps femoris, the semimembranosus, and the _____.
   Answer: semitendinosus
   Page Ref: 364

24) The antagonists to the hamstrings regarding movements of the lower leg is the _____.
   Answer: quadriceps femoris
   Page Ref: 364

25) The muscle that helps expel urine during urination, that helps propel semen along the urethra, and that assists in the erection of the penis is the _____ muscle.
   Answer: bulbospongiosus
   Page Ref: 332

26) The "saw-toothed" muscle that abducts and upwardly rotates the scapula is the _____.
   Answer: serratus anterior
   Page Ref: 335

27) In RICE therapy, the "C" stands for _____.
   Answer: compression
   Page Ref: 374

28) The muscle in the rotator cuff whose tendon is most commonly damaged in sports injuries involving repetitive shoulder motions is the _____ muscle.
   Answer: suprapinatus
   Page Ref: 337

29) The biceps brachii inserts onto the _____ and the bicipital aponeurosis.
   Answer: radial tuberosity
   Page Ref: 341

30) The action of the biceps brachii is to _____ the forearm.
   Answer: flex
   Page Ref: 341

31) The carpal tunnel is formed anteriorly by the _____ and posteriorly by the carpal bones.
Answer: flexor retinaculum
Page Ref: 350

32) The largest muscle mass and chief extensor of the vertebral column is the _____ group.
Answer: erector spinae
Page Ref: 353

33) The psoas major and iliacus both insert onto the _____ of the _____.
Answer: lesser trochanter; femur
Page Ref: 359

34) The four muscles of the quadriceps femoris are the _____ , the _____ , the _____ , and the
_____ .
Answer: rectus femoris; vastus lateralis; vastus medialis; vastus intermedius
Page Ref: 364

35) The calcaneal tendon provides the insertion for the plantaris, the _____ , and the _____ .
Answer: soleus; gastrocnemius
Page Ref: 368

ESSAY. Write your answer in the space provided or on a separate sheet of paper.

1) Identify the anatomical parts corresponding to the generic components of a lever system. Describe the arrangement of these parts in first, second, and third class lever systems.
   Answer: The bone is the lever; the joint is the fulcrum; the muscle contraction pulling on its insertion point is the effort; the weight of the part to be moved is the resistance. A first class lever has the fulcrum between the effort and the resistance; a second class lever has the resistance in the middle; the third class lever has the effort in the middle. In all cases, the lever moves around the fulcrum.
   Page Ref: 303–305

2) Discuss the roles of prime movers, antagonists, synergists, and fixators in movement.
   Answer: The prime mover contracts to cause a particular action. The antagonist causes the opposite action, and so, must relax while the prime mover contracts. Synergists prevent unwanted movements during an action, while fixators stabilize the origin of the prime mover. Both allow the prime mover to work more efficiently.
   Page Ref: 305–306

3) Roger, a right–handed pitcher, made several quick, hard throws from the pitcher's mound to first base. Next thing he knew, he was in severe pain and out of the lineup for a few days. He told reporters he was out with a "pulled hamstring," but you suspect he meant a "pulled groin." What is the difference between the two, and how do these injuries commonly occur?

Answer: Both occur with quick movements. A pulled groin involves the iliopsoas and/or adductors (needed for rotation toward first base). Pulled hamstrings involve biceps femoris, semimembranosus, or semitendinosus pulling from their origins on the ischial tuberosity. Pain would be anteromedial for a groin pull, and lateroposterior for a hamstring pull.

Page Ref: 358, 363

4) Elaine has had three children, none of them easy deliveries. Lately she is concerned that every time she coughs or sneezes suddenly, she wets herself. Fearing the prospect of adult diapers, she asks her doctor for advice. The doctor explains what she thinks has happened and suggests Kegel exercises. What explanation has the doctor most likely provided. What will Kegel exercises do to help Elaine?

Answer: The levator ani muscle has probably been damaged and the coccygeus weakened. Kegel exercises alternately contract and relax these muscles to strengthen them and allow them to better prevent stress incontinence.

Page Ref: 330

5) Chuck has a rotator cuff injury. What muscles and associated structures might be involved, and what sorts of activities might have led up to this injury. What movements might be inhibited by this injury?

Answer: The tendons of the subscapularis, supraspinatus, infraspinatus, and teres minor make up the rotator cuff. Any activity involving these muscles could be the problem—from throwing baseballs to shoveling snow. Inhibited movements depend on specific muscle involved—medial and lateral rotation, adduction, abduction, or extension of arm.

Page Ref: 337

6) Carolyn is doing jumping jacks. What muscles and actions are involved in the movements of the upper and lower extremities?

Answer: Deltoid for abduction of arm; latissimus dorsi and pectoralis major for adduction of arm (include other muscles of rotator cuff as desired); triceps brachii and anconeus for keeping forearm extended. Gluteus medius and minimus, tensor fasciae latae for abduction of thigh; adductor magnus, longus, and brevis, pectineus, and gracilis for adduction of thigh; quadriceps femoris for keeping leg extended; gluteus maximus for keeping thigh extended (include other muscles as desired).

Page Ref: 338, 341, 359

7) Name the three groups of muscles constituting the intrinsic muscles of the hand. Briefly describe their structures and functions.

Answer: 1. Thena—four muscles that act on the thumb and form the lateral rounded contour of the palm

2. Hypothenar—three muscles that act on the little finger and form the medial rounded contour of the palm

3. Intermediate—12 muscles acting on all digits except the thumb; subgrouped as lumbricals, palmar interossei, and dorsal interossei, and located between metacarpals; needed for all phalangeal movements

Page Ref: 350

8) Bill hasn't been able to run for about three months due to his very hectic schedule. Because he had always run ten miles at a time, he saw no reason not to resume that mileage since he had not suffered any injuries, but was only busy. The next day he complained of sore shins. What is the likely cause of this pain?

Answer: Bill most likely has shinsplints, which are probably due to tendinitis of the anterior compartment muscles and periositis, or possibly due to stress fractures of the tibia.

Page Ref: 366

9) Paul, who is 45 years old, had been on a new regimen of low--fat diet and daily walking, and had lost 75 pounds. After some abdominal surgery, he couldn't walk for exercise for about six weeks. During that time, he lost interest in the diet and exercise program, and after about six months had gained back some of the weight. He bought new walking shoes and started walking again, but now complains that he can barely walk due to pain in his heels. What is the likely cause of Paul's problem?

Answer: Paul most likely has plantar fasciitis, which is an inflammation of the plantar aponeurosis at its origin on the calcaneus. The tissue has become less elastic. Possibly due to the extra weight, or possibly poor fitting shoes, or possibly altered gait due to surgery.

Page Ref: 371

10) Name and describe the locations and actions of the muscles typically used in breathing.

Answer: The diaphragm forms the floor of the thoracic cavity. It flattens during inspiration to increase the size of the thoracic cavity. The external intercostals between the ribs increase the lateral and anteroposterior dimensions of the thorax. Internal intercostals between ribs pull ribs together in the opposite movement during expiration to decrease the size of the thoracic cavity. The diaphragm relaxes during expiration to form a dome and decrease the size of the thoracic cavity.

Page Ref: 328

CHAPTER 12   Nervous Tissue

MULTIPLE CHOICE. Choose the one alternative that best completes the statement or answers the question.

1) Small masses of neuron cell bodies located outside the CNS are called:
    A) interneurons.
    B) plexuses.
    C) nerves.
    D) ganglia.
    E) nuclei.

    Answer: D
    Page Ref: 379

2) Effectors in the autonomic nervous system would include the:
    A) brain.
    B) spinal cord.
    C) cardiac muscle.
    D) skeletal muscles.
    E) Both C and D are correct.

    Answer: C
    Page Ref: 379

3) Efferent neurons transmit impulses from:
    A) the CNS to effectors.
    B) receptors to the CNS.
    C) the CNS to receptors.
    D) effectors to the CNS.
    E) between the brain and the spinal cord only.

    Answer: A
    Page Ref: 380

4) Neuroglia in the central nervous system that produce the myelin sheath are the:
    A) astrocytes.
    B) oligodendrocytes.
    C) microglia.
    D) ependymal cells.
    E) Schwann cells.

    Answer: B
    Page Ref: 384

5) Neuroglia that are positioned between neurons and capillaries to form part of the blood–brain barrier are the:

   A) astrocytes.

   B) oligodendrocytes.

   C) microglia.

   D) ependymal cells.

   E) Schwann cells.

Answer: A
Page Ref: 384

6) The part of the nervous system that is considered voluntary is the:

   A) sympathetic nervous system.

   B) parasympathetic nervous system.

   C) central nervous system.

   D) somatic nervous system.

   E) enteric nervous system.

Answer: D
Page Ref: 380

7) Secretions of the gastrointestinal tract and contraction of smooth muscle in the walls of the gastrointestinal tract are monitored by the:

   A) sympathetic nervous system.

   B) parasympathetic nervous system.

   C) central nervous system.

   D) somatic nervous system.

   E) enteric nervous system.

Answer: E
Page Ref: 380

8) Nissl bodies are:

   A) the microtubules involved in fast axonal transport.

   B) clusters of rough ER in the cell body.

   C) gaps in the myelin sheath.

   D) clusters of cell bodies in the CNS.

   E) clusters of cell bodies in the PNS.

Answer: B
Page Ref: 381

9) Synaptic vesicles store:

   A) glycogen for energy production.

   B) lipofuscin.

   C) neurotransmitter.

   D) calcium ions.

   E) enzymes fore degrading neurotransmitter.

   Answer: C
   Page Ref: 381

10) **ALL** of the following are **TRUE** regarding axons **EXCEPT:**

   A) their plasma membranes are called axolemmas.

   B) the trigger zone is located on the axon hillock.

   C) multipolar neurons have multiple axons.

   D) multiple neurotransmitters may be released from a single axon.

   E) slow axonal transport conveys axoplasm from the cell body toward the axon terminals.

   Answer: C
   Page Ref: 381

11) Most neurons are:

   A) autonomic neurons.

   B) motor neurons.

   C) interneurons.

   D) afferent neurons.

   E) all classes of neurons are equally numerous.

   Answer: C
   Page Ref: 383

12) The trigger zone on a unipolar neuron is at the:

   A) tip of the dendrite.

   B) tip of the axon.

   C) cell body.

   D) junction of the axon and dendrite.

   E) junction with adjacent neuroglia.

   Answer: D
   Page Ref: 383

13) The function of Schwann cells is to:

   A) form the myelin sheaths of neurons in the PNS.

   B) form the myelin sheaths of neurons in the CNS.

   C) act as part of the blood–brain barrier.

   D) act as interneurons.

   E) produce cerebrospinal fluid.

   Answer: A
   Page Ref: 384

14) Membrane proteins called G proteins may be important in the activities of:

   A) voltage–gated ion channels.

   B) ligand–gated ion channels.

   C) mechanically gated ion channels.

   D) a presynaptic neuron's release of neurotransmitter into the synaptic cleft.

   E) electric synapses.

   Answer: B
   Page Ref: 389

15) The Nodes of Ranvier are:

   A) sites of neurotransmitter storage.

   B) where the nucleus of a neuron is located.

   C) gaps in the myelin sheath.

   D) sites of myelin production.

   E) sites of neurotransmitter production.

   Answer: C
   Page Ref: 384

16) The branch of a neuron that carries a nerve impulse away from the cell body is the:

   A) axon.

   B) dendrite.

   C) perikaryon.

   D) Nissl body.

   E) Node of Ranvier.

   Answer: A
   Page Ref: 381

17) **ALL** of the following are **TRUE** concerning action potentials **EXCEPT**:
   A) according to the all–or–none principle, all action potentials fired by a given neuron are of the same amplitude.
   B) during depolarization, sodium ion inactivation gates close a few 10,000ths of a second after the activation gates open.
   C) after–hyperpolarization is due to rapid outflow of potassium ions.
   D) the threshold of a given neuron varies considerably depending on local conditions.
   E) once threshold is reached, both sodium ion and potassium ion voltage–gated channels open.

   Answer: D
   Page Ref: 392

18) Afferent nerves conduct nerve impulses from:
   A) the central nervous system to effectors.
   B) effectors to the central nervous system.
   C) receptors to the central nervous system.
   D) the central nervous system to receptors.
   E) one effector to another.

   Answer: C
   Page Ref: 379

19) The absolute refractory period is the time:
   A) it takes a neurotransmitter to diffuse across a synaptic cleft.
   B) it takes to reach threshold via temporal summation.
   C) following birth when neurons can still reproduce.
   D) between injury to an axon and recovery of function.
   E) following an action potential during which a second action potential cannot be initiated regardless of stimulus strength.

   Answer: E
   Page Ref: 394

20) During the depolarization phase of an action potential, which of the following is the primary activity?
   A) Potassium ions are flowing into the cell.
   B) Potassium ions are flowing out of the cell.
   C) Sodium ions are flowing into the cell.
   D) Sodium ions are flowing out of the cell.
   E) Neurotransmitter is diffusing into the cell.

   Answer: C
   Page Ref: 392

21) During the depolarization phase of an action potential, which of the following situations exists?

   A) The inside of the membrane is becoming more negative with respect to the outside.

   B) The inside of the membrane is becoming more positive with respect to the outside.

   C) The membrane is becoming less permeable to all ions.

   D) The membrane potential remains constant.

   E) The threshold is changing.

   Answer: B
   Page Ref: 392

22) During the repolarization phase of an action potential, which of the following is the primary activity

   A) Potassium ions are flowing into the cell.

   B) Potassium ions are flowing out of the cell.

   C) Sodium ions are flowing into the cell.

   D) Sodium ions are flowing out of the cell.

   E) The membrane is impermeable to all ions.

   Answer: B
   Page Ref: 393

23) During the repolarization phase of an action potential, which of the following situations exists?

   A) The inside of the membrane is becoming more negative with respect to the outside.

   B) The inside of the membrane is becoming more positive with respect to the outside.

   C) The membrane is becoming less permeable to all ions.

   D) The membrane potential remains constant.

   E) The threshold is changing.

   Answer: A
   Page Ref: 393

24) When ion movements across the membrane occur during the depolarization and repolarization phases of an action potential, they are moving by:

   A) primary active transport.

   B) secondary active transport.

   C) exocytosis.

   D) filtration.

   E) simple diffusion.

   Answer: E
   Page Ref: 392

25) The after–hyperpolarization that follows an action potential occurs due to a rapid:

    A) outflow of sodium ions.

    B) outflow of potassium ions.

    C) influx of sodium ions.

    D) influx of potassium ions.

    E) release of neurotransmitter.

Answer: B
Page Ref: 393

26) The factor most affecting the rate of impulse conduction is the:

    A) length of the axon.

    B) site of initial stimulation.

    C) rate of axonal transport.

    D) number of neuroglia associated with it.

    E) presence or absence of a myelin sheath.

Answer: E
Page Ref: 395

27) The term *saltatory conduction* refers to:

    A) "leaping" of an action potential across a synapse.

    B) movement of sodium ions into the cell during depolarization.

    C) one–way conduction of a nerve impulse across a synapse.

    D) conduction of a nerve impulse along a myelinated axon.

    E) action of the sodium–potassium pump.

Answer: D
Page Ref: 395

28) **ALL** of the following are **TRUE** concerning graded potentials **EXCEPT**:

    A) they involve mainly voltage–gated ion channels.

    B) they may be hyperpolarizing or depolarizing.

    C) they do not exhibit a refractory period.

    D) their amplitude depends of the strength of the stimulus.

    E) they arise mainly in dendrites and on cell bodies.

Answer: A
Page Ref: 396

29) The effect of a neurotransmitter on the postsynaptic cell occurs when the neurotransmitter:
    A) diffuses into the postsynaptic cell.
    B) flows along the postsynaptic cell membrane into transverse tubules.
    C) is broken down by enzymes in the synaptic cleft.
    D) actively transports sodium ions into the postsynaptic cell.
    E) binds to specific receptors on the postsynaptic cell membrane.

    Answer: E
    Page Ref: 397

30) The voltage across a neuron's membrane has changed from its resting potential of –70mV to –80mV. Which of the following is most likely to be **TRUE** regarding this situation?
    A) The neuron has bound a neurotransmitter that opens ligand–gated sodium ion channels.
    B) The neuron has bound a neurotransmitter that opens ligand–gated chloride ion channels.
    C) Large pores have opened in the membrane to allow release of large intracellular anions.
    D) The sodium/potassium pump has ceased functioning.
    E) Additional myelin has been added to the membrane to provide greater electrical insulation.

    Answer: B
    Page Ref: 399

31) The voltage across a neuron's membrane has changed from its resting potential of –70mV to –60mV. Which of the following is most likely to be **TRUE** regarding this situation?
    A) The membrane has bound an excitatory neurotransmitter.
    B) The membrane has bound an inhibitory neurotransmitter.
    C) An anesthetic drug has been applied to the neuron.
    D) Voltage–gated potassium ion channels have been opened.
    E) The metabolic activities of the cell have caused production of more anions that are now trapped inside the cell.

    Answer: A
    Page Ref: 399

32) What would happen to a postsynaptic neuron that binds a neurotransmitter that closes potassium ion channels?
   A) An EPSP would result because potassium ions are positively charged, and as they accumulate inside the cell, the membrane moves closer to threshold.
   B) An EPSP would result because the sodium/potassium pump would work to force potassium ions out of the cell, and sodium ions would be brought in as a result.
   C) An IPSP would result because potassium ions are negatively charged, and as they accumulate inside the cell, the membrane becomes more hyperpolarized.
   D) There would be no change in membrane potential because the membrane potential is dependent only on the opening and closing of sodium ion channels.
   E) There would be no change in membrane potential because there would be an increase in production of intracellular anions to compensate for the added potassium ions.

Answer: A
Page Ref: 399

33) A neurotransmitter that allows sodium ions to leak into a postsynaptic neuron causes:
   A) excitatory postsynaptic potentials.
   B) inhibitory postsynaptic potentials.
   C) no changes in resting potential.
   D) an alteration of the membrane threshold.
   E) damage to the myelin sheath.

Answer: A
Page Ref: 399

34) Diazepam is a GABA *agonist*. This means that it:
   A) breaks down GABA inside neuroglia.
   B) counteracts the effects of GABA.
   C) enhances the action of GABA.
   D) stimulates skeletal muscle movement.
   E) stimulates pain receptors.

Answer: C
Page Ref: 402

35) When depolarization reaches the axon terminal of a presynaptic neuron, the next event is:
   A) immediate release of neurotransmitter.
   B) uptake of neurotransmitter from the synaptic cleft.
   C) diffusion of calcium ions out of the cell.
   D) diffusion of calcium ions into the cell.
   E) active transport of calcium ions out of the cell.

Answer: D
Page Ref: 397

36) Most excitatory neurons in the CNS communicate via the neurotransmitter:
    A) acetylcholine.
    B) epinephrine.
    C) GABA.
    D) glutamate.
    E) dopamine.

    Answer: D
    Page Ref: 402

37) A neurotransmitter that allows negatively charged chloride ions to enter the postsynaptic cell causes:
    A) excitatory postsynaptic potentials because the membrane would begin to depolarize as the inside becomes more negative.
    B) inhibitory postsynaptic potentials because the membrane would become hyperpolarized as the inside becomes more negative.
    C) no change in resting potential because only sodium and potassium ions are involved in maintaining resting potential.
    D) immediate cell death as chloride blocks the action of ATP.
    E) inactivation of the enzymes that break down the neurotransmitter.

    Answer: B
    Page Ref: 399

38) A drug that is an *MAO inhibitor* would:
    A) block the action of acetylcholine.
    B) increase the effects of catecholamines by inhibiting their breakdown.
    C) reduce the effects of catecholamines by promoting their breakdown.
    D) block the manufacture of acetylcholine.
    E) block the manufacture of epinephrine.

    Answer: B
    Page Ref: 402

39) The neurotransmitter that is not synthesized in advanced and packaged into synaptic vesicles is:
    A) acetylcholine.
    B) GABA.
    C) nitric oxide.
    D) dopamine.
    E) epinephrine.

    Answer: C
    Page Ref: 402

40) The plasma membrane of a neuron is more permeable to potassium ions than to sodium ions because the membrane has:

   A) more voltage–gated sodium ion channels.

   B) more ligand–gated potassium ion channels.

   C) more potassium leakage channels.

   D) fewer voltage–gated sodium ion channels.

   E) more carrier molecules for potassium ions.

   Answer: C
   Page Ref: 390

41) Nitric oxide is thought to work by:

   A) opening voltage–gated sodium ion channels.

   B) opening ligand–gated potassium ion channels.

   C) opening ligand–gated chloride ion channels.

   D) preventing the breakdown of catecholamines.

   E) activating an enzyme for production of cyclic GMP.

   Answer: E
   Page Ref: 402

42) Regarding a neuron at rest, **ALL** of the following conditions exist **EXCEPT**:

   A) there are relatively more sodium ions in the extracellular fluid than in the intracellular fluid.

   B) there are relatively more potassium ions in the intracellular fluid than in the extracellular fluid.

   C) most intracellular anions cannot leave the intracellular fluid.

   D) the sodium / potassium active transport pump is operating.

   E) the membrane is relatively more permeable to sodium ions than to potassium ions.

   Answer: E
   Page Ref: 390

43) The threshold of a neuron is the:

   A) time between binding of the neurotransmitter and firing of an action potential.

   B) voltage at which the inflow of sodium ions causes reversal of the resting potential.

   C) total number of sodium ions that enters the cell before sodium inactivation gates close.

   D) total amount of neurotransmitter it takes to cause an action potential.

   E) voltage across the resting cell membrane.

   Answer: B
   Page Ref: 391

44) Parkinson's disease occurs when there has been degeneration of the axons containing:
   A) acetylcholine.
   B) GABA.
   C) endorphins.
   D) dopamine.
   E) epinephrine.

   Answer: D
   Page Ref: 402

45) Endorphins and enkephalins are neuropeptides that:
   A) induce pain.
   B) relieve pain.
   C) block the action of serotonin.
   D) are not stored in synaptic vesicles.
   E) regulate water balance.

   Answer: B
   Page Ref: 403

46) An neuronal circuit in which one presynaptic neuron stimulates a group of neurons, each of which then synapses with a common postsynaptic cell is a:
   A) converging circuit.
   B) diverging circuit.
   C) reverberating circuit.
   D) parallel after-discharge circuit.
   E) temporal summation circuit.

   Answer: D
   Page Ref: 404

47) The neuroglia that seem to exert and inhibitory effect on neurogenesis in the CNS are the:
   A) astrocytes.
   B) microglia.
   C) ependymal cells.
   D) Schwann cells.
   E) oligodendrocytes.

   Answer: E
   Page Ref: 405

48) Wallerian degeneration is degeneration of:

A) neuroglia in the blood–brain barrier.

B) Schwann cells.

C) the myelin sheath in multiple sclerosis.

D) unnecessary neurons during fetal development.

E) the distal fragment of a severed neuronal process and its myelin sheath.

Answer: E
Page Ref: 406

49) Following injury to a peripheral neuron, chromatolysis occurs, which is:

A) release of neurotransmitter from remaining synaptic vesicles.

B) breakup of the Nissl bodies.

C) degeneration of the myelin sheath.

D) reproduction of the local neuroglia.

E) degeneration of the distal fragment of a severed neuronal process and its myelin sheath.

Answer: B
Page Ref: 405

50) Prozac is an antidepressant drug that works by inhibiting the reuptake of:

A) acetylcholine.

B) GABA.

C) serotonin.

D) dopamine.

E) nitric oxide.

Answer: C
Page Ref: 399

MATCHING. Choose the item in column 2 that best matches each item in column 1.

Choose the item from column 2 that best matches each item in column 1.

1) Column 1: neuronal process that
conducts impulses away from
the cell body

Column 2: axon

Answer: axon

Page Ref: 381

2) Column 1: neuronal process that
conducts impulses toward the
cell body

Column 2: dendrite

Answer: dendrite

Page Ref: 381

3) Column 1: location of the nucleus of a
            neuron
   Column 2: cell body
   Answer: cell body
   Page Ref: 381

4) Column 1: storage sites for
            neurotransmitter
   Column 2: synaptic vesicles
   Answer: synaptic vesicles
   Page Ref: 381

5) Column 1: provide framework along
            which fast axonal transport
            occurs
   Column 2: microtubules
      Foil: plexuses
   Answer: microtubules
   Page Ref: 381

6) Column 1: substance that provides
            electrical insulation and
            increases propagation speed
   Column 2: myelin
   Answer: myelin
   Page Ref: 384

7) Column 1: unmyelinated areas of a
            myelinated axon
   Column 2: Nodes of Ranvier
   Answer: Nodes of Ranvier
   Page Ref: 384

8) Column 1: encloses the myelin sheath of
            axons in the PNS
   Column 2: neurolemma
   Answer: neurolemma
   Page Ref: 384

9) Column 1: site of protein synthesis in
      neurons
   Column 2: Nissl bodies
   Answer: Nissl bodies
   Page Ref: 381

10) Column 1: site at which nerve impulses
       are initiated in most neurons
    Column 2: trigger zone
    Answer: trigger zone
    Page Ref: 381

MATCHING. Choose the item in column 2 that best matches each item in column 1.

Choose the item from column 2 that best matches each item in column 1.

1) Column 1: a depolarizing graded
      potential
   Column 2: EPSP
   Answer: EPSP
   Page Ref: 399

2) Column 1: a hyperpolarizing graded
      potential
   Column 2: IPSP
   Answer: IPSP
   Page Ref: 399

3) Column 1: time required for release,
      diffusion, and binding of a
      neurotransmitter
   Column 2: synaptic delay
   Answer: synaptic delay
   Page Ref: 397

4) Column 1: ionic currents in cytosol open
      voltage–gated sodium ion
      channels at Nodes Ranvier
   Column 2: saltatory conduction
   Answer: saltatory conduction
   Page Ref: 395

5) Column 1: time when voltage–gated K$^+$ channels are still open and Na$^+$ channels are in resting state

Column 2: relative refractory period

Answer: relative refractory period

Page Ref: 392

6) Column 1: integration of inputs from several presynaptic neurons

Column 2: spatial summation

Answer: spatial summation

Page Ref: 399

7) Column 1: integration of inputs from rapid firing of single presynaptic neuron

Column 2: temporal summation

Answer: temporal summation

Page Ref: 399

8) Column 1: critical membrane potential at which voltage–gated Na$^+$ channels open rapidly

Column 2: threshold

Answer: threshold

Page Ref: 391

9) Column 1: time when Na$^+$ activation gates are open or inactivating and when K$^+$ channels are open

Column 2: absolute refractory period

Answer: absolute refractory period

Page Ref: 392

10) Column 1: sequence of events that reverse then restore resting potential

Column 2: action potential

Answer: action potential

Page Ref: 391

TRUE/FALSE. Write 'T' if the statement is true and 'F' if the statement is false.

1) Mature neurons normally do not undergo mitosis.

Answer: TRUE
Page Ref: 405

2) A nerve is the same thing as a neuron.

Answer: FALSE
Page Ref: 378

3) At rest, a neuron's cell membrane is slightly more positively charged inside than outside.

Answer: FALSE
Page Ref: 389

4) Dendrites are usually not myelinated.

Answer: TRUE
Page Ref: 381

5) Acetylcholine acts as an excitatory neurotransmitter on the heart.

Answer: FALSE
Page Ref: 401

6) A resting neuron cell membrane is more permeable to sodium ions than to potassium ions.

Answer: FALSE
Page Ref: 390

7) Exocytosis of synaptic vesicles is triggered by an increase in the concentration of calcium ions inside a presynaptic neuron.

Answer: TRUE
Page Ref: 397

8) A neuron cell membrane can be hyperpolarized either by an influx of negatively charged ions or by an outflow of positively charged ions.

Answer: TRUE
Page Ref: 399

9) An action potential becomes weaker and slower as it nears the end of an axon.

Answer: FALSE
Page Ref: 391

10) Saltatory conduction occurs on myelinated axons, but not on unmyelinated axons.

Answer: TRUE
Page Ref: 394

11) Leakage channels in a plasma membrane are always open.

Answer: TRUE
Page Ref: 387

12) The neurolemma is seen only around axons in the PNS.

Answer: TRUE
Page Ref: 384

13) Depolarization occurs due to outflow of potassium ions.

Answer: FALSE
Page Ref: 393

14) Cardiac muscle and glands are effectors for the autonomic nervous system.

Answer: TRUE
Page Ref: 380

15) The autonomic nervous system stimulates skeletal muscles.

Answer: FALSE
Page Ref: 380

SHORT ANSWER. Write the word or phrase that best completes each statement or answers the question.

1) The two principal divisions of the nervous system are the _____ , and the _____ .
Answer: central nervous system; peripheral nervous system
Page Ref: 379

2) Neurons that serve the integrative function of the nervous system are called _____ .
Answer: interneurons (association neurons)
Page Ref: 379

3) The _____ nervous system provides involuntary regulation of the gastrointestinal tract.
Answer: enteric
Page Ref: 380

4) _____ neurons transmit nerve impulses from receptors to the central nervous system.
Answer: Afferent
Page Ref: 379

5) Motor neurons that conduct impulses from the CNS to smooth and cardiac muscle belong to the _____ nervous system.
Answer: autonomic
Page Ref: 380

6) Neuoglia that produce the myelin sheath in the central nervous system are the _____.
   Answer: oligodendrocytes
   Page Ref: 333

7) The nucleus of a neuron is located in the _____ of a neuron.
   Answer: cell body
   Page Ref: 381

8) Nerve impulses are conducted toward the cell body by a neuronal process called a(n) _____.
   Answer: dendrite
   Page Ref: 381

9) Neurons having one main axon and one main dendrite are classified structurally as being _____.
   Answer: bipolar
   Page Ref: 383

10) The outer nucleated cytoplasmic layer of a Schwann cell is the _____.
    Answer: neurolemma
    Page Ref: 384

11) White matter looks white in color due to the presence of _____.
    Answer: myelin
    Page Ref: 384

12) A cluster of neuron cell bodies within the CNS is called a(n) _____.
    Answer: nucleus
    Page Ref: 385

13) The effectors for general somatic efferent neurons are _____.
    Answer: skeletal muscles
    Page Ref: 380

14) Phagocytic neuroglia are the _____.
    Answer: microglia
    Page Ref: 386

15) Ion channels in a plasma membrane that are always open are called _____ channels.
    Answer: leakage
    Page Ref: 387

16) A membrane whose polarization is more negative than the resting level is said to be _____.
Answer: hyperpolarized
Page Ref: 390

17) Ion channels in a plasma membrane that open in response to changes in membrane potential are called _____ channels.
Answer: voltage-gated
Page Ref: 387

18) Recovery of the resting potential due to opening of voltage-gated potassium ion channels and closing of voltage-gated sodium ion channels is called _____.
Answer: repolarization
Page Ref: 345

19) Impulse conduction that appears to jump from one Node of Ranvier to the next is called _____ conduction.
Answer: saltatory
Page Ref: 395

20) Ion channels in a plasma membrane that open or close in response to a specific chemical stimulus are called _____ channels.
Answer: ligand-gated
Page Ref: 387

21) Ion channels in a plasma membrane that open in response to vibration or pressure are called _____ channels.
Answer: mechanically gated
Page Ref: 389

22) At rest, the extracellular fluid around a neuron's plasma membrane is especially rich in positively charged _____ ions.
Answer: sodium
Page Ref: 390

23) In the cytosol, the predominant cation is _____.
Answer: potassium
Page Ref: 390

24) A neurotransmitter that causes hyperpolarization of the membrane is said to cause a(n) _____ postsynaptic potential.
Answer: inhibitory
Page Ref: 399

25) The critical membrane potential at which a neuron must generate an action potential is called
_____.

Answer: threshold

Page Ref: 391

26) The after–hyperpolarization phase of an action potential is due to rapid outflow of _____.

Answer: potassium ions

Page Ref:

27) A neuronal circuit in which a postsynaptic neuron receives input from several different sources is called a(n) _____ circuit.

Answer: converging

Page Ref: 404

28) A neurotransmitter that is excitatory for skeletal muscle but inhibitory for cardiac muscle is
_____.

Answer: acetylcholine

Page Ref: 401

29) A highly reactive free radical that acts as a neurotransmitter that is formed on demand is
_____.

Answer: nitric oxide

Page Ref: 402

30) A group of neuropeptides that suppress the release of Substance P is the _____.

Answer: enkephalins (or endorphins)

Page Ref: 403

31) The site of functional contact between two neurons or between a neuron and an effector is called a(n) _____.

Answer: synapse

Page Ref: 381

32) The capability of the nervous system to change based on experience is called _____.

Answer: plasticity

Page Ref: 404

33) A pathological condition in which there is progressive destruction of the myelin sheath is
_____.

Answer: multiple sclerosis

Page Ref: 406

34) Epinephrine, norepinephrine, and dopamine belong to a group of biogenic amines called _____.

Answer: catecholamines

Page Ref: 402

35) The most common inhibitory neurotransmitter in the brain is the amino acid _____.
Answer: GABA

Page Ref: 402

ESSAY. Write your answer in the space provided or on a separate sheet of paper.

1) Axon X has a diameter of 1.0 μm, is 10 cm long, and is unmyelinated. Axon Y has a diameter of 10 μm, is 25 cm long, and is myelinated. Axon Z is 2.5 μm in diameter, is 2.5 cm long, and is myelinated. Rank these axons in orders of fastest to slowest conduction rate. Explain your answer.

Answer: Y–X–Z. Axon Y is fastest due to myelin sheath and largest diameter. Axon X is slowest due to smallest diameter and no myelin sheath. The length of the axon is irrelevent to the conduction rate.

Page Ref: 395–396

2) Describe the advantages of electrical synapses over chemical synapses. Where do they commonly occur?

Answer: Seen in smooth and cardiac muscle and in the developing embryo, electrical synapses provide faster communication, allow for synchronous activity of many neurons or muscle fibers, and allow two–way transmission. Chemical synapses suffer a synaptic delay and provide for only one–way impulse conduction.

Page Ref: 397

3) Describe the characteristics of the neuron cell membrane and its environment that contribute to the existence of a resting potential.

Answer: Sodium and chloride ions predominate in the ECF, while potassium, organic phosphates, and amino acids predominate in the ICF. The membrane is moderately permeable to potassium, but only slightly permeable to sodium. Any sodium that leaks in is removed via active transport pumps, which pump out three sodium ions for each two potassium ions imported. Anions in the ICF are generally too large to escape. The net effect is an accumulation of positive charges outside, while the inner surface of the membrane becomes more negatively charged.

Page Ref: 389

4) Describe the phases of an action potential. including all appropriate ion movements and the mechanisms by which such movements occur.

Answer: 1. Depolarization—graded potential brings the membrane to threshold and voltage-gated sodium ion channels open; sodium rushes in by diffusion and creates positive feedback situation; sodium inactivation gates close just after activation gates open
2. Repolarization—voltage-gated potassium ion channels open as soon as sodium ions channels are closing; potassium diffuses out to restore resting potential; voltage-gated sodium ion channels revert to resting state
3. After–hyperpolarization—may occur as large outflow of potassium passes normal resting potential

Page Ref: 391

5) Describe the means by which a neurotransmitter may be removed from the synaptic cleft.

Answer: 1. simple diffusion away from cleft
2. inactivation by enzymes
3. uptake into presynaptic neuron or into neighboring neuroglia

Page Ref: 399

6) Bacteria produce a toxin that causes a flaccid paralysis. How might this toxin cause its effects?

Answer: It could block ACh release, increase acetylcholinesterase production, or block receptors so ACh cannot bind.

Page Ref: 401

7) Bacteria produce a toxin that causes all skeletal muscles to contract at the same time. How might this toxin cause its effects?

Answer: It could block action of acetylcholinesterase, mimic the action of ACh on postsynaptic receptors, or block glycine release (allows antagonists to contract with prime movers).

Page Ref: 401

8) Kevin reached into his snowblower while it was still running and partially severed three fingers on his right hand. After lengthy surgery to reattach the fingers, he has regained much of his motor ability, but little of the sensory functions. What factors affect the regeneration of Kevin's neurons?

Answer: First, the cell bodies must be intact. Since the cell bodies are all in or near the CNS, Kevin's injury didn't involve the cell bodies. The fact that PNS neurons were involved increases the chances of regeneration. The Schwann cells must be functional. The gap between severed pieces cannot be too large or fill too rapidly with collagen fibers.

Page Ref: 405

9) Predict the effects on levels of excitability of A) increased extracellular concentrations of sodium ions, and B) increased extracellular concentrations of potassium ions. Explain your answers.

Answer: Many answers could be acceptable, depending on what you expect your students to know at this point —i.e., the answers do not necessarily have to be absolutely correct as long as the students are thinking about the right things. Students should mention increases in concentration gradients and possible changes in resting potential. You might also expect comments about ion movements through leakage channels.

Page Ref: 389

10) You need to develop a drug that will block the transmission of impulses across a chemical synapse. By what possible mechanisms could this drug work?

Answer: The drug could block release of the neurotransmitter, block the binding of the neurotransmitter to the postsynaptic cell, or promote removal of the neurotransmitter from the synaptic cleft.

Page Ref: 401

CHAPTER 13   The Spinal Cord and Spinal Nerves

MULTIPLE CHOICE. Choose the one alternative that best completes the statement or answers the question.

1) What would normally be found within the central canal of the spinal cord?
   A) blood
   B) myelin
   C) cerebrospinal fluid
   D) air
   E) gray matter

   Answer: C
   Page Ref: 417

2) The filum terminale is:
   A) the roots of spinal nerves hanging inferiorly from the inferior end of the spinal cord in the vertebral column.
   B) an indentation on the dorsal side of the spinal cord.
   C) the tapered end of the spinal cord.
   D) an extension of the pia mater that anchors the spinal cord to the coccyx.
   E) where the cell bodies of sensory neurons are located.

   Answer: D
   Page Ref: 414

3) The cauda equina is:
   A) the roots of spinal nerves hanging inferiorly from the inferior end of the spinal cord in the vertebral column.
   B) an indentation on the dorsal side of the spinal cord.
   C) the tapered end of the spinal cord.
   D) an extension of the pia mater that anchors the spinal cord to the coccyx.
   E) where the cell bodies of sensory neurons are located.

   Answer: A
   Page Ref: 414

4) The posterior root ganglion is:
   A) the roots of spinal nerves hanging inferiorly from the inferior end of the spinal cord in the vertebral column.
   B) an indentation on the dorsal side of the spinal cord.
   C) the tapered end of the spinal cord.
   D) an extension of the pia mater that anchors the spinal cord to the coccyx.
   E) where the cell bodies of sensory neurons are located.

   Answer: E
   Page Ref: 414

5) What would normally be found immediately surrounding central canal of the spinal cord?
   A) white matter
   B) gray matter
   C) cerebrospinal fluid
   D) the pia mater
   E) the dura mater

   Answer: B
   Page Ref: 417

6) Cerebrospinal fluid normally circulates in the:
   A) epidural space.
   B) subdural space.
   C) subarachnoid space.
   D) ascending tracts.
   E) descending tracts.

   Answer: C
   Page Ref: 413

7) In the adult, the spinal cord extends from the medulla to the:
   A) coccyx.
   B) sacral promontory.
   C) point of attachment of the most inferior pair of ribs.
   D) sacral hiatus.
   E) upper border of vertebra L2.

   Answer: E
   Page Ref: 414

8) Spinal nerves are considered mixed, which means that:
   A) they contain both nerves and tracts.
   B) they contain both gray and white matter.
   C) they contain both afferent and efferent nerves.
   D) they use multiple types of neurotransmitters.
   E) a single nerve arises from multiple segments of the spinal cord.

   Answer: C
   Page Ref: 427

9) The part of a spinal nerve that contains only efferent fibers is the:
   A) dorsal root.
   B) ventral root.
   C) dorsal ramus.
   D) ventral ramus.
   E) plexus.

   Answer: B
   Page Ref: 414

10) To do a lumbar puncture, the needle is inserted into the:
    A) central canal.
    B) sacral plexus.
    C) nucleus pulposus.
    D) subarachnoid space.
    E) gray commissure.

    Answer: D
    Page Ref: 414

11) The nerve that stimulates the diaphragm to contract arises from the:
    A) cervical plexus.
    B) lumbar plexus.
    C) brachial plexus.
    D) sacral plexus.
    E) intercostal nerves.

    Answer: A
    Page Ref: 429

12) The nerve that stimulates the diaphragm to contract is the:

    A) median nerve.

    B) phrenic nerve.

    C) sciatic nerve.

    D) radial nerve.

    E) second intercostal nerve.

Answer: B
Page Ref: 429

13) The sacral plexus is the origin of the:

    A) axillary nerve.

    B) obturator nerve.

    C) femoral nerve.

    D) sciatic nerve.

    E) Both C and D are correct.

Answer: D
Page Ref: 439

14) **ALL** of the following arise from the brachial plexus **EXCEPT** the:

    A) axillary nerve.

    B) phrenic nerve.

    C) radial nerve.

    D) long thoracic nerve.

    E) median nerve.

Answer: B
Page Ref: 431

15) The endoneurium is the:

    A) lining of the central canal of the spinal cord.

    B) space between the pia mater and the spinal cord.

    C) connective tissue surrounding an individual axon.

    D) connective tissue surrounding an entire nerve.

    E) group of neurons forming a spinal tract.

Answer: C
Page Ref: 426

16) Spinal nerves emerge from the vertebral column via:

   A) vertebral bodies.

   B) intervertebral discs.

   C) intervertebral foramina.

   D) vertebral foramina.

   E) the central canal.

   Answer: C
   Page Ref: 426

17) Fat is normally found in the:

   A) epidural space.

   B) subdural space.

   C) central canal.

   D) subarachnoid space.

   E) filum terminale.

   Answer: A
   Page Ref: 412

18) The spinal cord passes through the:

   A) vertebral bodies.

   B) intervertebral discs.

   C) intervertebral foramina.

   D) vertebral foramen.

   E) All of the above except the intervertebral foramina.

   Answer: D
   Page Ref: 414

19) The spinal cord is suspended in the middle of its dural sheath by:

   A) ascending spinal tracts.

   B) the cauda equina.

   C) cerebrospinal fluid.

   D) denticulate ligaments.

   E) epidural fat.

   Answer: D
   Page Ref: 414

20) The diameter of the spinal cord is slightly larger in the:
    A) cervical and thoracic regions.
    B) cervical and lumbar regions.
    C) cervical and sacral regions.
    D) thoracic and lumbar regions.
    E) lumbar and sacral regions.

Answer: B
Page Ref: 414

21) The subdural space normally contains:
    A) fat.
    B) interstitial fluid.
    C) cerebrospinal fluid.
    D) blood.
    E) air.

Answer: B
Page Ref: 412

22) Which of the following is **TRUE** about the arachnoid?
    A) It is the most superficial of the meninges.
    B) It is made of mesothelium.
    C) It contains cerebrospinal fluid.
    D) It lines the central canal.
    E) It is avascular.

Answer: E
Page Ref: 412

23) The highly vascular, innermost layer of the meninges is the:
    A) dura mater.
    B) arachnoid.
    C) pia mater.
    D) gray commissure.
    E) conus medullaris.

Answer: C
Page Ref: 412

24) The nerves to and from the lower limbs arise from the:

A) intercostal region.

B) filum terminale.

C) dura mater.

D) brachial plexus.

E) lumbar enlargement.

Answer: E
Page Ref: 414

25) Integration of incoming and outgoing information is the function of:

A) gray matter.

B) white matter.

C) dorsal and ventral rami.

D) meninges.

E) posterior root ganglia.

Answer: A
Page Ref: 416

26) Ascending tracts contain:

A) motor neurons.

B) sensory neurons.

C) cerebrospinal fluid.

D) only cell bodies.

E) only unmyelinated axons.

Answer: B
Page Ref: 417

27) The spinothalamic tracts convey:

A) motor impulses to skeletal muscles.

B) sensory impulses regarding proprioception.

C) sensory impulses regarding discriminative touch.

D) sensory impulses regarding vibration.

E) sensory impulses regarding temperature.

Answer: E
Page Ref: 418

28) The posterior column tracts convey **ALL** of the following **EXCEPT:**

   A) sensory impulses regarding pain.

   B) sensory impulses regarding proprioception.

   C) sensory impulses regarding discriminative touch.

   D) sensory impulses regarding vibration.

   E) sensory impulses regarding two-point discrimination.

   Answer: A
   Page Ref: 418

29) Which of the following lists the anatomical features in correct order from outermost to innermost?

   A) dura mater, epidural space, arachnoid, subdural space, pia mater, subarachnoid space

   B) pia mater, epidural space, dura mater, subdural space, arachnoid, subarachnoid space

   C) arachnoid, subarachnoid space, pia mater, epidural space, dura mater, subdural space

   D) epidural space, dura mater, subdural space, arachnoid, subarachnoid space, pia mater

   E) dura mater, epidural space, subdural space, arachnoid, subarachnoid space, pia mater

   Answer: D
   Page Ref: 412

30) Voluntary skeletal muscle movements are stimulated via the:

   A) spinothalamic tracts.

   B) posterior column tracts.

   C) corticospinal tracts.

   D) vestibulospinal tract.

   E) tectospinal tract.

   Answer: C
   Page Ref: 418

31) The spinal cord is continuous with the:

   A) occipital bone.

   B) cerebral cortex.

   C) medulla oblongata.

   D) thalamus.

   E) coccyx.

   Answer: C
   Page Ref: 414

32) **ALL** of the following would be examples of autonomic reflexes **EXCEPT**:

   A) raising heart rate as blood pressure drops.

   B) contraction of smooth muscle in the wall of the gastrointestinal tract to push food along.

   C) secretion of hormones from the adrenal medulla during stress.

   D) contraction of the quadriceps femoris when the patellar tendon is stretched.

   E) dilation of blood vessels in the skin when body temperature increases.

   Answer: D
   Page Ref: 418

33) Cell bodies of motor neurons to skeletal muscles are located in the:

   A) anterior gray horns.

   B) lateral gray horns.

   C) anterior white columns.

   D) posterior white columns.

   E) central canal.

   Answer: A
   Page Ref: 417

34) **ALL** of the following are **TRUE** for the stretch reflex **EXCEPT**:

   A) it is a contralateral reflex arc.

   B) the receptors in the arc are called muscle spindles.

   C) it is a monosynaptic reflex arc.

   D) the sensory neuron synapses with a motor neuron in the anterior gray horn of the spinal cord.

   E) the effectors in the arc are skeletal muscles.

   Answer: A
   Page Ref: 420

35) Which of the following lists the components of a reflex arc in the correct order of functioning?

   A) receptor, motor neuron, integrating center, sensory neuron, effector

   B) motor neuron, receptor, integrating center, sensory neuron, effector

   C) receptor, sensory neuron, effector, motor neuron, integrating center

   D) receptor, sensory neuron, integrating center, motor neuron, effector

   E) effector, sensory neuron, integrating center, motor neuron, receptor

   Answer: D
   Page Ref: 419

36) The flexor reflex is considered to be an intersegmental reflex because it:

A) involves reciprocal innervation.

B) is a contralateral reflex.

C) con occur in any region of the spinal cord.

D) always occurs following the same sequence of events.

E) involves one sensory neuron activating interneurons in different segments of the spinal cord.

Answer: E
Page Ref: 423

37) The contralateral reflex that helps you maintain your balance when the flexor reflex is initiated is the:

A) stretch reflex.

B) tendon reflex.

C) crossed extensor reflex.

D) abdominal reflex.

E) patellar reflex.

Answer: C
Page Ref: 423

38) Clark has fallen off his horse and landed on his head. He now can breathe only with the aid of a respirator. This is most likely because he has:

A) damaged the spinal cord above the level of C3.

B) punctured his lungs via broken vertebrae and ribs.

C) severed the intercostal nerves innervating the thoracic structures.

D) crushed the centers in the brain that regulate breathing.

E) ruptured the upper air passages as his head compressed onto his neck.

Answer: A
Page Ref: 429

39) A friend has a pain in his back and wants to know why, when he presses on a certain spot, his knee gives out from under him. The most likely reason is that he is pressing on the:

A) tibial portion of the sciatic nerve.

B) common peroneal portion of the sciatic nerve.

C) femoral nerve.

D) phrenic nerve.

E) blood vessels supplying the lower extremity.

Answer: C
Page Ref: 436

40) In the tendon reflex, the tendon organs sense changes in:

   A) muscle stretch.

   B) muscle contraction or passive stretch.

   C) blood flow to the tendon.

   D) the concentration of neurotransmitter.

   E) the angle of a joint.

   Answer: B
   Page Ref: 423

41) In the tendon reflex, the sensory neuron:

   A) directly stimulates a prime mover.
   B) stimulates an inhibitory motor neuron to the antagonist muscle and an excitatory motor neuron to the prime mover.
   C) stimulates an inhibitory motor neuron to the prime mover and an excitatory motor neuron to the antagonist muscle.
   D) synapses with only one motor neuron.
   E) stimulates the tendon organ to lengthen the tendon.

   Answer: C
   Page Ref: 423

42) In an adult, curling under of all the toes in response to gentle stroking of the lateral outer margin of the sole is:

   A) normal.

   B) a positive Babinski sign.

   C) indicative of damage to the corticospinal tract.

   D) Both A and B are correct.

   E) Both B and C are correct.

   Answer: A
   Page Ref: 426

43) The branch of a spinal nerve that supplies the vertebrae and blood vessels of the spinal cord is the:

   A) anterior ramus.

   B) posterior ramus.

   C) meningeal branch.

   D) rami communicantes.

   E) endoneurium.

   Answer: C
   Page Ref: 428

44) The branches of spinal nerves that form networks called plexuses are the:

A) dorsal roots.

B) ventral roots.

C) posterior rami.

D) anterior rami.

E) rami communicantes.

Answer: D
Page Ref: 427

45) Inability to abduct and adduct the fingers and atrophy of the interosseous muscles of the hand indicates injury to the:

A) axillary nerve.

B) phrenic nerve.

C) long thoracic nerve.

D) median nerve.

E) ulnar nerve.

Answer: E
Page Ref: 431

46) Inability to adduct the leg indicates injury to the:

A) femoral nerve.

B) pudendal nerve.

C) obturator nerve.

D) deep peroneal nerve.

E) tibial nerve.

Answer: C
Page Ref: 436

47) The gastrocnemius and soleus are stimulated by the:

A) obturator nerve.

B) median nerve.

C) superficial peroneal nerve.

D) deep peroneal nerve.

E) tibial nerve.

Answer: E
Page Ref: 439

48) The plexus from which the sciatic nerve arises is located:

 A) between the psoas major and quadratus lumborum muscles.

 B) anterior to the sacrum.

 C) posterior to the sacrum.

 D) in the obturator foramen.

 E) between the gluteus maximus and gluteus medius muscles.

Answer: B
Page Ref: 439

49) The one cranial nerve that has a dermatome is the:

 A) optic.

 B) vagus.

 C) trigeminal.

 D) facial.

 E) glossopharyngeal.

Answer: C
Page Ref: 441

50) The polio virus typically attacks:

 A) posterior root ganglia.

 B) neurons in the anterior gray horns of the spinal cord.

 C) only sensory neurons.

 D) only interneurons.

 E) the connective tissues surrounding neurons.

Answer: B
Page Ref: 442

MATCHING. Choose the item in column 2 that best matches each item in column 1.

Choose the item from column 2 that best matches each item in column 1.

1) Column 1: phrenic nerve

 Column 2: diaphragm

 Answer: diaphragm
 Page Ref: 429

2) Column 1: tibial nerve

 Column 2: gastrocnemius

 Answer: gastrocnemius
 Page Ref: 439

3) Column 1: femoral nerve
   Column 2: extensors of leg
   Answer: extensors of leg
   Page Ref: 436

4) Column 1: obturator nerve
   Column 2: adductors of leg
   Answer: adductors of leg
   Page Ref: 436

5) Column 1: intercostal nerves
   Column 2: abdominal muscles
   Answer: abdominal muscles
   Page Ref: 428

6) Column 1: axillary nerve
   Column 2: deltoid
   Answer: deltoid
   Page Ref: 432

7) Column 1: radial nerve
   Column 2: triceps brachii
   Answer: triceps brachii
   Page Ref: 432

8) Column 1: median nerve
   Column 2: flexors of forearm
   Answer: flexors of forearm
   Page Ref: 432

9) Column 1: deep peroneal nerve
   Column 2: tibialis anterior
   Answer: tibialis anterior
   Page Ref: 439

10) Column 1: pudendal nerve
    Column 2: muscles of perineum
    Answer: muscles of perineum
    Page Ref: 439

MATCHING. Choose the item in column 2 that best matches each item in column 1.

Choose the item from column 2 that best matches each item in column 1.

1) Column 1: tough, outermost layer of
   meninges
   Column 2: dura mater
   Answer: dura mater
   Page Ref: 412

2) Column 1: avascular, middle layer of
   meninges
   Column 2: arachnoid
   Answer: arachnoid
   Page Ref: 412

3) Column 1: highly vascular, innermost
   layer of meninges
   Column 2: pia mater
   Answer: pia mater
   Page Ref: 412

4) Column 1: contains fat and connective
   tissue
   Column 2: epidural space
   Answer: epidural space
   Page Ref: 412

5) Column 1: contains interstitial fluid
   Column 2: subdural space
   Answer: subdural space
   Page Ref: 412

6) Column 1: contains cerebrospinal fluid
   Column 2: subarachnoid space
   Answer: subarachnoid space
   Page Ref: 412

7) Column 1: tapered end of spinal cord
   below the lumbar enlargement
   Column 2: conus medullaris
   Answer: conus medullaris
   Page Ref: 414

8) Column 1: extension of the pia mater attaching the spinal cord to the coccyx

Column 2: filum terminale

Answer: filum terminale

Page Ref: 414

9) Column 1: axons conveying sensory information to the brain

Column 2: ascending tracts

Answer: ascending tracts

Page Ref: 417

10) Column 1: axons conveying motor impulses from the brain to effectors

Column 2: descending tracts

Answer: descending tracts

Page Ref: 417

TRUE/FALSE. Write 'T' if the statement is true and 'F' if the statement is false.

1) Descending spinal tracts have a sensory function.

Answer: FALSE
Page Ref: 418

2) The epidural space normally contains cerebrospinal fluid.

Answer: FALSE
Page Ref: 412

3) The filum terminale is all the roots of spinal nerves that angle inferiorly from the end of the spinal cord.

Answer: FALSE
Page Ref: 414

4) The femoral nerve is the largest nerve in the body.

Answer: FALSE
Page Ref: 439

5) The arachnoid is the middle meninx.

Answer: TRUE
Page Ref: 412

6) The flexor reflex is a contralateral reflex.

Answer: FALSE
Page Ref: 423

7) The endoneurium is the lining of the central canal of the spinal cord.

Answer: FALSE
Page Ref: 427

8) The lumbar plexus lies between the psoas major and quadratus lumborum muscles.

Answer: TRUE
Page Ref: 436

9) A spinal tap is done to remove cerebrospinal fluid from the central canal of the spinal cord.

Answer: FALSE
Page Ref: 414

10) The anterior gray horns contain cell bodies of somatic motor neurons that stimulate skeletal muscles.

Answer: TRUE
Page Ref: 417

11) The stretch reflex is an example of an ipsilateral monosynaptic reflex arc.

Answer: TRUE
Page Ref: 420

12) The sensory receptors in the stretch reflex arc are called muscle spindles.

Answer: TRUE
Page Ref: 420

13) The median nerve stimulates the flexors of the forearm.

Answer: TRUE
Page Ref: 432

14) The spinal cord extends from the medulla to the coccyx.

Answer: FALSE
Page Ref: 414

15) The sciatic nerve arises from the lumbar plexus.

Answer: FALSE
Page Ref: 439

SHORT ANSWER. Write the word or phrase that best completes each statement or answers the question.

1) The innermost of the meninges is the _____.
Answer: pia mater
Page Ref: 412

2) Cerebrospinal fluid circulates in the _____ space.
Answer: subarachnoid
Page Ref: 414

3) In the adult, the spinal cord extends from the medulla to the _____ vertebra.
Answer: second lumbar
Page Ref: 414

4) The avascular layer of the meninges is the _____.
Answer: arachnoid
Page Ref: 412

5) The extensions of the pia mater that suspend the spinal cord in the middle of the dural sheath are called _____.
Answer: denticulate ligaments
Page Ref: 414

6) The cell bodies of peripheral sensory neurons are located in swellings known as _____.
Answer: posterior (dorsal) root ganglia
Page Ref: 414

7) Motor neuron axons are contained in the _____ root of a spinal nerve.
Answer: ventral
Page Ref: 414

8) Bundles of axons in the spinal cord having a common origin or destination and carrying similar information are called _____.
Answer: tracts
Page Ref: 417

9) Sensory spinal tracts are also known as _____ tracts.
Answer: ascending
Page Ref: 417

10) Proprioception and discriminative touch are some of the sensory inputs transmitted by the sensory tracts known as the _____ tract.

Answer: posterior column

Page Ref: 418

11) The indirect descending pathways include the rubrospinal, tectospinal, and _____ tracts.

Answer: vestibulospinal

Page Ref: 418

12) Changes in the internal or external environment are sensed by the component of a reflex arc known as the _____.

Answer: receptor

Page Ref: 419

13) Reflexes involving smooth muscle, cardiac muscle, and glands are called _____ reflexes.

Answer: autonomic (visceral)

Page Ref: 419

14) In a somatic reflex, the effector is a(n) _____.

Answer: skeletal muscle

Page Ref: 419

15) A neural circuit which simultaneously causes contraction of one muscle and relaxation of its antagonists is called _____.

Answer: reciprocal innervation

Page Ref: 420

16) The reflex that operates as a feedback mechanism to control muscle tension is called the _____ reflex.

Answer: tendon

Page Ref: 421

17) The connective tissue covering a whole nerve is called the _____.

Answer: epineurium

Page Ref: 427

18) The anterior rami of spinal nerves (except T2–T12) form networks called _____.

Answer: plexuses

Page Ref: 428

19) The phrenic nerve stimulates the _____.
    Answer: diaphragm
    Page Ref: 429

20) There are _____ pairs of spinal nerves.
    Answer: 31
    Page Ref: 426

21) Wrist drop, the inability to extend the wrist and fingers, results from damage to the _____ nerve, which arises from the _____ plexus.
    Answer: radial (or axillary); brachial
    Page Ref: 431

22) The branch of a spinal nerve containing the autonomic components is the _____.
    Answer: rami communicantes
    Page Ref: 427

23) The ventral rami of spinal nerves T2–T12 are known as _____ nerves.
    Answer: intercostal
    Page Ref: 428

24) The phrenic nerve arises from the _____ plexus.
    Answer: cervical
    Page Ref: 429

25) The plexus that passes superior to the first rib posterior to the clavicle is the _____ plexus.
    Answer: brachial
    Page Ref: 431

26) The entire nerve supply to the shoulder and upper limb is provided by the _____ plexus.
    Answer: brachial
    Page Ref: 432

27) The obturator nerve arises from the _____ plexus.
    Answer: lumbar
    Page Ref: 436

28) The largest nerve in the body is the _____ nerve.
    Answer: sciatic
    Page Ref: 439

29) The area of skin providing sensory input to one pair of spinal nerves is called a(n) _____.

Answer: dermatome

Page Ref: 441

30) The tibial and common peroneal nerves are branches of the _____ nerve.

Answer: sciatic

Page Ref: 439

ESSAY. Write your answer in the space provided or on a separate sheet of paper.

1) Doctors suspect that Ginny, age 15, has meningitis, and want to do a spinal tap. What is meningitis? Describe the procedure to be performed on Ginny. What is the purpose of this procedure?

Answer: Meningitis is an inflammation of the coverings of the brain and spinal cord. Doctors will insert a needle between vertebrae L3 and L4 or between L4 and L5 into the subarachnoid space to withdraw a sample of CSF for diagnostic purposes.

Page Ref: 414

2) Describe the cross-sectional anatomy of the spinal cord.

Answer: The spinal cord is slightly flattened in its anterior-posterior dimension. It has two grooves—anterior median fissure and shallower posterior median sulcus. The central canal contains CSF. The gray commissure surrounds the central canal, and contains gray horns (anterior, posterior, lateral), together forming an "H" arrangement. White matter surrounds the gray and is subdivided into columns (anterior, posterior, lateral). The anterior white commissure is anterior to the gray commissure.

Page Ref: 417

3) Describe the gross external anatomy of the spinal cord.

Answer: The spinal cord is roughly cylindrical, but slightly flattened anterior/posterior. It extends from the medulla to the superior border of L2 (16"–18") and is approximately 2 cm in diameter. There is a cervical enlargement from C4–T1 and a lumbar enlargement from T9–T12. The conus medullaris is the tapered inferior end. The filum terminale is an extension of the pia mater that anchors the cord to the coccyx. The cauda equina is the roots of spinal nerves angling inferiorly in the vertebral canal from the end of the spinal cord. 31 pairs of spinal nerves leave the cord at regular intervals.

Page Ref: 414

4) Identify the components of a spinal reflex arc, and describe the function of each.

Answer: 1. receptor—responds to specific changes in environment by producing graded potential
2. sensory neuron—conducts impulse from receptor to integrating center in gray matter of spinal cord
3. integrating center—site of synapse between sensory and other neurons; decision-making area in gray matter of spinal cord
4. motor neuron—conducts impulse from integrating center to effector
5. effector—responds to motor nerve impulse; either muscle or gland

Page Ref: 419

5) One of the effects of long-term untreated syphilis is sclerosis of the posterior column tracts. Predict the signs and symptoms a patient with this condition might exhibit.

Answer: Posterior column tracts carry sensations of proprioception, so ataxia results. Discriminative touch and two point discrimination are affected, so a patient would have an inability to distinguish what part of the body is being touched. There would also be disturbances in perception of pressure and vibration.

Page Ref: 418

6) A lesion has formed in the anterior gray horns in the segment of the spinal cord from which spinal nerves L1 –L4 arise. Predict the possible effects such a lesion might have on body function, and explain your answer.

Answer: Anterior gray horns contain motor neurons to skeletal muscles, so paralysis of whatever muscles are served by the affected neurons is likely. Most likely lower limbs served by nerves from the lumbar and/or sacral plexuses would be affected.

Page Ref: 417

7) Rosa's doctor asks her to sit on the examining table and dangle her legs over the edge. He then takes a small rubber hammer and taps just above her tibial tuberosity. Rosa's leg kicks forward. Explain what has happened.

Answer: The doctor is eliciting a stretch reflex in Rosa's patellar tendon/quadriceps femoris. Tapping the tendon stretches the muscle, causing muscle spindles to recognize change in length and notify a sensory neuron, which sends the message via a monosynaptic reflex to the integrating center and motor neuron, which triggers a contraction in the quadriceps to extend the leg (ipsilateral reflex arc).

Page Ref: 420

8) Name and describe the locations of the four major plexuses of spinal nerves. Name a major nerve arising from each.

Answer: 1. Cervical—alongside C1 –C4—phrenic

2. Brachial —inferior and lateral to C4 –T1 and superior to rib posterior to clavicle — axillary, ulnar, radial, median

3. Lumbar—lateral to L1 –L4 passing obliquely posterior to psoas major and anterior to quadratus lumborum—femoral

4. Sacral—anterior to sacrum—sciatic

Page Ref: 429-440

9) George is 80 years old and has just developed painful blisters that seem to start abruptly at the anterior midline, circle around his waist on his right side, and stop equally abruptly on the posterior midline. What is probably wrong with George, and what accounts for the pattern of lesions?

Answer: George has shingles (herpes zoster). He probably had chickenpox as a child and some viruses stayed latent in his posterior root ganglia in his thoracic region. With age, his immunity to the virus has fallen off, and the virus has reactivated to travel via fast axonal transport to the skin surface. Lesions only appear on areas of skin served by the affected nerves (dermatomes).

Page Ref: 441-442

10) On observing a person walking along the sidewalk, you notice that the person's right foot seems to go limp every time he takes a step. Offer a plausible neurological reason to explain this phenomenon.

Answer: The person possibly has foot drop caused by damage to the common peroneal branch of the sciatic nerve, which causes the inability to dorsiflex the foot. Other explanations may be acceptable.

Page Ref: 439

CHAPTER 14   The Brain and Cranial Nerves

MULTIPLE CHOICE. Choose the one alternative that best completes the statement or answers the question.

1) The cavities within the brain are called:
   A) sulci.
   B) choroid plexuses.
   C) nuclei.
   D) ventricles.
   E) commissures.

   Answer: D
   Page Ref: 449

2) Fine control of body coordination and balance is a function of the:
   A) cerebellum.
   B) hypothalamus.
   C) thalamus.
   D) pituitary gland.
   E) reticular activating system.

   Answer: A
   Page Ref: 458

3) The falx cerebri is:
   A) the deep groove between the precentral and postcentral gyri.
   B) the lobe of the cerebrum not visible on the surface.
   C) an extension of the dura matter separating the cerebral hemispheres.
   D) an extension of the dura matter separating the cerebellar hemispheres.
   E) an extension of the dura matter separating the cerebrum from the cerebellum.

   Answer: C
   Page Ref: 448

4) The brain requires such a large percentage of the body's total blood flow because:
   A) it is such a large percentage of the body's total weight.
   B) its cells are always dividing to replace old cells.
   C) no glucose, the brain's exclusive energy source, is stored.
   D) it needs the heat to supply an alternative energy source.
   E) the movement of the blood stimulates the growth the neuronal cytoplasmic extensions.

   Answer: C
   Page Ref: 447

5) Paired masses of gray matter within the white matter of the cerebrum that are rich in dopamine and are involved in maintenance of muscle tone are the:

A) corpora quadrigemina.

B) basal ganglia.

C) mammillary bodies.

D) substantia nigra.

E) supraoptic nuclei.

Answer: B
Page Ref: 465

6) The type of neuroglia that wrap around capillaries in the blood–brain barrier are the:

A) astrocytes.

B) Schwann cells.

C) oligodendrocytes.

D) microglia.

E) ependymal cells.

Answer: A
Page Ref: 448

7) The main relay center for conducting information between the spinal cord and the cerebrum is the:

A) thalamus.

B) insula.

C) corpus callosum.

D) cerebellar peduncles.

E) tentorium cerebelli.

Answer: A
Page Ref: 460

8) The blood–brain barrier does not prevent passage of:

A) any hormones.

B) most bacteria.

C) vitamins.

D) red blood cells.

E) lipid-soluble substances.

Answer: E
Page Ref: 448

9) The brain stem is made up of the:
   A) cerebellum, pons, and hypothalamus.
   B) medulla oblongata, thalamus, and midbrain.
   C) medulla oblongata, hypothalamus, and pons.
   D) medulla oblongata, pons, and midbrain.
   E) midbrain, hypothalamus, and thalamus.

   Answer: D
   Page Ref: 452

10) Which of the following is **NOT TRUE** for cerebrospinal fluid?
    A) It acts as a shock absorber for the brain.
    B) It may contain white blood cells.
    C) It is a medium for exchange of nutrients and wastes.
    D) It acts as a neurotransmitter in the brain.
    E) It is produced by filtration and secretion in choroid plexuses.

    Answer: D
    Page Ref: 449

11) Superior to the hypothalamus and between the halves of the thalamus is the:
    A) subthalamus.
    B) third ventricle.
    C) fourth ventricle.
    D) superior sagittal sinus.
    E) midbrain.

    Answer: B
    Page Ref: 449

12) The function of a choroid plexus is to:
    A) receive sensations from the viscera.
    B) send motor impulses to the diaphragm.
    C) produce cerebrospinal fluid.
    D) reabsorb cerebrospinal fluid.
    E) transmits impulses from one cerebral hemisphere to the other.

    Answer: C
    Page Ref: 449

13) The function of arachnoid villi is to:

   A) reabsorb cerebrospinal fluid.

   B) produce cerebrospinal fluid.

   C) hold the meninges onto the brain.

   D) provide nourishment for neurons in the CNS.

   E) conduct impulses from one cerebral hemisphere to the other.

   Answer: A
   Page Ref: 450

14) The blood–CSF barrier is composed of:

   A) astrocytes.

   B) oligodendrocytes.

   C) myelin.

   D) dense irregular connective tissue.

   E) ependymal cells.

   Answer: E
   Page Ref: 450

15) The median and lateral apertures are the connection between the:

   A) right and left cerebral hemispheres.

   B) right and left cerebellar hemispheres.

   C) fourth ventricle and subarachnoid space.

   D) third and fourth ventricles.

   E) lateral ventricles and third ventricle.

   Answer: D
   Page Ref: 450

16) If a blockage occurred in the interventricular foramina, what would be the likely result?

   A) hydrocephalus.

   B) anosmia.

   C) blindness.

   D) deafness.

   E) encephalitis.

   Answer: A
   Page Ref: 450

17) The pneumotaxic and apneustic centers are located in the:

   A) medulla oblongata.

   B) pons.

   C) cerebellum.

   D) hypothalamus.

   E) cerebral cortex.

   Answer: B
   Page Ref: 455

18) The function of the corpora quadrigemina is to:

   A) control reflex movements of the body in response to visual and auditory stimuli.

   B) produce cerebrospinal fluid.

   C) set the basic pattern of breathing.

   D) produce hormones that control the anterior pituitary gland.

   E) control blood pressure.

   Answer: A
   Page Ref: 457

19) White fibers that transmit impulses between corresponding gyri in opposite cerebral hemispheres are called:

   A) association fibers.

   B) projection fibers.

   C) commissural fibers.

   D) ganglia.

   E) choroid plexuses.

   Answer: C
   Page Ref: 465

20) Damage to the cerebellum would result in:

   A) loss of memory.

   B) uncoordinated movement.

   C) inability to dream.

   D) altered pituitary function.

   E) uncontrollable body temperature.

   Answer: B
   Page Ref: 458

21) The hippocampus is most important for:

    A) conversion of short-term to long-term memory.

    B) production of cerebrospinal fluid.

    C) maintenance of posture.

    D) setting the basic pattern of breathing.

    E) controlling blood pressure.

Answer: A
Page Ref: 467

22) The reason hydrocephalus is so dangerous is that:

    A) too many toxic products flood the brain.

    B) excess cerebrospinal fluid puts pressure on neurons, damaging them.

    C) the brain dehydrates.

    D) bacteria can grow more easily in accumulated fluid.

    E) it causes excessive release of hormones from the hypothalamus.

Answer: B
Page Ref: 450

23) Between the foramen magnum and the pons is the:

    A) pituitary gland.

    B) hypothalamus.

    C) cerebellum.

    D) medulla oblongata.

    E) midbrain.

Answer: D
Page Ref: 452

24) Which of the following combinations of cranial nerves cause movements of the eyeball?

    A) optic, trochlear, and abducens.

    B) optic, oculomotor, and trochlear.

    C) optic, oculomotor, and abducens.

    D) trochlear, oculomotor, and abducens.

    E) trochlear, oculomotor, and trigeminal.

Answer: D
Page Ref: 475-476

25) Impulses from proprioceptors, such as muscle spindles, are relayed from the medulla to the cerebellum by neurons in the:

   A) intermediate mass.

   B) olive.

   C) circumventricular organs.

   D) superior cerebellar peduncles.

   E) corpora quadrigemina.

   Answer: B
   Page Ref: 453

26) The left side of the cerebrum controls skeletal muscles on the right side of the body because motor neurons cross from left to right in the:

   A) precentral gyrus.

   B) cerebellum.

   C) medulla oblongata.

   D) hypothalamus.

   E) thalamus.

   Answer: C
   Page Ref: 453

27) The pneumotaxic and apneustic areas help control:

   A) heart rate.

   B) blood pressure.

   C) breathing.

   D) skeletal movements.

   E) extracellular fluid volume.

   Answer: C
   Page Ref: 455

28) The cerebral aqueduct passes through the:

   A) longitudinal fissure.

   B) midbrain.

   C) infundibulum.

   D) medulla.

   E) cerebrum.

   Answer: B
   Page Ref: 455

29) A sudden noise occurs behind you and you turn around in response. This is a reflex, which is the responsibility of the:

   A) substantia nigra.

   B) medial lemniscus.

   C) superior colliculi.

   D) inferior colliculi.

   E) basal ganglia.

   Answer: D
   Page Ref: 457

30) Cranial nerve number VIII conveys sensory information about:

   A) visual stimuli.

   B) facial expression.

   C) taste.

   D) equilibrium.

   E) smell.

   Answer: D
   Page Ref: 477

31) The flocculonodular lobe of he cerebellum is concerned with the:

   A) regulation of blood pressure.

   B) sense of smell.

   C) regulation of the pineal gland.

   D) regulation of breathing.

   E) sense of equilibrium.

   Answer: E
   Page Ref: 457

32) The right and left portions of the thalamus are connected by the:

   A) intermediate mass.

   B) infundibulum.

   C) corpus callosum.

   D) mammillary bodies.

   E) cerebral aqueduct.

   Answer: A
   Page Ref: 460

33) The hypothalamo–hypophyseal tract is made up of axons from the:
   A) geniculate nuclei.
   B) mammillary bodies.
   C) paraventricular and supraoptic nuclei.
   D) substantia nigra.
   E) pneumotaxic and apneustic centers.

   Answer: C
   Page Ref: 460

34) The satiety center causes:
   A) sexual arousal.
   B) arousal from sleep.
   C) secretion of hormones from the posterior pituitary.
   D) stimulation of the thirst center.
   E) inhibition of the feeding center.

   Answer: E
   Page Ref: 462

35) Sensory impulses related to equilibrium are carried by a branch of the same nerve that conveys sensory impulses associated with:
   A) vision.
   B) hearing.
   C) smell.
   D) taste.
   E) visceral pain.

   Answer: B
   Page Ref: 477

36) The superior sagittal sinus is normally filled with:
   A) air.
   B) blood.
   C) cerebrospinal fluid.
   D) gray matter.
   E) interstitial fluid.

   Answer: B
   Page Ref: 450

37) Releasing hormones that control the anterior pituitary gland are produced by the:

    A) pineal gland.

    B) thalamus.

    C) hypothalamus.

    D) medulla oblongata.

    E) corpus callosum.

    Answer: C
    Page Ref: 462

38) Patterns of sleep and established by the:

    A) suprachiasmatic nucleus of the hypothalamus.

    B) substantia nigra of the midbrain.

    C) corpora quadrigemina of the midbrain.

    D) decussation of pyramids in the medulla.

    E) arbor vitae of the cerebellum.

    Answer: A
    Page Ref: 463

39) The cerebral hemispheres are connected internally by the:

    A) intermediate mass.

    B) basal ganglia.

    C) corpus callosum.

    D) arachnoid villi.

    E) habenular nuclei.

    Answer: C
    Page Ref: 463

40) The diameter of blood vessels is controlled by centers located in the:

    A) thalamus.

    B) midbrain.

    C) cerebellum.

    D) medulla oblongata.

    E) occipital lobe of the cerebrum.

    Answer: D
    Page Ref: 453

41) The primary motor area of the cerebral cortex is located in the:

   A) precentral gyrus.

   B) postcentral gyrus.

   C) temporal lobe.

   D) occipital lobe.

   E) insula.

   Answer: A
   Page Ref: 469

42) The primary visual area and visual association area of the cerebral cortex are both located in the:

   A) frontal lobe.

   B) temporal lobe.

   C) parietal lobe.

   D) insula.

   E) occipital lobe.

   Answer: E
   Page Ref: 469

43) A patient has had a cerebrovascular accident involving the middle region of the temporal cerebral cortex. Which of the following would most likely be a problem for this patient?

   A) recognizing friends and family.

   B) identifying foods by taste.

   C) determining the relationships between body parts.

   D) determining whether a sound is speech, music, or noise.

   E) translating thoughts into speech.

   Answer: D
   Page Ref: 469

44) Damage to the cribriform plate of the ethmoid bone would most likely result in loss of:

   A) vision.

   B) sensations to the side of the face.

   C) the sense of smell.

   D) the ability to speak.

   E) equilibrium.

   Answer: C
   Page Ref: 475

45) Slowing of the heart rate and secretion of digestive fluids are motor functions of cranial nerve:

   A) V.
   B) VII.
   C) VIII.
   D) X.
   E) XII.

   Answer: D
   Page Ref: 478

46) Movement of the tongue during speech and swallowing is a motor function of the:

   A) abducens nerve.
   B) facial nerve.
   C) hypoglossal nerve.
   D) glossopharyngeal nerve.
   E) vagus nerve.

   Answer: C
   Page Ref: 479

47) Cranial nerve VII is the:

   A) trigeminal nerve.
   B) facial nerve.
   C) abducens nerve.
   D) glossopharyngeal nerve.
   E) accessory nerve.

   Answer: B
   Page Ref: 477

48) The cranial nerve that terminates in the lateral geniculate nucleus of the thalamus is the:

   A) accessory nerve.
   B) trigeminal nerve.
   C) vagus nerve.
   D) olfactory nerve.
   E) optic nerve.

   Answer: E
   Page Ref: 475

49) The ophthalmic, maxillary, and mandibular are all branches of the:
   A) trigeminal nerve.
   B) vagus nerve.
   C) facial nerve.
   D) hypoglossal nerve.
   E) abducens nerve.

   Answer: A
   Page Ref: 476

50) Secretion of saliva is stimulated by cranial nerve:
   A) XII.
   B) IV.
   C) V.
   D) IX.
   E) X.

   Answer: D
   Page Ref: 478

MATCHING. Choose the item in column 2 that best matches each item in column 1.

Choose the best item from column 2 that best matches each item in column 1.

1) Column 1: hypothalamus
   Column 2: satiety center
   Answer: satiety center
   Page Ref: 462

2) Column 1: pons
   Column 2: pneumotaxic center
   Answer: pneumotaxic center
   Page Ref: 455

3) Column 1: medulla oblongata
   Column 2: cardiovascular center
   Answer: cardiovascular center
   Page Ref: 453

4) Column 1: midbrain
   Column 2: corpora quadrigemina
   Answer: corpora quadrigemina
   Page Ref: 457

5) Column 1: thalamus
   Column 2: geniculate nuclei
   Answer: geniculate nuclei
   Page Ref: 460

6) Column 1: limbic system
   Column 2: olfactory bulbs
   Answer: olfactory bulbs
   Page Ref: 467

7) Column 1: cerebellum
   Column 2: vermis
   Answer: vermis
   Page Ref: 457

8) Column 1: epithalamus
   Column 2: habenular nuclei
   Answer: habenular nuclei
   Page Ref: 463

9) Column 1: basal ganglia
   Column 2: globus pallidus
   Answer: globus pallidus
   Page Ref: 465

10) Column 1: temporal lobe of cerebrum
    Column 2: primary olfactory area
    Answer: primary olfactory area
    Page Ref: 468

MATCHING. Choose the item in column 2 that best matches each item in column 1.

Choose the best item from column 2 that best matches each item in column 1.

1) Column 1: olive
   Column 2: medulla oblongata
   Answer: medulla oblongata
   Page Ref: 453

2) Column 1: apneustic area
   Column 2: pons
   Answer: pons
   Page Ref: 455

3) Column 1: substantia nigra
   Column 2: midbrain
   Answer: midbrain
   Page Ref: 457

4) Column 1: arbor vitae
   Column 2: cerebellum
   Answer: cerebellum
   Page Ref: 457

5) Column 1: intermediate mass
   Column 2: thalamus
   Answer: thalamus
   Page Ref: 403

6) Column 1: supraoptic nuclei
   Column 2: hypothalamus
   Answer: hypothalamus
   Page Ref: 460

7) Column 1: putamen
   Column 2: basal ganglia
   Answer: basal ganglia
   Page Ref: 465

8) Column 1: hippocampus
   Column 2: limbic system
   Answer: limbic system
   Page Ref: 467

9) Column 1: primary visual area
   Column 2: occipital lobe of cerebrum
   Answer: occipital lobe of cerebrum
   Page Ref: 468

10) Column 1: primary motor area

   Column 2: frontal lobe of cerebrum

   Answer: frontal lobe of cerebrum

   Page Ref: 469

TRUE/FALSE. Write 'T' if the statement is true and 'F' if the statement is false.

1) The brain stem consists of the thalamus and the hypothalamus.

   Answer: FALSE
   Page Ref: 452

2) The falx cerebri is an extension of the dura mater that separates the cerebral hemispheres.

   Answer: TRUE
   Page Ref: 446

3) Cerebrospinal fluid is produced by arachnoid villi.

   Answer: FALSE
   Page Ref: 450

4) The fourth ventricle is located between the brain stem and the cerebellum.

   Answer: TRUE
   Page Ref: 449

5) The adult brain consumes about 20% of the oxygen used at rest.

   Answer: TRUE
   Page Ref: 447

6) The rate and force of heartbeat are regulated by the cardiovascular center in the pons.

   Answer: FALSE
   Page Ref: 453

7) The medullary rhythmicity center regulates heart rate.

   Answer: FALSE
   Page Ref: 453

8) The reticular activating system is responsible for maintaining consciousness.

   Answer: TRUE
   Page Ref: 457

9) Association fibers transmit nerve impulses between the brain and the spinal cord.

   Answer: FALSE
   Page Ref: 465

10) The pineal gland is located in the sella turcica of the sphenoid bone.

Answer: FALSE
Page Ref: 463

11) The mammillary bodies are part of the hypothalamus.

Answer: TRUE
Page Ref: 460

12) The hypothalamus produces hormones that regulate secretion of hormones from the anterior pituitary gland.

Answer: TRUE
Page Ref: 462

13) The limbic system includes parts of the cerebellum.

Answer: FALSE
Page Ref: 467

14) The primary motor area of the cerebrum is located in the occipital lobe.

Answer: FALSE
Page Ref: 469

15) Cranial nerve I passes through the cribriform plate of the ethmoid bone.

Answer: TRUE
Page Ref: 475

SHORT ANSWER. Write the word or phrase that best completes each statement or answers the question.

1) The cranial meninges include the outer _____ , the middle _____ , and the inner _____ .
Answer: dura mater; arachnoid; pia mater
Page Ref: 446

2) The large, dural venous sinus extending over the top of the brain is the _____ .
Answer: superior sagittal sinus
Page Ref: 450

3) The neuropeptides produced by the hypothalamus that are released as hormones from the posterior pituitary gland are _____ and _____ .
Answer: oxytocin; antidiuretic hormone
Page Ref: 462

4) Cranial nerve V is the _____ nerve.
Answer: trigeminal
Page Ref: 475

5) The nuclei in the medulla oblongata that adjust the basic rhythm of breathing are called the
_____.

Answer: medullary rhythmicity center

Page Ref: 453

6) Cerebrospinal fluid flows from the fourth ventricle through the lateral and median apertures
into the _____.

Answer: subarachnoid space

Page Ref: 453

7) The superior sagittal sinus contains _____.

Answer: venous blood

Page Ref: 450

8) The superior and inferior colliculi are the rounded elevations that make up the _____ of the
midbrain.

Answer: corpora quadrigemina

Page Ref: 457

9) The _____ is responsible for maintaining consciousness and for awakening from sleep.

Answer: reticular activating center

Page Ref: 457

10) The superior cerebellar peduncles connect the _____ and the _____.

Answer: cerebellum; midbrain

Page Ref: 457

11) The ventricles of the brain normally are filled with _____.

Answer: cerebrospinal fluid

Page Ref: 449

12) Networks of capillaries involved in the production of cerebrospinal fluid are called _____.

Answer: choroid plexuses

Page Ref: 449

13) The main brain region that regulates posture and balance is the _____.

Answer: cerebellum

Page Ref: 458

14) Small brain regions in the walls of the third and fourth ventricles that can monitor chemical changes in blood because they lack a blood–brain barrier are called the _____.
Answer: circumventricular organs
Page Ref: 463

15) Raising osmotic pressure in the extracellular fluid stimulates the thirst center located in the _____.
Answer: hypothalamus
Page Ref: 462

16) Control of the ANS is an important function of the area of the diencephalon called the _____.
Answer: hypothalamus
Page Ref: 460

17) The brain stem consists of the _____ , the _____ , and the _____.
Answer: medulla oblongata; pons; midbrain
Page Ref: 452

18) The areas of the hypothalamus that regulate eating behavior are the _____ center, which is responsible for hunger sensations, and the _____ center that is stimulated when enough food has been ingested.
Answer: feeding; satiety
Page Ref: 462

19) The _____ are part of the epithalamus involved in olfaction.
Answer: habenular nuclei
Page Ref: 463

20) The red nucleus is a region of the _____ that is involved in coordinating muscular movements.
Answer: midbrain
Page Ref: 457

21) The pineal gland secretes the hormone _____ that functions to _____.
Answer: melatonin; promote sleepiness (and help set biological clock)
Page Ref: 463

22) The upfolds of cerebral tissue are known as _____ or _____.
Answer: gyri; convolutions
Page Ref: 463

23) The largest portion of the diencephalon is the _____.
    Answer: thalamus
    Page Ref: 460

24) The infundibulum is a stalklike structure that attaches the _____ to the _____.
    Answer: pituitary; hypothalamus
    Page Ref: 460

25) The postcentral gyrus of the cerebrum contains the primary _____ area.
    Answer: somatosensory
    Page Ref: 463

26) The part of the diencephalon that is functionally linked to the basal ganglia is the _____.
    Answer: subthalamus
    Page Ref: 465

27) The region/lobe of the cerebrum that cannot be seen from the exterior surface of the brain is the _____.
    Answer: insula
    Page Ref: 465

28) The caudate nucleus and the lentiform nucleus form the _____ of the basal ganglia.
    Answer: corpus striatum
    Page Ref: 465

29) Bruising of the brain due to trauma in which there is leakage of blood and possible tearing of the pia mater is called a(n) _____.
    Answer: contusion
    Page Ref: 468

30) The substantia nigra is particularly rich in the neurotransmitter _____.
    Answer: dopamine
    Page Ref: 457

ESSAY. Write your answer in the space provided or on a separate sheet of paper.

1) Describe the structure and function of the blood-brain barrier.

    Answer: The barrier is formed by capillaries whose endothelial cells have tight junctions and a continuous basement membrane. Astroytes also press against the capillaries to help control what can leave the blood and enter the brain. Small molecules and lipid-soluble substances pass easily; water-soluble substances may pass via carrier. Large molecules typically do not pass at all.
    Page Ref: 449

2) A patient is experiencing smell sensations that are not real. She is subsequently diagnosed with a brain tumor. Where would you predict the tumor to be located? Why was she experiencing false sensations of smell? Explain your answers.

Answer: The tumor is likely in any of the olfactory regions of the brain—e.g., olfactory bulbs or primary olfactory area on the medial aspect of the temporal lobe. False smell sensations are likely forms of seizures that result from pressure created by the tumor on sensory olfactory neurons or neurons in the association areas related to smell.

Page Ref: 468

3) Several patients were admitted to the emergency rooms of several hospitals in a large urban area exhibiting effects of damage to the substantia nigra by an illegal drug. What would you expect these effects to be? Explain your answer.

Answer: Symptoms similar to Parkinson's Disease (inability to control skeletal movements, etc.) would result, due to loss of dopamine-producing cells. The substantia nigra would be unable to contribute to the activities of the basal ganglia, cerebellum, and cerebrum.

Page Ref: 457

4) Explain why a crushing injury to the occipital bone is often fatal.

Answer: The crushing of the bone also crushes the brainstem, particularly the medulla oblongata. Damage to important nuclei regulating vital functions, such as respiration, heart rate and force of contraction, and diameter of blood vessels, may result in death.

Page Ref: 453

5) Mrs. Booth is suffering the effects of a stroke. She has some paralysis of muscles on her right side and is experiencing some problems speaking. What is the most likely location of her brain injury? Explain your answer.

Answer: The most likely location is the left frontal lobe around the junction of the precentral gyrus and the lateral cerebral sulcus. The primary motor area has been affected (precentral gyrus,) as well as Broca's speech area (lateral cerebral sulcus). The right-sided paralysis and loss of speech indicates left-sided brain damage, since the left side of the premotor area controls the right side of the body and most people's speech area is on the left side.

Page Ref: 469

6) Mr. Dodge was crossing the road and was hit by a car. When he fell, he hit the back of his head on the pavement. He never lost consciousness, and there was no discernible damage. However, the next day he suddenly lost his color vision. What do you think has happened? Explain your answer.

Answer: Damage (perhaps a small clot) to part of the primary visual area in the occipital lobe is most likely. Students may suggest other plausible answers.

Page Ref: 468

7) Identify and describe the roles of the components of the brain involved in coordination of movement.

Answer: The following areas should be included: cerebellum, substantia nigra and red nucleus of midbrain, basal ganglia of cerebrum, subthalamus, and ventral nuclei of thalamus. The premotor area should be included as a motor association area.

Page Ref: 457–470

8) Describe the structural and functional relationship between the hypothalamus and the pituitary gland.

Answer: The hypothalamus releases regulatory hormones into the capillary networks in the median eminence to increase or decrease hormone production and secretion from the anterior pituitary. Axons from the paraventricular and supraoptic nuclei extend through the infundibulum to the posterior pituitary. Their cell bodies produce oxytocin or antidiuretic hormone, which is stored and released from the axons which form the posterior pituitary.

Page Ref: 462

9) Your A&P I professor has told you during her discussion of the hypothalamus that "from this day forward until the end of A&P II, you must never forget the hypothalamus!" Why do you suppose she has made such a big deal out of such a small region of the brain? Be specific in your response, and use the Table of Contents of your text, if necessary.

Answer: It controls the ANS, which regulates smooth and cardiac muscle and secretion from many glands. Therefore, it regulates cardiovascular, digestive, and excretory activities. It regulates the pituitary gland, which itself regulates many other glands and organs. It regulates emotional behavior, including those behavior patterns associated with sexual arousal. It regulates eating behavior and fluid balance. All of these topics are generally covered subsequent to the introduction of the hypothalamus, and mostly in A&P II.

Page Ref: 460–463

10) Identify and describe the anatomical origins of those cranial nerves with exclusively or mainly sensory functions.

Answer: 1. Cranial nerve I (olfactory)—smell—nasal mucosa
2. Cranial nerve II (optic)—vision—retina of eye
3. Cranial nerve VIII (vestibulocochlear)—hearing and equilibrium—spiral organ of ear for hearing, and semicircular canals, utricle, and saccule of ear for equilibrium

Page Ref: 475, 477

CHAPTER 15   Sensory, Motor, and Integrative Systems

MULTIPLE CHOICE. Choose the one alternative that best completes the statement or answers the question.

1) The degree of muscled stretch is monitored by:
   A) tendon organs.
   B) Merkel discs.
   C) joint kinesthetic receptors.
   D) muscle spindles.
   E) lamellated corpuscles.

   Answer: D
   Page Ref: 492

2) The function of tendon organs is to monitor the:
   A) change in angle at joints.
   B) degree of muscle stretch.
   C) force of muscle contraction.
   D) change in angle between tendon and muscle.
   E) heat generated by muscle contraction.

   Answer: C
   Page Ref: 493

3) A sensory neuron's receptive field is the:
   A) range of stimuli within a modality to which the neuron can respond.
   B) area of skin that is served by a particular sensory neuron.
   C) part of the neuron that is able to respond to the sensation.
   D) range of strengths of possible generator potentials for a particular neuron.
   E) all the different modalities to which a sensory neuron can respond.

   Answer: C
   Page Ref: 486

4) Light is an appropriate stimulus for:
   A) thermoreceptors.
   B) mechanoreceptors.
   C) chemoreceptors.
   D) photoreceptors.
   E) Both A and D are correct.

   Answer: D
   Page Ref: 488

5) The conscious awareness and interpretation of sensations is called:
   A) modality.
   B) transduction.
   C) reception.
   D) perception.
   E) conduction.

   Answer: D
   Page Ref: 485

6) Precise location and identification of specific sensations occurs in the:
   A) spinal cord.
   B) thalamus.
   C) brain stem.
   D) cerebral cortex.
   E) All of the above.

   Answer: D
   Page Ref: 485

7) One is generally unaware of changes in blood pressure because:
   A) there are no receptors that monitor such changes.
   B) the input never reaches the thalamus or cerebral cortex.
   C) changes in blood pressure do not involve the brain at all.
   D) the body only senses changes to its external environment.
   E) there are no lamellated corpuscles in blood vessels.

   Answer: B
   Page Ref: 485

8) **ALL** of the following are considered *general* senses **EXCEPT**:
   A) smell.
   B) vibration.
   C) pain.
   D) thermal sensations.
   E) joint and muscle position sense.

   Answer: A
   Page Ref: 486

9) Which of the following is **NOT** considered a *special* sense?

   A) smell

   B) vision

   C) pain

   D) taste

   E) equilibrium

Answer: C
Page Ref: 486

10) A stimulus that elicits a receptor potential causes:

   A) direct release of neurotransmitter via exocytosis from synaptic vesicles.

   B) conduction of a nerve impulse along a first–order sensory nerve fiber.

   C) initiation of an action potential in the receptor.

   D) a subthreshold generator potential.

   E) reuptake of neurotransmitter from the extracellular fluid.

Answer: A
Page Ref: 486

11) For a sensation to arise, which of the following occurs first?

   A) triggering of an action potential in a first–order neuron

   B) integration of input by the cerebral cortex

   C) stimulation of an interneuron

   D) exocytosis of neurotransmitter molecules from a receptor

   E) transduction of a stimulus to a graded potential by a receptor.

Answer: E
Page Ref: 486

12) A generator potential would be produced by **ALL** of the following **EXCEPT**:

   A) Pacinian corpuscles.

   B) Merkel discs.

   C) tendon organs.

   D) Meissner corpuscles.

   E) taste buds.

Answer: E
Page Ref: 486

13) Exteroreceptors include receptors for **ALL** of the following **EXCEPT**:
   A) vision.
   B) joint position.
   C) taste.
   D) smell.
   E) touch.

   Answer: B
   Page Ref: 488

14) **ALL** of the following are **TRUE** for pain receptors **EXCEPT**:
   A) pain receptors are called nociceptors.
   B) pain receptors are sensitive to all stimuli.
   C) pain receptors are free nerve endings.
   D) pain receptors are rapidly adapting receptors.
   E) pain receptors are found in almost all body tissues.

   Answer: D
   Page Ref: 491

15) **ALL** of the following would be sensed by mechanoreceptors **EXCEPT**:
   A) hearing.
   B) pressure.
   C) touch.
   D) equilibrium.
   E) light.

   Answer: E
   Page Ref: 488

16) Which of the following would be sensed by chemoreceptors?
   A) light
   B) hydrogen ion concentration in blood
   C) smell
   D) pain
   E) Both B and C are correct.

   Answer: E
   Page Ref: 488

17) During a maintained, constant stimulus, a generator potential or a receptor potential decreases in amplitude in a phenomenon known as:

A) adaptation.

B) transduction.

C) propagation.

D) perception.

E) integration.

Answer: A
Page Ref: 488

18) Tactile sensations other than itch and tickle are detected by:

A) free nerve endings.

B) encapsulated mechanoreceptors.

C) special senses.

D) encapsulated proprioceptors.

E) nociceptors.

Answer: B
Page Ref: 489

19) Receptors for discriminative touch that are located in the stratum basale of the epidermis are the:

A) Meissner corpuscles.

B) Pacinian corpuscles.

C) Ruffini corpuscles.

D) Merkel discs.

E) intrafusal muscle fibers.

Answer: D
Page Ref: 489

20) Receptors for pressure that are widely distributed in the subcutaneous tissue and the submucosal tissues are the:

A) Meissner corpuscles.

B) Pacinian corpuscles.

C) Ruffini corpuscles.

D) Merkel discs.

E) intrafusal muscle fibers.

Answer: B
Page Ref: 489

21) Cold receptors are located in the:
    A) subcutaneous layer.
    B) reticular layer of the dermis.
    C) stratum basale of the epidermis.
    D) dermal papillae.
    E) hair follicles.

Answer: C
Page Ref: 490

22) Intrafusal muscle fibers contract when stimulated by:
    A) alpha motor neurons.
    B) upper motor neurons.
    C) gamma motor neurons.
    D) third–order neurons.
    E) interneurons.

Answer: C
Page Ref: 492

23) The brain sets an overall level of muscle tone by adjusting:
    A) the angles at joints.
    B) the tension on a tendon.
    C) the amount of actin and myosin in muscle fibers.
    D) the conduction speed along type Ia sensory fibers.
    E) how vigorously a muscle spindle responds to stretching.

Answer: E
Page Ref: 492

24) The afferent part of stretch reflexes is provided by:
    A) muscle spindles.
    B) tendon organs.
    C) joint kinesthetic receptors.
    D) lamellated corpuscles.
    E) type II cutaneous mechanoreceptors.

Answer: A
Page Ref: 493

25) The dendrites of type Ib sensory fibers of tendon organs entwine around and among:

A) intrafusal muscle fibers.

B) extrafusal muscle fibers.

C) collagen fibers.

D) gamma motor neurons.

E) alpha motor neurons.

Answer: C
Page Ref: 493

26) **ALL** of the following are types of joint kinesthetic receptors **EXCEPT**:

A) Pacinian corpuscles.

B) Ruffini corpuscles.

C) "tendon organs" in ligaments.

D) free nerve endings.

E) intrafusal muscle fibers.

Answer: E
Page Ref: 494

27) Second-order neurons conduct nerve impulses from:

A) the PNS to the CNS.

B) the spinal cord to the brain stem.

C) the spinal cord and brain stem to the thalamus.

D) the thalamus to the postcentral gyrus of the cerebral cortex.

E) upper motor neurons to lower motor neurons.

Answer: C
Page Ref: 495

28) The primary somatosensory area of the cerebral cortex is located in the:

A) thalamus.

B) occipital lobe.

C) precentral gyrus.

D) postcentral gyrus.

E) hippocampus.

Answer: D
Page Ref: 495

29) Third–order sensory neurons in the posterior column–medial lemniscus pathway extend from the:

    A) skin to posterior root ganglia.

    B) posterior root ganglia to the posterior gray horn of the spinal cord.

    C) spinal cord to the medulla oblongata.

    D) medulla oblongata to the thalamus.

    E) thalamus to the somatosensory area of the cerebral cortex.

    Answer: E
    Page Ref: 495

30) Injury to lower motor neurons results in:

    A) kinesthesia.

    B) spastic paralysis.

    C) flaccid paralysis.

    D) coma.

    E) long–term potentiation.

    Answer: C
    Page Ref: 500

31) **ALL** of the following are indirect (extrapyramidal) motor tracts **EXCEPT** the:

    A) rubrospinal tract.

    B) tectospinal tract.

    C) vestibulospinal tract.

    D) corticobulbar tract.

    E) lateroreticulospinal tract.

    Answer: D
    Page Ref: 501

32) Long–term potentiation is a phenomenon that occurs in:

    A) formation of short–term memories.

    B) transition from NREM to REM sleep.

    C) conversion of short–term to long–term memory.

    D) destruction of neurons by the rubella virus.

    E) recovery of reflex activity following spinal shock.

    Answer: C
    Page Ref: 506

33) The cell bodies of first–order neurons in the posterior column–medial lemniscus pathway to the cortex are located in the:

A) posterior root ganglia of spinal nerves.

B) medulla.

C) medial lemniscus.

D) anterior gray horns of the spinal cord.

E) precentral gyrus.

Answer: A
Page Ref: 495

34) The medial lemniscus is a projection tract of second–order neurons extending from the:

A) posterior root ganglia to the medulla.

B) proprioceptors to the anterior gray horns of the spinal cord.

C) thalamus to the postcentral gyrus of the cerebral cortex.

D) upper motor neurons to the lower motor neurons.

E) medulla to the thalamus.

Answer: E
Page Ref: 495

35) The distinct quality that makes one sensation different from others is called its:

A) perception.

B) receptive field.

C) receptor potential.

D) generator potential.

E) modality.

Answer: E
Page Ref: 485

36) Conversion of a stimulus into a graded potential is called:

A) stimulation.

B) perception.

C) conduction.

D) transduction.

E) translation.

Answer: D
Page Ref: 486

37) First-order sensory neurons conduct impulses from:

A) the spinal cord to the brain stem.

B) the thalamus to the somatosensory cortex.

C) the CNS to an effector.

D) a receptor to the CNS.

E) one part of the spinal cord to another.

Answer: D
Page Ref: 486

38) The reason visceral pain is referred to surface structures is that:

A) there are no nociceptors in internal organs, so visceral sensory neurons must stimulate somatic sensory neurons to get a response.

B) Substance P is produced only in second–order sensory neurons that are used for both visceral and somatic sensations.

C) the affected organ has been removed, so the brain localizes the pain in the nearest remaining structure.

D) neurotransmitters released at the site of injury diffuse through the interstitial fluid to surface structures, triggering impulses there.

E) sensory neurons for both visceral pain and surface structures enter the same segment of the spinal cord, and surface sensations are better localized by the brain.

Answer: E
Page Ref: 491

39) Muscle spindles are located:

A) interspersed within skeletal muscle fibers.

B) at the junction of tendon and muscle.

C) at the junction of tendon and bone.

D) within the articular capsule.

E) in the cerebellum.

Answer: A
Page Ref: 492

40) Tendon organs are located:

A) interspersed within skeletal muscle fibers.

B) at the junction of tendon and muscle.

C) at the junction of tendon and bone.

D) within the articular capsule.

E) in the cerebellum.

Answer: B
Page Ref: 493

41) Joint kinesthetic receptors are located:

   A) interspersed within skeletal muscle fibers.

   B) at the junction of tendon and muscle.

   C) at the junction of tendon and bone.

   D) within the articular capsule.

   E) in the cerebellum.

   Answer: D
   Page Ref: 494

42) Cell bodies for upper motor neurons are located in the:

   A) precentral and postcentral gyri of the cerebral cortex.

   B) cerebellum.

   C) thalamus.

   D) anterior gray horns of the spinal cord.

   E) connective tissues surrounding skeletal muscles.

   Answer: A
   Page Ref: 499

43) Lower motor neurons whose cell bodies are in nuclei in the brain stem stimulate:

   A) upper motor neurons.

   B) interneurons.

   C) movements of the face and head.

   D) movements of limbs.

   E) parts of the cerebellum.

   Answer: C
   Page Ref: 500

44) The stage of deep sleep dominated by delta waves on an EEG, and during which events such as bed–wetting and sleepwalking occur is:

   A) REM sleep.

   B) Stage 1 NREM sleep.

   C) Stage 2 NREM sleep.

   D) Stage 3 NREM sleep.

   E) Stage 4 NREM sleep.

   Answer: E
   Page Ref: 505

45) The internal capsule of the cerebrum contains:

A) axons of upper motor neurons.

B) cell bodies of lower motor neurons.

C) axons of second–order sensory neurons.

D) axons of lower motor neurons.

E) cell bodies of first–order sensory neurons.

Answer: A
Page Ref: 499

46) Motor neurons that form the so–called *final common pathway* are the:

A) upper motor neurons.

B) interneurons.

C) lower motor neurons.

D) first–order neurons.

E) third order–neurons.

Answer: C
Page Ref: 499

47) Skilled movements of the limbs, hands and feet are controlled by motor neurons of the:

A) posterior columns.

B) anterior spinothalamic tract.

C) corticobulbar tract.

D) tectospinal tract.

E) lateral corticospinal tract.

Answer: E
Page Ref: 500

48) Axons passing through the cerebral peduncles and terminating in the nine pairs of cranial nerves in the pons and medulla belong to the:

A) posterior columns.

B) anterior spinothalamic tract.

C) corticobulbar tract.

D) tectospinal tract.

E) lateral corticospinal tract.

Answer: C
Page Ref: 500

49) Fred has a tumor that is interfering only with the lateral white columns of the spinal cord in his thoracic region. Which of the following is most likely to result?

A) flaccid paralysis of limbs, hands, and feet

B) spastic paralysis of limbs, hands, and feet

C) flaccid paralysis of facial muscles

D) spastic paralysis of facial muscles

E) loss of sensation in the extremities

Answer: A
Page Ref: 500

50) Monitoring intention for movement and sending out corrective signals to coordinate movement are important functions of:

A) the primary somatosensory area.

B) first–order neurons.

C) third–order neurons.

D) the thalamus.

E) the cerebellum.

Answer: E
Page Ref: 502

MATCHING. Choose the item in column 2 that best matches each item in column 1.

Choose the item from column 2 that best matches each item in column 1.

1) Column 1: conveys nerve impulses for sensations of discriminative touch, stereognosis, and conscious proprioception
Column 2: posterior column
Answer: posterior column
Page Ref: 498

2) Column 1: conveys nerve impulses for pain and thermal sensations
Column 2: lateral spinothalamic tract
Answer: lateral spinothalamic tract
Page Ref: 498

3) Column 1: conveys nerve impulses for itch, tickle, pressure, and crude touch sensations
Column 2: anterior spinothalamic tract
Answer: anterior spinothalamic tract
Page Ref: 498

4) Column 1: conveys nerve impulses for subconscious proprioception to allow coordination of skilled movements and maintenance of posture and balance

   Column 2: spinocerebellar tract

   Answer: spinocerebellar tract

   Page Ref: 498

5) Column 1: direct pathway that conveys motor impulses to muscles performing precise, voluntary movements of the limbs, hands, and feet

   Column 2: lateral corticospinal tract

   Answer: lateral corticospinal tract

   Page Ref: 501

6) Column 1: conveys motor impulses to muscles performing precise, voluntary movements of the head and neck

   Column 2: corticobulbar tract

   Answer: corticobulbar tract

   Page Ref: 501

7) Column 1: conveys motor impulses to muscles needed for maintaining balance in response to head movements

   Column 2: vestibulospinal tract

   Answer: vestibulospinal tract

   Page Ref: 501

8) Column 1: indirect pathway that conveys motor impulses to muscles involved in precise movements of the limbs, hands, and feet

   Column 2: rubrospinal tract

   Answer: rubrospinal tract

   Page Ref: 501

9) Column 1: indirect pathway that conveys motor impulses to muscles that move the head and eyes in response to visual stimuli

Column 2: tectospinal tract

Answer: tectospinal tract

Page Ref: 501

10) Column 1: conveys motor impulses to facilitate flexor reflexes and decrease muscle tone in muscles of the axial skeleton

Column 2: lateral reticulospinal tract

Answer: lateral reticulospinal tract

Page Ref: 501

MATCHING. Choose the item in column 2 that best matches each item in column 1.

Choose the item from column 2 that best matches each item in column 1.

1) Column 1: type I cutaneous mechanoreceptors (Merkel discs)

Column 2: discriminative touch

Answer: discriminative touch

Page Ref: 489

2) Column 1: type II cutaneous mechanoreceptors (Ruffini corpuscles)

Column 2: heavy, continuous touch

Answer: heavy, continuous touch

Page Ref: 489

3) Column 1: lamellated (Pacinian) corpuscles

Column 2: pressure and high-frequency vibration

Answer: pressure and high-frequency vibration

Page Ref: 489

4) Column 1: thermoreceptors

Column 2: warm and cold stimuli

Answer: warm and cold stimuli

Page Ref: 488

5) Column 1: nociceptors

   Column 2: pain

   Answer: pain

   Page Ref: 488

6) Column 1: muscle spindles

   Column 2: rate and degree of change in
   muscle length

   Answer: rate and degree of change in muscle length

   Page Ref: 492

7) Column 1: tendon organs

   Column 2: force of muscle contraction

   Answer: force of muscle contraction

   Page Ref: 493

8) Column 1: joint kinesthetic receptors

   Column 2: acceleration and deceleration
   of joint movement

   Answer: acceleration and deceleration of joint movement

   Page Ref: 494

9) Column 1: photoreceptors

   Column 2: light

   Answer: light

   Page Ref: 488

10) Column 1: chemoreceptors

    Column 2: smell and taste stimuli

    Answer: smell and taste stimuli

    Page Ref: 488

TRUE/FALSE. Write 'T' if the statement is true and 'F' if the statement is false.

1) Information concerning body position and equilibrium is transmitted by interoreceptors.

   Answer: FALSE
   Page Ref: 488

2) Tactile sensations and pain sensations are examples of modalities categorized as special senses.

   Answer: FALSE
   Page Ref: 486

3) Pain receptors are called nociceptors.

Answer: TRUE
Page Ref: 491

4) Sensory neurons that propagate impulses from the PNS into the CNS are called first-order neurons.

Answer: TRUE
Page Ref: 486

5) Kinesthesia is the perception of body movements.

Answer: TRUE
Page Ref: 492

6) Nociceptors are rapidly adapting receptors.

Answer: FALSE
Page Ref: 491

7) Joint kinesthetic receptors are located at the junction of a tendon with a muscle.

Answer: FALSE
Page Ref: 494

8) Pain sensations in an amputated limb are called referred pain.

Answer: FALSE
Page Ref: 491

9) Cell bodies of first-order neurons conveying sensations of conscious proprioception are located in the posterior root ganglia of spinal nerves.

Answer: TRUE
Page Ref: 495

10) Cell bodies of direct pathway upper motor neurons are located in the precentral and postcentral gyri of the cerebral cortex.

Answer: TRUE
Page Ref: 499

11) Destruction of certain basal ganglia connections results in abnormal muscle rigidity.

Answer: TRUE
Page Ref: 502

12) The corticobulbar and corticospinal tracts are somatic sensory pathways.

Answer: FALSE
Page Ref: 500

13) As a person ages, the average amount of time spent sleeping increases.

Answer: FALSE
Page Ref: 505

14) Awakening from sleep is a major role of the cerebellum.

Answer: FALSE
Page Ref: 502

15) Most dreaming occurs during REM sleep.

Answer: TRUE
Page Ref: 505

SHORT ANSWER. Write the word or phrase that best completes each statement or answers the question.

1) A sense organ transduces a stimulus into a _____.
Answer: graded potential
Page Ref: 486

2) The portion of a receptor that is capable of responding to stimulation is called the _____.

Answer: receptive field
Page Ref: 486

3) Receptors of discriminative touch located in the dermal papillae of hairless skin are called _____.

Answer: corpuscles of touch (Meissner corpuscles)
Page Ref: 489

4) The perception of body movements is called _____.
Answer: kinesthesia
Page Ref: 492

5) Long-term potentiation is a phenomenon believed to occur in a region of the cerebrum known as the _____.
Answer: hippocampus
Page Ref: 506

6) The special cells that make up a muscle spindle are called _____.
Answer: intrafusal muscle fibers
Page Ref: 492

7) The ability to recognize by "feel" the size, shape, and texture of an object is called _____.
Answer: stereognosis
Page Ref: 495

8) _____ is the conscious or unconscious awareness of external or internal stimuli.
Answer: Sensation
Page Ref: 485

9) Each specific type of sensation is called a sensory _____.
Answer: modality
Page Ref: 485

10) Muscle tone is regulated by the brain as it adjusts the level of sensitivity of receptors called _____ to the degree of muscle stretching.
Answer: muscle spindles
Page Ref: 492

11) Receptors that provide information concerning body position and movement are classified as _____.
Answer: proprioceptors
Page Ref: 488

12) _____ initiate reflexes that cause muscle relaxation to decrease muscle tension before damage occurs.
Answer: Tendon organs
Page Ref: 493

13) The proprioceptors present in and around the articular capsules of synovial joints are called _____.
Answer: joint kinesthetic receptors
Page Ref: 494

14) A decrease in sensitivity to a long-term stimulus is called _____.
Answer: adaptation
Page Ref: 488

15) _____ neurons conduct impulses from the spinal cord and brain stem to the thalamus.
Answer: Second-order
Page Ref: 495

16) A projection tract of sensory neurons that extends from the medulla to the thalamus is the
_____.

Answer: medial lemniscus

Page Ref: 495

17) Visceral pain that is perceived as localized in the skin served by the same segment of the
spinal cord is called _____.

Answer: referred pain

Page Ref: 491

18) The axons of first–order neurons transmitting impulses of conscious proprioception form the
spinal tracts known as the _____.

Answer: posterior columns

Page Ref: 495

19) Axons of second–order neurons in the anterolateral pathways synapse with third–order
neurons in the _____.

Answer: thalamus

Page Ref: 495

20) The region of the cerebral cortex that provides the major control for initiation of voluntary
movements is the _____.

Answer: primary motor area (precentral gyrus)

Page Ref: 499

21) _____ are the only neurons that carry information from the CNS to skeletal muscle
fibers.

Answer: Lower motor neurons

Page Ref: 499

22) Most upper motor neurons _____ (or cross over) to the contralateral side of the medulla.

Answer: decussate

Page Ref: 499

23) Skilled movements of the limbs, hands, and feet are controlled by motor neurons of the
_____ tracts.

Answer: lateral corticospinal

Page Ref: 500

24) Awakening from sleep involves increased activity in fibers known as the _____ that
project from the brain stem through the thalamus to the cerebral cortex.

Answer: reticular activating system

Page Ref: 503

25) Damage to lower motor neurons produces _____ paralysis of muscles on the same side of the body.

Answer: flaccid

Page Ref: 500

26) The medical term for jerky, uncoordinated movements is _____.

Answer: ataxia

Page Ref: 508

27) Most upper motor neurons synapse with _____, which then synapse with lower motor neurons.

Answer: interneurons

Page Ref: 499

28) The _____ of the cerebrum help program habitual or automatic movement sequences, such as swinging the arms while walking.

Answer: basal ganglia

Page Ref: 502

29) Output from the basal ganglia comes mainly from the region known as the _____.

Answer: globus pallidus

Page Ref: 502

30) Delta waves on an EEG are characteristic of stage _____ of NREM sleep.

Answer: four

Page Ref: 505

ESSAY. Write your answer in the space provided or on a separate sheet of paper.

1) You are sitting on a sunny Florida beach during spring break among thousands of other students. Identify the modalities of the many sensations you perceive while on this beach. What types of receptors allow you to perceive these sensations?

Answer: Thermoreceptors sense the warmth of the sun of the skin. Chemoreceptors sense the smells of the ocean and sunscreen, etc. Various mechanoreceptors sense the sounds of the ocean and crowd and the feel of the sand against the skin. Photoreceptors sense the light of the sun. Nociceptors sense the pain of the sunburn.

Page Ref: 485–494

2) While walking along a Florida beach as the sun is setting, you see a flash of fireworks off to your left. You turn to look and, in doing so, step on a piece of broken seashell in the sand. You begin hopping on one foot and remarking on the pain. Identify and describe the major somatic sensory and motor pathways involved in this scenario.

Answer: The tectospinal tracts mediate the head–turning in response to the visual stimulus of the fireworks. Flexor and extensor reflexes are mediated by the lateral and medial reticulospinal tracts. Pain is transmitted via the lateral spinothalamic tract. Input for balance and coordination involve the spinocerebellar and posterior column tracts.

Page Ref: 498; 501

3) A paramedic team arrives on the scene of an accident in which a man is found with his foot twisted and crushed beneath his overturned car. Subsequently, the man's lower leg and foot must be amputated. Weeks after the amputation, the man continues to feel extreme pain in his foot, even though it is no longer there. What is this phenomenon called, and why is it occurring?

Answer: This is phantom limb sensation. In one explanation, the cerebral cortex is interpreting impulses arising in the proximal portions of the severed sensory neurons that previously carried impulses from the foot as coming from the nonexistent extremity. Another explanation suggests that neuron networks in the brain that were involved in sensations from the limb before the amputation continue to generate sensations after the amputation.

Page Ref: 491

4) Describe the possible relationships between sensory receptors and first–order sensory neurons.

Answer: Receptors for general senses could be free or encapsulated nerve endings of first–order sensory neurons in which stimuli elicit generator potentials. Receptors for the special senses consist of separate cells in which stimuli elicit receptor potentials that trigger exocytosis of neurotransmitter that diffuses across a synapse to initiate nerve impulses in a first–order neuron.

Page Ref: 487

5) Compare short–term memory vs. long–term memory with regard to specific changes that are thought to occur in the brain.

Answer: Short–term memory may depend on forming new synapses and reverberating circuits. Long–term memory is thought to involve high–frequency stimulation within the hippocampus at glutamate synapses. Nitric oxide and other neurotransmitters may be involved. Neurons develop new presynaptic terminals, larger synaptic end bulbs, and more dendritic branches. Enhanced facilitation occurs. DNA and RNA are possibly involved.

Page Ref: 505–506

6) Describe the role of the reticular activating system in sleep, arousal, and consciousness.

Answer: A variety of sensory stimuli feed into the RAS, which feeds into the thalamus and cerebral cortex to increase neuronal activity, causing arousal from sleep and maintaining consciousness. During periods of high ATP use, adenosine accumulates and binds to A1 receptors, inhibiting cholinergic neurons in the RAS, and inducing sleep.

Page Ref: 503–504

7) You are sitting on a sunny Florida beach. Describe the anatomical structures that must be present and the physiological events that must occur in order for you to perceive the warmth of the sun.

Answer: Thermoreceptors must be present to sense the thermal stimuli. The stimulus must occur within the receptor's receptive field. The stimuli are transduced into graded potentials that eventually reach threshold to trigger nerve impulses in a first–order neuron, which transmits the information to the CNS via the neurons of the spinothalamic tract. The primary somatosensory area then must interpret the information provided by these neurons.

Page Ref: 486; 495

8) Two children were born in England who lacked nociceptors. What effects would this have on the lives of these children? Explain your answer.

Answer: Lack of pain sensations would require careful monitoring by parents and the children themselves for tissue damage (or the potential thereof...). The question might be expanded to include speculation about the social/behavioral effects of this condition.

Page Ref: 491

9) A well-known musician suffered nearly complete destruction of the hippocampus due to a viral infection. Predict the effects of this damage. Explain your answer.

Answer: Students should describe the role of the hippocampus on conversion of short–term to long–term memory. The patient would be unable to form new memories. The question could be expanded to include the potential social/behavioral consequences of this condition.

Page Ref: 447

10) A patient is exhibiting tremors of the hands while sitting still. Propose where the neurological problem might be. Explain your answer.

Answer: The most likely answer would involve damage to the basal ganglia, particularly those portions involved in inhibition of unnecessary movements. Other answers may be acceptable.

Page Ref: 502

CHAPTER 16   The Special Sense

MULTIPLE CHOICE. Choose the one alternative that best completes the statement or answers the question.

1) In the process of forming an image on the retina, convergence occurs to allow:
   A) a change in shape of the lens.
   B) three dimensional image formation.
   C) refraction of light rays.
   D) focusing of light through the center of the lens.
   E) production of new photoreceptors.

   Answer: B
   Page Ref: 525

2) New olfactory receptors are produced by reproduction of:
   A) olfactory hairs.
   B) gustatory hairs.
   C) basal stem cells.
   D) supporting cells.
   E) filiform papillae.

   Answer: C
   Page Ref: 512

3) The sites of olfactory transduction are the olfactory hairs, which are:
   A) cilia projecting from the dendrites of first–order neurons.
   B) microvilli on the axons of first–order neurons.
   C) columnar epithelial cells in the nasal mucosa.
   D) mucus–producing cells in the nasal epithelium.
   E) projection tracts between the thalamus and the temporal lobe.

   Answer: A
   Page Ref: 512

4) The retina is held in place by the:
   A) optic disc.
   B) vitreous body.
   C) ciliary muscle.
   D) bipolar neurons.
   E) iris.

   Answer: B
   Page Ref: 523

5) Photoreceptors are located in the:
   A) choroid.
   B) cornea.
   C) iris.
   D) retina.
   E) Both C and D are correct.

   Answer: D
   Page Ref: 521

6) Strong odors may stimulate tear production by the lacrimal glands due to stimulation of cranial nerve:
   A) I.
   B) II.
   C) V.
   D) VII.
   E) X.

   Answer: D
   Page Ref: 513

7) G proteins activated by binding of odorant molecules to olfactory receptors cause:
   A) exocytosis of neurotransmitter.
   B) activation of adenylate cyclase.
   C) influx of calcium ions.
   D) bending of olfactory hairs.
   E) hyperpolarization of olfactory neurons.

   Answer: B
   Page Ref: 513

8) The auditory (Eustachian) tube connects the:
   A) middle ear and inner ear.
   B) external ear and middle ear.
   C) middle ear and nasopharynx.
   D) cochlea and vestibule.
   E) inner ear and primary auditory area of the cerebrum.

   Answer: C
   Page Ref: 532

9) The ossicles are the major structures of the:

    A) external ear.

    B) middle ear.

    C) vestibule.

    D) cochlea.

    E) auditory regions of the cerebrum.

Answer: B
Page Ref: 532

10) The primary function of the utricle and saccule is to:

    A) transduce sound waves into generator potentials.

    B) monitor static equilibrium.

    C) monitor dynamic equilibrium.

    D) cause movements of the ossicles.

    E) produce endolymph in the cochlea.

Answer: B
Page Ref: 538

11) The receptors in the utricle and saccule are stimulated when:

    A) endolymph flows over the spiral organ.

    B) the otoliths bend stereocilia in response to gravity.

    C) the tympanic membrane vibrates.

    D) perilymph bends hair cells.

    E) the stapes pushes into the oval window.

Answer: B
Page Ref: 541

12) First-order olfactory neurons synapse with second-order neurons in the:

    A) olfactory epithelium.

    B) cribriform plate.

    C) olfactory tract.

    D) temporal lobe.

    E) olfactory bulbs.

Answer: E
Page Ref: 514

13) The threshold is the lowest for which of the primary tastes?
   A) sweet.
   B) sour.
   C) salty.
   D) bitter.
   E) All taste receptors have equal thresholds.

   Answer: D
   Page Ref: 515

14) In order for a substance to be tasted, it must be:
   A) a partially denatured protein.
   B) of a pH below 7.
   C) an ionic compound.
   D) dissolved in saliva.
   E) Both C and D are correct.

   Answer: D
   Page Ref: 514

15) The receptors on the tip of the tongue are most sensitive to:
   A) sweet.
   B) sour.
   C) salty.
   D) bitter.
   E) None of these; there are no taste buds at the tip of the tongue.

   Answer: A
   Page Ref: 515

16) The primary gustatory area of the cerebrum is in the:
   A) parietal lobe.
   B) frontal lobe.
   C) temporal lobe.
   D) occipital lobe.
   E) midbrain.

   Answer: A
   Page Ref: 516

17) The lacrimal apparatus produces:

   A) sweat.

   B) sebum.

   C) aqueous humor.

   D) tears.

   E) Both C and D are correct.

   Answer: D
   Page Ref: 517

18) Which of the following is **NOT** one of the extrinsic muscles that move the eyeball?

   A) medial rectus

   B) inferior oblique.

   C) lateral rectus.

   D) superior rectus.

   E) levator palpebrae superioris.

   Answer: E
   Page Ref: 517

19) Olfactory sensations reach the brain via:

   A) cranial nerve I.

   B) cranial nerve II.

   C) cranial nerve VII.

   D) cranial nerve VIII.

   E) spinal nerves C1.

   Answer: A
   Page Ref: 514

20) Most impulses related to gustatory sensations arising on the tongue are conveyed to the brain via:

   A) cranial nerve I.

   B) cranial nerve II.

   C) cranial nerve VII.

   D) cranial nerve VIII.

   E) spinal nerves C1.

   Answer: C
   Page Ref: 516

21) The fibrous tunic of the eyeball includes the:

A) tarsal plate and conjunctiva.

B) choroid and ciliary body.

C) choroid and sclera.

D) conjunctiva and sclera.

E) cornea and sclera.

Answer: E
Page Ref: 517

22) "Bloodshot eyes" are the result of dilation of blood vessels in the:

A) lens.

B) cornea.

C) sclera.

D) conjunctiva.

E) iris.

Answer: D
Page Ref: 517

23) The curved, avascular, transparent, fibrous coat covering the iris is the:

A) cornea.

B) sclera.

C) lens.

D) uvea.

E) pupil.

Answer: A
Page Ref: 517

24) The function of the ciliary processes is to:

A) alter the shape of the lens.

B) prevent objects from falling into the eye.

C) produce aqueous humor.

D) change the diameter of the pupil.

E) transduce light stimuli into nerve impulses.

Answer: C
Page Ref: 519

25) Parasympathetic neurons stimulate:

A) isomerization of retinal.

B) bipolar neurons in the retina.

C) production of new proteins in the lens.

D) constriction of the pupil.

E) dilation of the pupil.

Answer: D
Page Ref: 520

26) The only place in the body where blood vessels can be viewed directly is the:

A) conjunctiva.

B) anterior surface of the retina.

C) choroid.

D) tympanic membrane.

E) cornea.

Answer: B
Page Ref: 520

27) The central fovea is a small depression in the center of the:

A) macula lutea of the retina.

B) optic disc of the retina.

C) lens.

D) cornea.

E) vitreous body.

Answer: A
Page Ref: 521

28) The blind spot of the retina is so–called because:

A) only cones are found there.

B) only rods are found there.

C) there are no rods or cones there.

D) it is impossible for light rays to be focused on that spot.

E) inhibitory neurotransmitters are released from the receptors there.

Answer: C
Page Ref: 521

29) The lens is held in place by the:

A) choroid.

B) iris.

C) ciliary processes.

D) vitreous body.

E) suspensory ligaments.

Answer: E
Page Ref: 522

30) Which of the following occurs when dim light stimulates the eye?
A) Parasympathetic fibers stimulate contraction of the circular muscles of the iris to decrease pupil diameter.
B) Parasympathetic fibers stimulate contraction of the circular muscles of the iris to increase pupil diameter.
C) Sympathetic fibers stimulate contraction of the circular muscles of the iris to decrease pupil diameter.
D) Sympathetic fibers stimulate contraction of the radial muscles of the iris to decrease pupil diameter.
E) Sympathetic fibers stimulate contraction of the radial muscles of the iris to increase pupil diameter.

Answer: E
Page Ref: 520

31) Intraocular pressure is produced mainly by:

A) aqueous humor.

B) vitreous humor.

C) constriction of the pupil.

D) lacrimal secretions.

E) photopigments.

Answer: A
Page Ref: 522

32) The spaces anterior to the lens are filled with:

A) aqueous humor.

B) vitreous humor.

C) photoreceptors.

D) lacrimal gland secretions.

E) air.

Answer: A
Page Ref: 522

33) **ALL** of the following are **TRUE** regarding photoreceptors of the eye **EXCEPT:**

A) there are more cones than rods in the retina.

B) rods contain the photopigment rhodopsin.

C) cones respond best to bright light.

D) rods respond best to dim light.

E) there are no photoreceptors in the optic disc.

Answer: A
Page Ref: 520

34) The central fovea is:

A) where the optic nerve exits the back of the eye.

B) the area of highest visual acuity on the retina.

C) what secretes aqueous humor.

D) where the retinal artery branches.

E) where new photopigments are produced.

Answer: B
Page Ref: 521

35) The optic nerve is made up of the:

A) axons of the rods and cones.

B) axons of the bipolar cells.

C) axons of the ganglion cells.

D) dendrites of the bipolar cells.

E) dendrites of the ganglion cells.

Answer: C
Page Ref: 528

36) Nutrients are provided to the posterior surface of the retina by blood vessels in the darkly pigmented portion of the vascular tunic known as the:

A) choroid.

B) ciliary body.

C) iris.

D) sclera.

E) macula lutea.

Answer: A
Page Ref: 519

37) A scratch on the cornea most directly interferes with:
    A) accommodation.
    B) refraction.
    C) constriction of the pupil.
    D) convergence.
    E) transduction.

Answer: B
Page Ref: 523

38) For sharpest visual acuity, light rays must be refracted so that they:
    A) change wavelength to fall within the visible range.
    B) stimulate constriction of the pupil.
    C) turn photopigments in the lens into their colorless form.
    D) hit the melanin in the choroid.
    E) fall directly on the central fovea.

Answer: E
Page Ref: 524

39) Which of the following occurs when trying to focus on a close object?
    A) relaxation of the ciliary muscle to flatten the lens
    B) relaxation of the ciliary muscle to make the lens more convex
    C) contraction of the ciliary muscle to flatten the lens
    D) contraction of the ciliary muscle to make the lens more convex
    E) contraction of the ciliary muscle to increase the diameter of the pupil

Answer: D
Page Ref: 524

40) The middle ear is normally filled with:
    A) air.
    B) blood.
    C) endolymph.
    D) perilymph.
    E) cerumen.

Answer: A
Page Ref: 532

41) Which of the following lists the route of impulse transmission in the correct order?

   A) photoreceptors, ganglion cells, bipolar cells, optic nerve, optic chiasm, optic tract

   B) bipolar cells, ganglion cells, photoreceptors, optic nerve, optic tract, optic chiasm

   C) photoreceptors, bipolar cells, ganglion cells, optic nerve, optic tract, optic chiasm

   D) photoreceptors, bipolar cells, ganglion cells, optic nerve, optic chiasm, optic tract

   E) bipolar cells, ganglion cells, photoreceptors, optic nerve, optic chiasm, optic tract

   Answer: D
   Page Ref: 528

42) The characteristic shared by photopigments in rods and cones is that they all:

   A) contain the same opsin molecule.

   B) respond to the same wavelengths of light.

   C) contain retinal as the light–absorbing molecule.

   D) Both A and C are correct.

   E) A, B, and C are all correct.

   Answer: C
   Page Ref: 526

43) The neurotransmitter in rods is:

   A) acetylcholine.

   B) substance P.

   C) glutamate.

   D) dopamine.

   E) epinephrine.

   Answer: C
   Page Ref: 527

44) The role of the stapedius muscle is to:

   A) stabilize the tympanic membrane.

   B) connect the ossicles to the cochlea.

   C) flex the hair cells of the spiral organ.

   D) constrict the Eustachian tube.

   E) limit vibration of the stapes.

   Answer: E
   Page Ref: 532

45) Receptor potentials are produced when:

    A) the tympanic membrane moves the malleus.

    B) the stapes pushes into the oval window.

    C) perilymph moves in the scala vestibuli.

    D) stereocilia bend against the tectorial membrane.

    E) all of these generate receptor potentials.

Answer: D
Page Ref: 535

46) The function of *tip link* proteins in the stereocilia of the hair cells of the spiral organ is to:

    A) produce neurotransmitter molecules.

    B) open transduction channels.

    C) hold the hair cells into the tectorial membrane.

    D) link the tectorial and basilar membranes together.

    E) stimulate second-order neurons.

Answer: B
Page Ref: 535

47) First-order sensory neurons of the cochlear branch of the vestibulocochlear nerve terminate in the:

    A) thalamus.

    B) occipital lobe.

    C) basilar membrane.

    D) medulla oblongata.

    E) vestibular branch.

Answer: D
Page Ref: 535

48) What happens at the optic chiasm?

    A) Rods stimulate bipolar cells.

    B) The optic nerve exits the eye.

    C) Visual input is perceived.

    D) The optic nerves cross.

    E) Aqueous humor is reabsorbed.

Answer: D
Page Ref: 529

49) Presence of too much aqueous humor within the eye is dangerous because it:
    A) alters the refractive abilities of the eye by making the lens swell.
    B) put pressure on neurons in the retina, damaging them.
    C) causes blockage of the pupil.
    D) stimulates reabsorption of the vitreous body.
    E) pries the retina away from the back of the eye.

Answer: B
Page Ref: 542

50) Which of the following occurs in the hypermetropic eye?
    A) Light rays converge on the central fovea.
    B) Light rays converge in front of the central fovea.
    C) Light rays converge behind the central fovea.
    D) Intraocular pressure builds to damage neurons.
    E) The lens becomes cloudy.

Answer: C
Page Ref: 524

MATCHING. Choose the item in column 2 that best matches each item in column 1.

Choose the item from column 2 that best matches each item in column 1.

1) Column 1: tube within the temporal bone
          leading from the auricle to the
          eardrum
   Column 2: external auditory canal

   Answer: external auditory canal
   Page Ref: 531

2) Column 1: separates external auditory
          canal from the middle ear
   Column 2: tympanic membrane

   Answer: tympanic membrane
   Page Ref: 531

3) Column 1: ossicle attached to the
          internal surface of the
          eardrum
   Column 2: malleus

   Answer: malleus
   Page Ref: 532

4) Column 1: ossicle that fits into the oval
   window
   Column 2: stapes

   Answer: stapes

   Page Ref: 532

5) Column 1: tube that connects the middle
   ear with the nasopharynx
   Column 2: auditory tube

   Answer: auditory tube

   Page Ref: 532

6) Column 1: fluid that fills the bony
   labyrinth
   Column 2: perilymph

   Answer: perilymph

   Page Ref: 533

7) Column 1: fluid that fills the
   membranous labyrinth
   Column 2: endolymph

   Answer: endolymph

   Page Ref: 533

8) Column 1: contains the utricle and the
   saccule
   Column 2: vestibule

   Answer: vestibule

   Page Ref: 533

9) Column 1: contains the receptors for
   hearing
   Column 2: spiral organ

   Answer: spiral organ

   Page Ref: 534

10) Column 1: structure pulled by gravity
    over hair cells involved in
    static equilibrium
    Column 2: otolithic membrane

    Answer: otolithic membrane

    Page Ref: 541

MATCHING. Choose the item in column 2 that best matches each item in column 1.

Choose the item from column 2 that best matches each item in column 1.

1) Column 1: avascular, transparent part of
        fibrous tunic
   Column 2: cornea
        Foil: conjunctiva
   Answer: cornea
   Page Ref: 517

2) Column 1: the "white" of the eye
   Column 2: sclera
   Answer: sclera
   Page Ref: 517

3) Column 1: transparent, avascular protein
        structure that fine–tunes
        focusing of light rays
   Column 2: lens
   Answer: lens
   Page Ref: 522

4) Column 1: circular and radial muscles
        that help regulate the amount
        of light entering the posterior
        cavity
   Column 2: iris
   Answer: iris
   Page Ref: 519

5) Column 1: produces aqueous humor and
        alters the shape of the lens
   Column 2: ciliary body
   Answer: ciliary body
   Page Ref: 519

6) Column 1: jellylike substance in posterior
        cavity that helps hold retina
        flush against the eyeball
   Column 2: vitreous body
        Foil: aqueous humor
   Answer: vitreous body
   Page Ref: 523

7) Column 1: highly vascular, darkly
            pigmented portion of uvea
   Column 2: choroid

   Answer: choroid
   Page Ref: 519

8) Column 1: photoreceptors for vision in
            dim light
   Column 2: rods

   Answer: rods
   Page Ref: 520

9) Column 1: photoreceptors for color vision
            in bright light
   Column 2: cones

   Answer: cones
   Page Ref: 520

10) Column 1: the hole through which light
            passes to reach the lens,
            posterior cavity, and retina
    Column 2: pupil
        Foil: optic disc

    Answer: pupil
    Page Ref: 520

TRUE/FALSE. Write 'T' if the statement is true and 'F' if the statement is false.

1) The olfactory epithelium covers the inferior surface of the cribriform plate, the superior nasal conchae, and part of the middle nasal conchae.

   Answer: TRUE
   Page Ref: 512

2) A chemical must be dissolved in saliva to be tasted.

   Answer: TRUE
   Page Ref: 515

3) Axons of the olfactory tract terminate in the occipital lobe of the cerebrum.

   Answer: FALSE
   Page Ref: 514

4) The conjunctiva covers the cornea.

Answer: FALSE
Page Ref: 517

5) Olfactory receptors are rapidly adapting.

Answer: TRUE
Page Ref: 514

6) The ciliary muscle controls the diameter of the pupil.

Answer: FALSE
Page Ref: 519

7) The optic disc is the area of the retina with the greatest visual acuity.

Answer: FALSE
Page Ref: 521

8) Light must pass through the ganglion and bipolar cell layers of the retina before reaching the photoreceptor layer.

Answer: TRUE
Page Ref: 520

9) There are many more rods than cones in the retina.

Answer: TRUE
Page Ref: 520

10) The vitreous body is continually being produced and reabsorbed.

Answer: FALSE
Page Ref: 523

11) Cones have a higher threshold than rods.

Answer: TRUE
Page Ref: 520

12) The lens is highly vascular.

Answer: FALSE
Page Ref: 522

13) The malleus is attached to the internal surface of the tympanic membrane.

Answer: TRUE
Page Ref: 532

14) The basilar membrane separates the middle ear from the inner ear.

Answer: FALSE
Page Ref: 534

15) The utricle and saccule contain the receptors for static equilibrium.

Answer: TRUE
Page Ref: 538

SHORT ANSWER. Write the word or phrase that best completes each statement or answers the question.

1) New olfactory receptors are produced by the division of cells within the olfactory epithelium called _____.

Answer: basal stem cells
Page Ref: 512

2) The _____ have the primary role in maintenance of dynamic equilibrium.

Answer: semicircular ducts
Page Ref: 541

3) Axons of cranial nerve I terminate in paired masses of gray matter inferior to the frontal lobes of the cerebrum known as the _____.

Answer: olfactory bulbs
Page Ref: 514

4) The receptors for gustatory sensations are located in gustatory receptors known as _____.

Answer: taste buds
Page Ref: 514

5) The four primary tastes are _____ , _____ , _____ , and _____.

Answer: sweet; sour; salty; bitter
Page Ref: 515

6) The anatomical name for the eyelids is the _____.

Answer: palpebrae
Page Ref: 516

7) The shape of the lens is altered for near or far vision by the _____.

Answer: ciliary muscle
Page Ref: 519

8) The hole in the center of the iris is the _____.

Answer: pupil

Page Ref: 520

9) Photoreceptors called _____ are most important for seeing shades of gray in dim light, while _____ provide color vision in bright light.

Answer: rods; cones

Page Ref: 520

10) The mucous membrane lining the eyelids and covering part of the anterior surface of the eyeball is the _____.

Answer: conjunctiva

Page Ref: 517

11) The dense connective tissue making up the white part of the fibrous tunic is called the _____.

Answer: sclera

Page Ref: 517

12) The highly vascularized layer of the uvea that lines most of the internal surface of the sclera is the _____.

Answer: choroid

Page Ref: 519

13) Aqueous humor is secreted by blood capillaries located in the _____ of the vascular tunic.

Answer: ciliary processes

Page Ref: 519

14) In dim light, _____ neurons stimulate _____ muscles of the iris to contract, causing a(n) _____ in the diameter of the pupil.

Answer: sympathetic; radial; increase

Page Ref: 520

15) The jellylike substance filling the posterior cavity of the eye is the _____.

Answer: vitreous body

Page Ref: 523

16) Bending of light rays as they pass through different media is called _____.

Answer: refraction

Page Ref: 523

17) The site on the retina where the optic nerve exits the eyeball is the _____.

Answer: optic disc

Page Ref: 520

18) Reflection and scattering of light rays within the eyeball is prevented by the absorption of stray light rays by _____ in the choroid and pigment epithelium of the retina.

Answer: melanin

Page Ref: 520

19) Aqueous humor drains from the anterior chamber back into the blood via the _____.

Answer: scleral venous sinus (canal of Schlemm)

Page Ref: 522

20) The photopigment in rods is _____.

Answer: rhodopsin

Page Ref: 526

21) The first point of refraction as light passes into the eye is the _____.

Answer: cornea

Page Ref: 523

22) The external auditory canal and the middle ear are separated by the _____.

Answer: tympanic membrane

Page Ref: 531

23) The auditory ossicles are the _____ , the _____ , and the _____.

Answer: malleus; incus; stapes

Page Ref: 532

24) A refraction abnormality in which either the cornea or the lens has an irregular curvature is called _____.

Answer: astigmatism

Page Ref: 525

25) The light-absorbing portion of all visual photopigments is _____ , which is derived from vitamin _____.

Answer: retinal; A

Page Ref: 526

26) The membranous labyrinth of the vestibule consists of two sacs called the _____ and the _____.

Answer: utricle; saccule

Page Ref: 533

27) The conversion of *cis*-retinal to *trans*-retinal as it absorbs a photon of light is called _____.

Answer: isomerization

Page Ref: 526

28) The complete separation of *trans*-retinal from opsin is called _____.

Answer: bleaching

Page Ref: 527

29) The ligand in the outer segments of photoreceptor cells that holds ligand-gated sodium ion channels open in darkness to depolarize the membrane is _____.

Answer: cyclic GMP

Page Ref: 527

30) Specialized glands in the external auditory canal that secrete earwax are the _____.

Answer: ceruminous glands

Page Ref: 531

31) The fluid contained in the membranous labyrinth of the ear is called _____.

Answer: endolymph

Page Ref: 533

32) The organ of Corti is housed within the part of the inner ear called the _____.

Answer: cochlea

Page Ref: 534

33) The organ of Corti rests of the _____ , which separates the cochlear duct from the scala tympani.

Answer: basilar membrane

Page Ref: 534

34) Movement of hair cells of the spiral organ against the tectorial membrane causes bending of _____ , which produces receptor potentials that lead to generation of nerve impulses in cochlear nerve fibers.

Answer: stereocilia.

Page Ref: 535

35) The foot of the stapes fits into the _____.

Answer: oval window

Page Ref: 532

ESSAY. Write your answer in the space provided or on a separate sheet of paper.

1) You are at a restaurant with your 45–year–old friend, who has never worn glasses. As she is looking at the menu, you notice she is slowly moving the menu further away until her arm is completely outstretched. What is your friend's most likely vision problem? Explain the anatomical and physiological changes that have caused this problem to develop.

Answer: Your friend most likely has presbyopia, in which near–point accommodation has increased due to age–related loss of elasticity of the lens. Because the lens can't accommodate and refract light properly, the image does not fall in the appropriate spot on the retina.

Page Ref: 524

2) Describe the process of image formation on the retina.

Answer: 1) Refraction—bending of light as medium changes to focus light into central fovea
2) Accommodation of lens for near/distance vision —shape of lens changed by ciliary muscle to make light focus on retina
3) Constriction of pupil —ANS reflex to prevent scattering of light through edges of lens
4) Convergence of eyes—to focus both eyes on same object and provide binocular (3D) vision

Images are focused on the retina upside–down and mirror–image, and the brain then translates this information.

Page Ref: 523–525

3) Explain the process by which smell sensations are sensed and perceived.

Answer: Odorant molecules dissolve in mucus secreted by the olfactory epithelium and bind to receptors, triggering a generator potential. In some cases the binding activates a G protein in the plasma membrane that activates adenylate cyclase that opens sodium ion channels. Axons of the receptors (first–order neurons) transmit impulses via cranial nerve I through the olfactory foramina of the cribriform plate and terminate in the olfactory bulbs, where they synapse with second–order neurons. These axons form the olfactory tracts, which transmit impulses to the olfactory area in the temporal lobe. Other important brain areas include the limbic system, the hypothalamus, and the orbitofrontal area.

Page Ref: 513–514

4) Luis was in an automobile accident in which he suffered a severely broken nose when his head hit the dashboard. Now, months later, he says he has lost all his enthusiasm for food because "it doesn't have much taste." What has probably happened to Luis' sense of taste? Explain your answer.

Answer: Possibly as his nose was broken and pushed back into his face, axons of the olfactory nerves were damaged. Without being able to perceive the odor along with the taste of food, the perception of taste is altered and limited to the four basic tastes sensed by the taste buds.

Page Ref: 514

5) Describe the anatomical features that provide protection to the delicate neural portion of the retina and that ensure the retina is kept flat against the back of the eye.

Answer: The bony orbit provides protection to most of the eye. The sclera makes the eyeball rigid and, by its toughness, prevents foreign objects from entering the eye. Aqueous fluid creates intraocular pressure to support the eye from inside, and the vitreous body holds the retina flush against the back of the eye.

Page Ref: 517–520

6) Differentiate between static and dynamic equilibrium. Describe the structures and physiological mechanisms involved in receiving and transducing vestibular sensations.

Answer: Static equilibrium is the maintenance of body position relative to gravity. Hair cells in the maculae of the utricle and saccule bend as the otolithic membrane slides forward due to gravity. Receptor potentials are transmitted to cranial nerve VIII to the pons. Dynamic equilibrium is the maintenance of body position in response to movement. Endolymph flowing over hair cells in the cristae of semicircular ducts causes bending. Receptor potentials are passed to cranial nerve VIII to the pons.

Page Ref: 538–541

7) Blindness can occur for many reasons. Using your knowledge of the structure of the eye and the processing of light stimuli, predict where some of the potential trouble spots might be. Explain your answers.

Answer: Examples could include: loss of transparency of the cornea or lens (light can't pass); detachment of the retina (loss of photoreceptive and conductive function); no photoreceptors or pigments (no transduction); damage to the optic nerve (no conduction); damage to the visual pathway or visual cortex (no conduction or translation).

Page Ref: 517–529

8) Deafness can occur for many reasons. Using your knowledge of the structure of the ear and the processing of sound stimuli, predict where some of the potential trouble spots might be. Explain your answers.

Answer: Examples could include: blockage of the external auditory meatus (sound doesn't reach eardrum); hole in eardrum (incomplete vibrations); fusion of ossicles or paralysis of associated muscles (no transmission to inner ear); damage to hair cells of spiral organ (no receptors); damage to cranial nerve VIII (no conduction); brain damage in auditory areas (no translation).

Page Ref: 529–538

9) Your mother always told you to "eat your carrots" because they were "good for your eyes."
   Why was your mother right?

   Answer: Carrots contain carotenoids from which vitamin A derivatives can be made.
   Retinal—a vitamin A derivative—is the light–absorbing part of all visual
   photopigments. The isomerization of retinal in light is the first step in the chemical
   reaction that triggers the receptor potentials in photoreceptors.

   Page Ref: 526

10) Why does chronic exposure to loud sounds lead to deafness?

    Answer: Sound waves of loud sounds have a greater amplitude (intensity) than softer sounds.
    As these sound waves are translated into waves in the fluids of the inner ear, hair cells
    are destroyed by the extreme vibrations. The hair cells are not replaced, and sensitivity
    to the particular frequency (pitch) sensed by those hair cells is lost forever.

    Page Ref: 534

CHAPTER 17   The Autonomic Nervous System

MULTIPLE CHOICE. Choose the one alternative that best completes the statement or answers the question.

1) In the autonomic nervous system, all preganglionic fibers release the neurotransmitter:

   A) acetylcholine.

   B) norepinephrine.

   C) serotonin.

   D) dopamine.

   E) epinephrine.

   Answer: A
   Page Ref: 556

2) In the autonomic nervous system, most sympathetic postganglionic fibers release the neurotransmitter:

   A) acetylcholine.

   B) norepinephrine.

   C) serotonin.

   D) dopamine.

   E) glutamate.

   Answer: B
   Page Ref: 557

3) Terminal ganglia are where:

   A) the cell bodies for sympathetic preganglionic fibers are located.

   B) parasympathetic preganglionic fibers synapse with parasympathetic postganglionic fibers.

   C) the cell bodies of sensory neurons are located.

   D) sympathetic preganglionic fibers synapse with sympathetic postganglionic fibers.

   E) sympathetic preganglionic fibers synapse with parasympathetic postganglionic fibers.

   Answer: B
   Page Ref: 553

4) Most autonomic sensory neurons are associated with:
   A) exteroreceptors.
   B) interoreceptors.
   C) proprioceptors.
   D) special senses.
   E) somatic efferent neurons.

   Answer: B
   Page Ref: 548

5) To say that most organs served by the **ANS** have "dual innervation" means that:
   A) these organs release either acetylcholine or norepinephrine when stimulated.
   B) it takes two postganglionic neurons to achieve the desired response.
   C) the organs are innervated by both sympathetic and parasympathetic neurons.
   D) the organs have both alpha and beta receptors.
   E) both a preganglionic and postganglionic neuron go to the organ.

   Answer: C
   Page Ref: 549

6) An adrenergic neuron produces the neurotransmitter:
   A) serotonin.
   B) GABA.
   C) norepinephrine.
   D) acetylcholine.
   E) glycine.

   Answer: C
   Page Ref: 557

7) Which of the following is an example of an effector for a visceral efferent neuron?
   A) quadriceps femoris
   B) diaphragm
   C) extrinsic eye muscles
   D) smooth muscle in the wall of the small intestine
   E) All of the above are correct except the quadriceps femoris.

   Answer: D
   Page Ref: 549

8) A small–diameter, myelinated type B neuron that terminates in an autonomic ganglion is a(n):

A) autonomic sensory neuron.

B) preganglionic neuron.

C) postganglionic neuron.

D) somatic motor neuron.

E) adrenergic neuron.

Answer: B
Page Ref: 550

9) A small–diameter unmyelinated type C neuron that terminates in a visceral effector is a(n):

A) autonomic sensory neuron.

B) preganglionic neuron.

C) postganglionic neuron.

D) white ramus.

E) splanchnic nerve.

Answer: C
Page Ref: 550

10) Which of the following statements is **TRUE** regarding the autonomic nervous system?

A) Its sensory input includes impulses from interoreceptors.

B) Its preganglionic fibers release acetylcholine or norepinephrine.

C) Its postganglionic fibers release only acetylcholine.

D) Its effectors include some skeletal muscles.

E) The sympathetic division is the "energy conservation–restoration" system.

Answer: A
Page Ref: 548

11) The lateral gray horns of the thoracic spinal cord is the location of:

A) splanchnic nerves.

B) sympathetic chains.

C) synapses between preganglionic and postganglionic neurons.

D) cell bodies of some sympathetic preganglionic neurons.

E) cell bodies of some parasympathetic neurons.

Answer: D
Page Ref: 550

12) The term *craniosacral outflow* refers to:

A) release of acetylcholine from preganglionic neurons.

B) axons of parasympathetic postganglionic neurons.

C) axons of sympathetic postganglionic neurons.

D) axons of parasympathetic preganglionic neurons.

E) axons of sympathetic preganglionic neurons.

Answer: D
Page Ref: 552

13) Cell bodies of preganglionic neurons of the parasympathetic division are located in the nuclei of **ALL** of the following cranial nerves **EXCEPT**:

A) III.

B) V.

C) VII.

D) IX.

E) X.

Answer: B
Page Ref: 555

14) In which of the following would synapses between sympathetic preganglionic and postganglionic fibers occur?

A) ciliary ganglion

B) superior mesenteric ganglion

C) celiac ganglion

D) otic ganglion

E) Both B and C are correct.

Answer: E
Page Ref: 555

15) In which of the following would synapses between parasympathetic preganglionic and postganglionic fibers occur?

A) ciliary ganglion

B) superior mesenteric ganglion

C) celiac ganglion

D) otic ganglion

E) Both A and D are correct.

Answer: E
Page Ref: 555

16) Postganglionic axons from sympathetic trunk ganglia provide innervation to **ALL** of the following **EXCEPT** the:

A) heart.

B) parotid salivary glands.

C) spleen.

D) nasal mucosa.

E) smooth muscle in the eye.

Answer: C
Page Ref: 552

17) Sympathetic chains are:

A) preganglionic fibers that pass through sympathetic trunk ganglia and extend to prevertebral ganglia.

B) connections between sympathetic and parasympathetic ganglia.

C) fibers extending from sympathetic trunk ganglia to effectors.

D) the autonomic part of a spinal nerve.

E) axon collaterals of sympathetic fibers extending between sympathetic trunk ganglia.

Answer: E
Page Ref: 555

18) Which of the following responses is initiated by the sympathetic nervous system?

A) decreased heart rate

B) constriction of pupils

C) splitting glycogen to glucose by the liver

D) constriction of the bronchioles

E) decreased blood pressure

Answer: C
Page Ref: 560

19) Which of the following pairs of ganglia receive sympathetic preganglionic fibers?

A) vertebral chain and terminal ganglia

B) collateral and intramural ganglia

C) terminal and dorsal root ganglia

D) paravertebral and prevertebral ganglia

E) ciliary and otic ganglia

Answer: D
Page Ref: 552

20) The sympathetic ganglia that lie close to large abdominal arteries are the:

   A) prevertebral ganglia.

   B) paravertebral ganglia.

   C) terminal ganglia.

   D) sympathetic trunk ganglia.

   E) dorsal root ganglia.

   Answer: A
   Page Ref: 553

21) Sympathetic preganglionic fibers that pass through sympathetic trunk ganglia to synapse in prevertebral ganglia are called:

   A) white rami communicantes.

   B) gray rami communicantes.

   C) splanchnic nerves.

   D) sympathetic chains.

   E) anterior roots.

   Answer: C
   Page Ref: 555

22) Which of the following is a sympathetic ganglion?

   A) middle cervical ganglion

   B) ciliary ganglion

   C) otic ganglion

   D) submandibular ganglion

   E) pterygopalatine ganglion

   Answer: A
   Page Ref: 552

23) The superior mesenteric ganglion is the termination point for the:

   A) vagus nerve.

   B) greater splanchnic nerve.

   C) lesser splanchnic nerve.

   D) lowest splanchnic nerve.

   E) lumbar splanchnic nerve.

   Answer: C
   Page Ref: 555

24) The renal plexus is the termination point for the:

    A) vagus nerve.

    B) greater splanchnic nerve.

    C) lesser splanchnic nerve.

    D) lowest splanchnic nerve.

    E) lumbar splanchnic nerve.

    Answer: D
    Page Ref: 555

25) The inferior mesenteric ganglion is the termination point for the:

    A) vagus nerve.

    B) greater splanchnic nerve.

    C) lesser splanchnic nerve.

    D) lowest splanchnic nerve.

    E) lumbar splanchnic nerve.

    Answer: E
    Page Ref: 555

26) Sympathetic stimulation to the heart is provided by fibers from the:

    A) hypogastric ganglion.

    B) celiac ganglion.

    C) inferior cervical ganglion.

    D) pterygopalatine ganglion.

    E) submandibular ganglion.

    Answer: C
    Page Ref: 554

27) The structure containing sympathetic postganglionic fibers that connect sympathetic trunk ganglia to spinal nerves is the:

    A) sympathetic chain.

    B) anterior root.

    C) posterior root.

    D) white ramus communicans.

    E) gray ramus communicans.

    Answer: E
    Page Ref: 554

28) The solar plexus is another name for the:

    A) superior cervical ganglion.

    B) junction of sympathetic preganglionic fibers and the adrenal medulla.

    C) celiac ganglion.

    D) ciliary ganglion.

    E) junction of the vagus nerve with thoracic visceral effectors.

Answer: C
Page Ref: 553

29) The great splanchnic nerve terminates in the:

    A) celiac ganglion.

    B) superior mesenteric ganglion.

    C) inferior mesenteric ganglion.

    D) adrenal medulla.

    E) lumbar plexus.

Answer: A
Page Ref: 555

30) The ciliary ganglia are located:

    A) just inferior to each foramen ovale.

    B) near the ducts of the submandibular salivary glands.

    C) in the ciliary body of the uvea.

    D) lateral to the optic nerves near the posterior aspect of the orbit.

    E) lateral to the optic chiasm.

Answer: D
Page Ref: 555

31) The otic ganglia are located:

    A) just inferior to each foramen ovale.

    B) near the ducts of the submandibular salivary glands.

    C) in the ciliary body of the uvea.

    D) lateral to the optic nerves near the posterior aspect of the orbit.

    E) lateral to the optic chiasm.

Answer: A
Page Ref: 555

32) Parasympathetic stimulation to the nasal mucosa, pharynx, and lacrimal glands is provided by fibers arising from the:

   A) superior cervical ganglion.

   B) middle cervical ganglion.

   C) inferior cervical ganglion.

   D) pterygopalatine ganglion.

   E) submandibular ganglion.

Answer: D
Page Ref: 555

33) Parasympathetic preganglionic fibers traveling with cranial nerve III terminate in the:

   A) superior cervical ganglion.

   B) inferior cervical ganglion.

   C) ciliary ganglia.

   D) otic ganglia.

   E) submandibular ganglia.

Answer: C
Page Ref: 555

34) Parasympathetic stimulation to the liver, stomach, and gallbladder is provided by fibers traveling with the:

   A) vagus nerve.

   B) greater splanchnic nerve.

   C) less splanchnic nerve.

   D) white rami communicantes.

   E) gray rami communicantes.

Answer: A
Page Ref: 556

35) A major organ that receives sympathetic stimulation, but not parasympathetic stimulation is the:

   A) heart.

   B) liver.

   C) stomach.

   D) lung.

   E) kidney.

Answer: E
Page Ref: 560

36) The pelvic splanchnic nerves supply:
   A) parasympathetic stimulation to smooth muscle in the urinary bladder and reproductive organs.
   B) sympathetic stimulation to smooth muscle in the urinary bladder and reproductive organs.
   C) sympathetic preganglionic fibers to the renal plexus.
   D) sympathetic stimulation to the kidney.
   E) parasympathetic stimulation to the liver and pancreas.

Answer: A
Page Ref: 556

37) Acetylcholine exerts its effects on postsynaptic cells when it:
   A) is broken down by enzymes in the synaptic cleft, and the end-products diffuse into the postsynaptic cell.
   B) binds to specific receptors on the postsynaptic cell membrane and changes the permeability of the membrane to particular ions.
   C) diffuses into the postsynaptic cell and changes the pH of the intracellular fluid.
   D) actively transports ions from the synaptic cleft into the postsynaptic cell.
   E) blocks specific receptors to which other neurotransmitters could attach.

Answer: B
Page Ref: 556

38) Norepinephrine and epinephrine enter the bloodstream when sympathetic stimulation is provided to the:
   A) adrenal medulla.
   B) liver.
   C) brain.
   D) heart.
   E) kidneys.

Answer: A
Page Ref: 560

39) Because the principal active ingredient in tobacco is nicotine, you might expect smoking to enhance the effects of:
   A) acetylcholine of parasympathetic visceral effectors.
   B) acetylcholine on any postganglionic neurons.
   C) norepinephrine on the heart and blood vessels.
   D) norepinephrine on the limbic system.
   E) norepinephrine on most sympathetic visceral effectors.

Answer: B
Page Ref: 556

40) Cholinergic sympathetic postganglionic neurons stimulate the:

   A) adrenal medulla.

   B) basal ganglia.

   C) sweat glands.

   D) heart.

   E) walls of the gastrointestinal tract.

   Answer: C
   Page Ref: 556

41) Loss of control over bladder and bowel functions in situations involving so–called paradoxical fear is due to:

   A) the fight–or–flight response.

   B) failure of the sympathetic nervous system to respond.

   C) failure of the parasympathetic nervous system to respond.

   D) inability to produce adequate amounts of acetylcholine to maintain muscle tone.

   E) massive activation on the parasympathetic nervous system.

   Answer: E
   Page Ref: 561

42) You have just discovered that your pants were unzipped the entire time you gave a speech to your class. Which of the following responses would you most likely experience?

   A) increased parasympathetic stimulation to the iris

   B) increased parasympathetic stimulation to the stomach

   C) increased sympathetic stimulation to the heart

   D) decreased sympathetic stimulation to the bronchioles

   E) decreased sympathetic stimulation to the small intestine

   Answer: C
   Page Ref: 560

43) The lumbar region of the spinal cord is the location of cell bodies of:

   A) parasympathetic preganglionic fibers.

   B) parasympathetic postganglionic fibers.

   C) sympathetic preganglionic fibers.

   D) sympathetic postganglionic fibers.

   E) Both A and C are correct.

   Answer: C
   Page Ref: 550

44) Which of the following are found in the celiac ganglion?

   A) cell bodies of sympathetic preganglionic fibers.

   B) cell bodies of sympathetic postganglionic fibers.

   C) cell bodies of parasympathetic preganglionic fibers.

   D) cell bodies of parasympathetic postganglionic fibers.

   E) Both B and D are correct.

   Answer: B
   Page Ref: 555

45) You are just about to perform a clinical procedure for the first time and your palms begin to sweat. This is due to:

   A) increased sympathetic stimulation of sweat glands possessing alpha receptors.

   B) increased sympathetic stimulation of sweat glands possessing beta receptors.

   C) increased parasympathetic stimulation of sweat glands possessing nicotinic receptors.

   D) increased parasympathetic stimulation of sweat glands possessing muscarinic receptors.

   E) increased sympathetic stimulation of sweat glands possessing muscarinic receptors.

   Answer: A
   Page Ref: 560

46) Increased sympathetic stimulation increases the secretion of **ALL** of the following **EXCEPT**:

   A) glucagon.

   B) renin.

   C) epinephrine.

   D) insulin.

   E) norepinephrine.

   Answer: D
   Page Ref: 560

47) Fibers of the ANS traveling with cranial nerve X will stimulate which of the following responses?

   A) increased activity from salivary glands

   B) increased heart rate

   C) increased activity of sweat glands on the palms and soles

   D) decreased force of contraction of cardiac muscle

   E) dilation of blood vessels in the skeletal muscle of the torso

   Answer: D
   Page Ref: 560

48) Which of the following is stimulated by the parasympathetic nervous system?
   A) dilation of the bronchioles
   B) erection of the penis
   C) increased gluconeogenesis
   D) dilation of the pupil
   E) increased secretion by sweat glands in the palms and soles

   Answer: B
   Page Ref: 561

49) Which of the following are found in the otic ganglia?
   A) cell bodies of sympathetic preganglionic fibers.
   B) cell bodies of sympathetic postganglionic fibers.
   C) cell bodies of parasympathetic preganglionic fibers.
   D) cell bodies of parasympathetic postganglionic fibers.
   E) Both B and D are correct.

   Answer: D
   Page Ref: 555

50) The greater splanchnic nerve stimulates postganglionic fibers that provide:
   A) sympathetic stimulation to the liver and spleen.
   B) sympathetic stimulation to the urinary bladder and reproductive organs.
   C) parasympathetic stimulation to the liver and spleen.
   D) parasympathetic stimulation to the urinary bladder and reproductive organs.
   E) sympathetic stimulation to the adrenal medulla.

   Answer: A
   Page Ref: 555

MATCHING. Choose the item in column 2 that best matches each item in column 1.

Choose the item from column 2 that best matches each item in column 1.

1) Column 1: a prevertebral ganglion
             located just inferior to the
             diaphragm that receives the
             greater splanchnic nerve
   Column 2: celiac ganglion

   Answer: celiac ganglion
   Page Ref: 555

2) Column 1: a prevertebral ganglion located in the upper abdomen that receives the lesser splanchnic nerve

Column 2: superior mesenteric ganglion

Answer: superior mesenteric ganglion

Page Ref: 555

3) Column 1: one of the sympathetic trunk ganglia; postganglionic fibers leaving here serve the head

Column 2: superior cervical ganglion

Answer: superior cervical ganglion

Page Ref: 554

4) Column 1: one of the sympathetic trunk ganglia; postganglionic fibers leaving here serve the heart

Column 2: inferior cervical ganglion

Answer: inferior cervical ganglion

Page Ref: 554

5) Column 1: parasympathetic ganglion providing innervation to smooth muscle in the eyeball

Column 2: ciliary ganglion

Answer: ciliary ganglion

Page Ref: 555

6) Column 1: parasympathetic ganglion providing innervation to the pharynx and lacrimal glands

Column 2: pterygopalatine ganglion

Answer: pterygopalatine ganglion

Page Ref: 555

7) Column 1: parasympathetic ganglion receiving preganglionic fibers from cranial nerve VII

Column 2: submandibular ganglion

Answer: submandibular ganglion

Page Ref: 555

8) Column 1: parasympathetic ganglion receiving preganglionic fibers from cranial nerve IX and innervating the parotid glands

Column 2: otic ganglion

Answer: otic ganglion

Page Ref: 555

9) Column 1: one of a group of axons of the parasympathetic sacral outflow

Column 2: pelvic splanchnic nerve

Answer: pelvic splanchnic nerve

Page Ref: 555

10) Column 1: a prevertebral ganglion that receives the lower splanchnic nerve

Column 2: inferior mesenteric ganglion

Answer: inferior mesenteric ganglion

Page Ref: 555

MATCHING. Choose the item in column 2 that best matches each item in column 1.

Choose the item from column 2 that best matches each item in column 1.

1) Column 1: origin of sympathetic postganglionic fibers that innervate the heart

Column 2: middle cervical ganglion

Answer: middle cervical ganglion

Page Ref: 554

2) Column 1: contains axons of parasympathetic preganglionic fibers

Column 2: vagus nerve

Answer: vagus nerve

Page Ref: 555

3) Column 1: contain postganglionic fibers connecting ganglia of sympathetic trunk to spinal nerves

Column 2: gray rami communicantes

Answer: gray rami communicantes

Page Ref: 553

4) Column 1: receive sympathetic preganglionic fibers; located along either side of vertebral column

Column 2: sympathetic trunk ganglia

Answer: sympathetic trunk ganglia

Page Ref: 552

5) Column 1: receive sympathetic preganglionic fibers; located close to large abdominal arteries

Column 2: prevertebral ganglia

Answer: prevertebral ganglia

Page Ref: 553

6) Column 1: receive parasympathetic preganglionic fibers; located close to or within walls of visceral organs

Column 2: terminal ganglia

Answer: terminal ganglia

Page Ref: 553

7) Column 1: contain preganglionic fibers connecting anterior rami of spinal nerves with sympathetic trunk ganglia

Column 2: white rami communicantes

Answer: white rami communicantes

Page Ref: 553

8) Column 1: axon collaterals of
   preganglionic fibers along
   which sympathetic trunk
   ganglia are strung

   Column 2: sympathetic chains

   Answer: sympathetic chains

   Page Ref: 555

9) Column 1: site of synapses between
   splanchnic nerves of the
   thoracic region and
   postganglionic cell bodies

   Column 2: celiac ganglion

   Answer: celiac ganglion

   Page Ref: 553

10) Column 1: sympathetic preganglionic
    fibers that pass through
    sympathetic trunk ganglia
    and extend to prevertebral
    ganglia

    Column 2: splanchnic nerves

    Answer: splanchnic nerves

    Page Ref: 555

TRUE/FALSE. Write 'T' if the statement is true and 'F' if the statement is false.

1) The hypothalamus is an important regulator of ANS activity.

   Answer: TRUE
   Page Ref: 548

2) Most autonomic sensory neurons are associated with proprioceptors.

   Answer: FALSE
   Page Ref: 548

3) The cell bodies of some sympathetic preganglionic neurons are located in the brain stem.

   Answer: FALSE
   Page Ref: 550

4) Axons of preganglionic neurons are myelinated, but axons of postganglionic neurons are
   unmyelinated.

   Answer: FALSE
   Page Ref: 550

5) Prevertebral ganglia receive parasympathetic preganglionic fibers.

Answer: FALSE
Page Ref: 553

6) Terminal ganglia receive parasympathetic preganglionic fibers.

Answer: TRUE
Page Ref: 553

7) Sympathetic ganglia are the sites of synapses between sympathetic preganglionic and postganglionic neurons.

Answer: TRUE
Page Ref: 555

8) Axons of parasympathetic preganglionic neurons synapse with 20 or more postganglionic neurons.

Answer: FALSE
Page Ref: 553

9) Cholinergic neurons release norepinephrine and epinephrine.

Answer: FALSE
Page Ref: 556

10) All preganglionic neurons release the neurotransmitter acetylcholine.

Answer: TRUE
Page Ref: 556

11) Splanchnic nerves extend from prevertebral ganglia to their effectors.

Answer: FALSE
Page Ref: 555

12) All postganglionic neurons have nicotinic receptors.

Answer: TRUE
Page Ref: 556

13) Nicotinic receptors bind epinephrine.

Answer: FALSE
Page Ref: 556

14) Norepinephrine stimulates alpha receptors more strongly than beta receptors.

Answer: TRUE
Page Ref: 558

15) In the fight–or–flight response, the liver decreases its rate of glycogenolysis and lipolysis.

Answer: FALSE
Page Ref: 559

SHORT ANSWER. Write the word or phrase that best completes each statement or answers the question.

1) Effector tissues for autonomic motor neurons are _____ , _____ , and _____ .
Answer: cardiac muscle; smooth muscle; glands
Page Ref: 549

2) An autonomic motor neuron that extends from an autonomic ganglion to a visceral effector is called a(n) _____ neuron.
Answer: postganglionic
Page Ref: 550

3) An autonomic motor neuron that extends from the CNS to an autonomic ganglion is called a(n) _____ neuron.
Answer: preganglionic
Page Ref: 550

4) Stimulation of the posterolateral regions of the hypothalamus would result in a(n) _____ in blood pressure because this region controls the _____ division of the ANS.
Answer: increase; sympathetic
Page Ref: 562

5) Stimulation of the anteromedial regions of the hypothalamus would result in a(n) _____ in secretion and motility of the gastrointestinal tract because this region controls the _____ division of the ANS.
Answer: increase; parasympathetic
Page Ref: 562

6) The main integrating centers for autonomic reflexes are the spinal cord, the brain stem, and the _____ .
Answer: hypothalamus
Page Ref: 562

7) Secretion of saliva and gastric juice is increased by the _____ division of the ANS.
Answer: parasympathetic
Page Ref: 561

8) Ejaculation of semen is an effect of the _____ division of the ANS.

Answer: sympathetic

Page Ref: 561

9) Autonomic motor nerves innervating the arterioles of the kidney belong to the _____ division of the ANS.

Answer: sympathetic

Page Ref: 561

10) Sympathetic preganglionic fibers that connect the anterior ramus of a spinal nerve with sympathetic trunk ganglia are collectively called the _____.

Answer: white rami communicantes

Page Ref: 553

11) The effector for sympathetic postganglionic fibers leaving the middle and inferior cervical ganglia is the _____.

Answer: heart

Page Ref: 554

12) Secretion of insulin from the pancreas is increased by stimulation from the _____ division of the ANS.

Answer: parasympathetic

Page Ref: 560

13) Alpha and beta receptors are the receptors for the neurotransmitter _____.

Answer: epinephrine (and norepinephrine)

Page Ref: 558

14) Atropine is a drug that blocks _____ receptors.

Answer: muscarinic

Page Ref: 559

15) Monoamine oxidase inactivates _____.

Answer: epinephrine (and norepinephrine)

Page Ref: 558

16) Activation of β_3 receptors causes _____.

Answer: thermogenesis

Page Ref: 558

17) Parasympathetic cranial outflow has five components: four pairs of ganglia and the plexuses associated with the _____ nerve.

Answer: vagus

Page Ref: 555

18) Activation of the sympathetic division of the ANS also results in the release of hormones from the modified postganglionic cells of the _____.

Answer: adrenal medulla

Page Ref: 560

19) Cholinergic neurons release the neurotransmitter _____.

Answer: acetylcholine

Page Ref: 556

20) _____ acetylcholine receptors are present on the sarcolemma of skeletal muscle fibers.

Answer: Nicotinic

Page Ref: 558

21) Adrenergic neurons release the neurotransmitters _____ and _____.

Answer: epinephrine; norepinephrine

Page Ref: 557

22) _____ receptors for acetylcholine are present on both sympathetic and parasympathetic postganglionic neurons.

Answer: Nicotinic

Page Ref: 556

23) _____ receptors for acetylcholine are present on all effectors innervated by parasympathetic postganglionic neurons.

Answer: Muscarinic

Page Ref: 556

24) Adrenergic receptors on blood vessels serving the heart are classified as _____.

Answer: β_2

Page Ref: 558

25) Binding of epinephrine to beta receptors on cardiac muscle fibers causes _____.

Answer: increase in rate and force of contraction

Page Ref: 558

26) Binding of epinephrine to beta receptors on the juxtaglomerular cells of the kidneys results in secretion of _____.

Answer: renin

Page Ref: 558

27) The four cranial nerves that carry cranial parasympathetic outflow are the _____, the _____, the _____, and the _____.

Answer: vagus (X); oculomotor (III); facial (VII); glossopharyngeal (IX)

Page Ref: 555

28) Binding of epinephrine to beta receptors on hepatocytes results in _____.

Answer: (increased) glycogenolysis

Page Ref: 558

29) Parasympathetic postganglionic fibers extend to salivary glands from the _____ ganglia and the _____ ganglia.

Answer: submandibular; otic

Page Ref: 555

30) The greater splanchnic nerve enters the _____ ganglion.

Answer: celiac

Page Ref: 555

ESSAY. Write your answer in the space provided or on a separate sheet of paper.

1) Explain why the sympathetic division of the ANS has more widespread and longer-lasting effects than the parasympathetic division.

Answer: A single sympathetic preganglionic neuron synapses with 20 or more postganglionic neurons vs. about five for parasympathetic. The sympathetic neurotransmitters are broken down more slowly than acetylcholine, so postganglionic cells are stimulated longer. The sympathetic division also stimulates release of catecholamines from the adrenal medulla, thus enhancing the sympathetic effects via the endocrine system. Many more visceral effectors have receptors for catecholamines than for acetylcholine.

Page Ref: 559–560

2) Describe the possible ways in which sympathetic preganglionic neurons may connect with postganglionic neurons.

Answer: The axon may 1) synapse with postganglionic neurons in the first ganglion it reaches, 2) ascend or descend to higher or lower ganglia via sympathetic chains, or 3) continue without synapsing through sympathetic trunk ganglia to prevertebral ganglia via splanchnic nerves.

Page Ref: 553–554

3) Colette was so frightened by her ride on the new roller coaster at the amusement park that she discovered at the end of the ride that she had wet her pants. Explain the physiology behind this embarrassing occurrence.

Answer: This is an example of "paradoxical fear" resulting from massive activation of the parasympathetic division of the ANS. This increases parasympathetic tone in the urinary bladder and causes loss of control over urination.

Page Ref: 561

4) An autonomic neuron releases the neurotransmitter acetylcholine. What can you tell about this neuron's role in the ANS? What possible characteristics can be determined about the postsynaptic cell? Explain your answers.

Answer: The neuron could be a preganglionic neuron in either division of the ANS, a parasympathetic postganglionic neuron, or one of a few sympathetic postganglionic neurons. The postsynaptic cell must possess either nicotinic or muscarinic receptors in order to respond to acetylcholine. This effector cell could be either a postganglionic neuron of either division, a parasympathetic visceral effector, or one of the few sympathetic effectors stimulated by cholinergic neurons.

Page Ref: 556–557

5) A postsynaptic cell has beta receptors on its membrane. Assuming that these beta receptors bind an ANS neurotransmitter, what are the possible general characteristics and/or activities of the postsynaptic cell? Explain your answer.

Answer: Possession of beta receptors indicates responsiveness to norepinephrine or epinephrine. The cell must be an effector in the sympathetic ANS, since these neurotransmitters are released only by sympathetic postganglionic neurons. The cell could be part of most any visceral effector, and whether the cell is excited or inhibited depends on the specific type of beta receptor and the cell that possesses it.

Page Ref: 558

6) Explain how the ANS regulates blood flow during times of fight–or–flight vs. times of rest/repose.

Answer: The sympathetic ANS serves arterioles and veins in all areas. Increased vasoconstriction or vasodilation occurs with greater sympathetic stimulation depending on the type of receptor present on the smooth muscle cells of the vessel walls. In general, vasodilation occurs in those vessels serving the heart and those skeletal muscles crucial to fight or flight. Vasoconstriction occurs in those vessels serving areas less vital to fighting/fleeing —e.g., in skin, digestive organs, and the urinary system. Most vessels do not have parasympathetic innervation.

Page Ref: 561

7) What are splanchnic nerves?

Answer: Sympathetic splanchnic nerves are those that pass through sympathetic trunk ganglia of the abdominopelvic region to extend to and terminate in prevertebral ganglia. The parasympathetic division includes pelvic splanchnic nerves, which are the collective preganglionic outflow from the sacral region.

Page Ref: 555

8) Knowing that nicotine in tobacco products binds to nicotinic receptors, what effects would you expect to see in people who use tobacco products? Why?

Answer: One might expect an increase in responses from cells with nicotinic receptors. Nicotine mimics the action of acetylcholine on these receptors. All postganglionic ANS neurons and skeletal muscle fibers have nicotinic receptors, so an increase in muscle tone and ANS activity might be expected.

Page Ref: 556

9) Blood pressure is regulated by an autonomic reflex. What does this mean? What structures and responses are involved?

Answer: An autonomic reflex is an automatic and generally involuntary response to changes in the internal environment. The receptor (an interoreceptor) sends sensory information to the CNS. Most ANS reflexes, including regulation of blood pressure, are integrated in the hypothalamus or brain stem. Two motor neurons (preganglionic and postganglionic) would convey nerve impulses to the effectors, which include the heart (adjustment of rate and force of contraction) and blood vessels (adjust diameter).

Page Ref: 562

10) Predict the effects of a drug called "an MAO inhibitor." Explain your answer.

Answer: An MAO inhibitor inhibits the enzyme monoamine oxidase, which breaks down epinephrine and norepinephrine. If the enzyme is inhibited, then these neurotransmitters accumulate, thus enhancing the effects of most of the sympathetic ANS.

Page Ref: 558

CHAPTER 18   The Endocrine System

MULTIPLE CHOICE. Choose the one alternative that best completes the statement or answers the question.

1) Hormones secreted from the posterior pituitary gland are synthesized by the:
   A) anterior pituitary gland.
   B) thyroid gland.
   C) posterior pituitary gland.
   D) hypothalamus.
   E) pineal gland.

   Answer: D
   Page Ref: 578

2) Increasing the uptake of iodide by the thyroid gland and increasing the growth of the thyroid gland are two functions of:
   A) TRH.
   B) TSH.
   C) T_3.
   D) thyroglobulin.
   E) thyroid binding globulin.

   Answer: B
   Page Ref: 581

3) The main target for ADH is the:
   A) kidney.
   B) hypothalamus.
   C) uterus.
   D) adrenal cortex.
   E) posterior pituitary.

   Answer: A
   Page Ref: 579

4) The thyroid gland is located:

   A) under the sternum.

   B) behind and beneath the stomach.

   C) in the sella turcica of the sphenoid bone.

   D) in the neck, anterior to the trachea.

   E) in the roof of the third ventricle of the brain.

   Answer: D
   Page Ref: 581

5) The primary effect of T_3 and T_4 is to:

   A) decrease blood glucose.

   B) promote the release of calcitonin.

   C) promote heat–generating reactions.

   D) stimulate the uptake of iodide by the thyroid gland.

   E) promote excretion of sodium ions in urine.

   Answer: C
   Page Ref: 583

6) The mammary glands are an important target for:

   A) FSH.

   B) LH.

   C) oxytocin.

   D) prolactin.

   E) Both C and D are correct.

   Answer: E
   Page Ref: 577, 580

7) The interstitial cells of the testes are an important target for:

   A) FSH.

   B) LH.

   C) GnRH.

   D) oxytocin.

   E) Both A and B are correct.

   Answer: B
   Page Ref: 577

8) Hormones from the posterior pituitary are released in response to:
   A) releasing hormones from the hypothalamus.
   B) nerve impulses from the hypothalamus.
   C) permissive hormones from the pineal gland.
   D) renin from the kidneys.
   E) releasing hormones from the anterior pituitary.

   Answer: B
   Page Ref: 580

9) The innermost layer of the adrenal cortex is the:
   A) medulla.
   B) delta cells.
   C) zona glomerulosa.
   D) zona reticularis.
   E) zona fasciculata.

   Answer: D
   Page Ref: 589

10) The primary effect of calcitonin is to:
    A) increase blood glucose.
    B) decrease blood glucose.
    C) increase excretion of calcium ions in urine.
    D) increase blood calcium.
    E) decrease blood calcium.

    Answer: E
    Page Ref: 584

11) The stimulus for release of parathyroid hormone is:
    A) PRH.
    B) low levels of calcium ions in the blood.
    C) TSH.
    D) nerve impulses from the hypothalamus.
    E) calcitonin.

    Answer: B
    Page Ref: 585

12) Increased heart rate and force of contraction are effects of:
   A) ADH.
   B) insulin.
   C) cortisol.
   D) epinephrine.
   E) aldosterone.

   Answer: D
   Page Ref: 591

13) An increase in blood glucose and an anti–inflammatory effect are important effects of:
   A) epinephrine.
   B) glucagon.
   C) corticosterone.
   D) insulin.
   E) ADH.

   Answer: C
   Page Ref: 590

14) A primary effect of mineralocorticoids is to promote:
   A) increased urine production.
   B) excretion of potassium ions by the kidney.
   C) excretion of sodium ions by the kidney.
   D) decreased blood glucose.
   E) increased secretion of ACTH.

   Answer: B
   Page Ref: 589

15) The primary target for glucagon is the:
   A) liver.
   B) hypothalamus.
   C) adrenal cortex.
   D) pancreas.
   E) kidney.

   Answer: A
   Page Ref: 594

16) Osmoreceptors in the hypothalamus stimulate secretion of:

   A) renin from the kidney in response to low osmotic pressure.

   B) ADH from the hypothalamus in response to low osmotic pressure.

   C) ADH from the hypothalamus in response to high osmotic pressure.

   D) aldosterone from the kidney in response to low osmotic pressure.

   E) aldosterone from the adrenal cortex in response to low osmotic pressure.

   Answer: C
   Page Ref: 580

17) Increasing synthesis of the enzymes that run the active transport pump Na^+/K^+ ATPase is the major effect of:

   A) androgens.

   B) glucocorticoids.

   C) mineralocorticoids.

   D) thyroid hormones.

   E) insulin.

   Answer: D
   Page Ref: 583

18) Promotion of the formation of calcitriol is a major effect of:

   A) parathormone.

   B) aldosterone.

   C) calcitonin.

   D) TSH.

   E) cortisol.

   Answer: A
   Page Ref: 587

19) The primary source of estrogens after menopause is the:

   A) ovaries.

   B) uterus.

   C) hypothalamus.

   D) thyroid gland.

   E) zona reticularis of the adrenal cortex.

   Answer: E
   Page Ref: 592

20) The islets of Langerhans are the endocrine portion of the:
    A) adrenal cortex.
    B) adrenal medulla.
    C) anterior pituitary gland.
    D) posterior pituitary gland.
    E) pancreas.

    Answer: E
    Page Ref: 592

21) The only hormone that promotes anabolism of glycogen, fats, and proteins is:
    A) hGH.
    B) insulin.
    C) epinephrine.
    D) aldosterone.
    E) corticosterone.

    Answer: B
    Page Ref: 593

22) When a hormone that uses a second messenger binds to a target cell, the next thing that happens is that:
    A) phosphodiesterase is activated.
    B) a protein kinase is activated.
    C) a gene is activated in the nucleus.
    D) adenylate cyclase is activated by a G protein.
    E) voltage–regulated ion channels open in the plasma membrane.

    Answer: D
    Page Ref: 571

23) The compound that most often acts as a second messenger is:
    A) cholesterol.
    B) phosphodiesterase.
    C) cyclic AMP.
    D) COMT.
    E) CRH.

    Answer: C
    Page Ref: 571

24) When a steroid hormone binds to its target cell receptor, it:

A) causes the formation of cyclic AMP.

B) is converted into cholesterol, which acts as a second messenger.

C) causes the formation of releasing hormones.

D) turns specific genes of the nuclear DNA on or off.

E) alters the membrane's permeability to G proteins.

Answer: D
Page Ref: 570

25) Releasing and inhibiting hormones are produced by the:

A) posterior pituitary to control the anterior pituitary.

B) anterior pituitary to control the posterior pituitary.

C) hypothalamus to control the anterior pituitary.

D) hypothalamus to control the posterior pituitary.

E) pineal gland to control the hypothalamus.

Answer: C
Page Ref: 573

26) The role of somatostatin from the pancreas is to:

A) promote secretion of pancreatic digestive enzymes.

B) promote formation of calcitriol to facilitate calcium absorption from the gastrointestinal tract.

C) inhibit secretion of insulin and glucagon.

D) promote secretion of insulin and glucagon.

E) inhibit the activity of the adrenal cortex.

Answer: C
Page Ref: 595

27) Which of the following hormones is an example of a mitogenic hormone?

A) insulin

B) GHRH

C) leptin

D) epidermal growth factor

E) All of the above are correct.

Answer: D
Page Ref: 598

28) Diabetes insipidus results when:

   A) alpha cells of the pancreas are destroyed.

   B) beta cells of the pancreas are destroyed.

   C) the kidneys cannot respond to ADH.

   D) the kidneys cannot respond to aldosterone.

   E) beta cells of the pancreas are hypersecreting.

   Answer: C
   Page Ref: 603

29) Thyroglobulin is:

   A) the major component of colloid inside follicles.

   B) another name for thyroid hormone.

   C) the major stimulus for release of thyroid hormones.

   D) the protein that transports thyroxine in the blood.

   E) the protein that transports TSH to the thyroid gland.

   Answer: A
   Page Ref: 582

30) An increase in glycogenolysis by the liver is an important effect of:

   A) glucagon.

   B) insulin.

   C) PTH.

   D) aldosterone.

   E) Both A and B are correct.

   Answer: A
   Page Ref: 594

31) Long-term therapy with steroid drugs, such as cortisone, can cause osteoporosis and muscle wasting because of:

   A) increased blood glucose.

   B) increased protein catabolism.

   C) bacterial breakdown of bone and muscle.

   D) increased protein anabolism.

   E) increased excretion of calcium ions in urine.

   Answer: B
   Page Ref: 590

32) The primary stimulus for the release of insulin is:

   A) an elevated level of blood glucose.

   B) a decreased level of blood glucose.

   C) insulin releasing hormone.

   D) insulinlike growth factors.

   E) pancreatic stimulating hormone.

   Answer: A
   Page Ref: 594

33) Insulinlike growth factors are necessary for the full effect of:

   A) insulin.

   B) hGH.

   C) somatostatin.

   D) triiodothyronine.

   E) glucagon.

   Answer: B
   Page Ref: 575

34) The primary stimulus for release of cortisol and corticosterone is:

   A) ACTH.

   B) increased levels of blood glucose.

   C) the renin–angiotensin pathway.

   D) increased levels of sodium ions in the blood.

   E) increased levels of calcium ions in the blood.

   Answer: A
   Page Ref: 590

35) Paracrines are:

   A) local hormones that act on neighboring cells.

   B) local hormones that act on the cells that produced them.

   C) circulating hormones that are never broken down.

   D) the receptors for steroid hormones.

   E) inactive forms of circulating hormones.

   Answer: A
   Page Ref: 568

36) **ALL** of the following are lipid–soluble **EXCEPT**:

   A) triiodothyronine.

   B) nitric oxide.

   C) insulin.

   D) aldosterone.

   E) progesterone.

   Answer: C
   Page Ref: 569

37) Tyrosine is modified to produce **ALL** of the following **EXCEPT**:

   A) norepinephrine.

   B) TSH.

   C) thyroxine.

   D) dopamine.

   E) epinephrine.

   Answer: B
   Page Ref: 569

38) The specific effect of a water–soluble hormone on a target cell depends on the:

   A) particular gene that is activated.

   B) type of adenylate cyclase present.

   C) source of the phosphate for the phosphorylation reaction.

   D) extent to which the hormone can diffuse into the target cell.

   E) specific protein kinase activated.

   Answer: E
   Page Ref: 571

39) If hormone A stimulates up–regulation of receptors for hormone B, then hormone A has exerted a(n):

   A) permissive effect.

   B) synergistic effect.

   C) antagonistic effect.

   D) mitogenic effect.

   E) autocrinal effect.

   Answer: A
   Page Ref: 572

40) A hormone that counteracts the effects of both ADH and aldosterone is:

   A) thymosin.

   B) atrial natriuretic peptide.

   C) calcitonin.

   D) somatostatin.

   E) insulin.

   Answer: B
   Page Ref: 598

41) Suckling is an important stimulus for release of:

   A) oxytocin.

   B) DHEA.

   C) estrogen.

   D) FSH.

   E) LH.

   Answer: A
   Page Ref: 580

42) A chemical grouping of hormones derived from arachidonic acid is the:

   A) eicosanoids.

   B) biogenic amines.

   C) proteins.

   D) peptides.

   E) steroids.

   Answer: A
   Page Ref: 569

43) Which of the following hormones works by direct gene activation?

   A) ADH.

   B) hGH.

   C) insulin.

   D) cortisol.

   E) glucagon.

   Answer: D
   Page Ref: 569, 570

44) Protein anabolism is promoted by:

   A) insulin.

   B) somatotropin.

   C) triiodothyronine.

   D) cortisol.

   E) All of the above except cortisol.

   Answer: E
   Page Ref: 590

45) If the levels of PTH are high, one would expect to see:

   A) increased osteoblast activity.

   B) increased excretion of calcium ions in urine.

   C) increased excretion of phosphate ions in urine.

   D) decreased absorption of vitamin D.

   E) increased deposition of calcium ions in bone.

   Answer: C
   Page Ref: 585

46) Which of the following pairs of hormones are **NOT** antagonists?

   A) GHRH–somatostatin

   B) PTH–calcitonin.

   C) insulin–glucagon.

   D) aldosterone–atrial natriuretic peptide.

   E) aldosterone–ADH.

   Answer: E
   Page Ref: 580, 590, 572

47) A hormone that influences an endocrine gland other than its source is called a(n):

   A) autocrine.

   B) paracrine.

   C) eicosanoid.

   D) tropin.

   E) mitogen.

   Answer: D
   Page Ref: 575

48) Hypoglycemia is a stimulus for release of:
    A) ACTH.
    B) GHRH.
    C) insulin.
    D) Both A and B are correct.
    E) A, B, and C are all correct.

    Answer: D
    Page Ref: 576, 578

49) GnRH directly stimulates the release of:
    A) FSH.
    B) estrogen.
    C) testosterone.
    D) DHEA.
    E) All of these are correct.

    Answer: A
    Page Ref: 576

50) Sympathetic autonomic stimulation increases:
    A) glucagon secretion.
    B) secretion from chromaffin cells.
    C) insulin secretion.
    D) Both B and C are correct.
    E) Both A and B are correct.

    Answer: E
    Page Ref: 594, 591

MATCHING. Choose the item in column 2 that best matches each item in column 1.

Choose the item from column 2 that best matches each item in column 1.

1) Column 1: CRH
   Column 2: ACTH

   Answer: ACTH
   Page Ref: 578

2) Column 1: GnRH
   Column 2: FSH

   Answer: FSH
   Page Ref: 577

3) Column 1: TRH
   Column 2: TSH
   Answer: TSH
   Page Ref: 577

4) Column 1: high blood glucose
   Column 2: insulin
   Answer: insulin
   Page Ref: 594

5) Column 1: TSH
   Column 2: triiodothyronine
   Answer: triiodothyronine
   Page Ref: 584

6) Column 1: dehydration
   Column 2: ADH
   Answer: ADH
   Page Ref: 580

7) Column 1: low blood calcium
   Column 2: PTH
   Answer: PTH
   Page Ref: 585

8) Column 1: high blood calcium
   Column 2: calcitonin
   Answer: calcitonin
   Page Ref: 584

9) Column 1: angiotensin II
   Column 2: aldosterone
   Answer: aldosterone
   Page Ref: 589

10) Column 1: LH
    Column 2: testosterone
    Answer: testosterone
    Page Ref: 577

MATCHING. Choose the item in column 2 that best matches each item in column 1.

Choose the item from column 2 that best matches each item in column 1.

1) Column 1: somatotrophs
   Column 2: human growth hormone
   Answer: human growth hormone
   Page Ref: 576

2) Column 1: thyrotrophs
   Column 2: TSH
   Answer: TSH
   Page Ref: 577

3) Column 1: neurosecretory cells of the
   hypothalamus
   Column 2: ADH
   Answer: ADH
   Page Ref: 580

4) Column 1: follicular cells
   Column 2: thyroxine
   Answer: thyroxine
   Page Ref: 582

5) Column 1: chromaffin cells
   Column 2: epinephrine
   Answer: epinephrine
   Page Ref: 591

6) Column 1: zona glomerulosa cells
   Column 2: aldosterone
   Answer: aldosterone
   Page Ref: 586

7) Column 1: zona reticularis cells
   Column 2: DHEA
   Answer: DHEA
   Page Ref: 586

8) Column 1: zona fasciculata cells
   Column 2: cortisol

   Answer: cortisol
   Page Ref: 586

9) Column 1: corticotrophs
   Column 2: ACTH

   Answer: ACTH
   Page Ref: 578

10) Column 1: delta cells
    Column 2: somatostatin

    Answer: somatostatin
    Page Ref: 592

11) Column 1: beta cells
    Column 2: insulin

    Answer: insulin
    Page Ref: 592

12) Column 1: alpha cells
    Column 2: glucagon

    Answer: glucagon
    Page Ref: 592

TRUE/FALSE. Write 'T' if the statement is true and 'F' if the statement is false.

1) Some hormones are released by exocrine glands.

   Answer: FALSE
   Page Ref: 567

2) A cell can respond to a hormone only if it possesses receptors for that hormone.

   Answer: TRUE
   Page Ref: 568

3) If there is an overproduction of human growth hormone, one would expect to see the effect of up-regulation on target tissues.

   Answer: FALSE
   Page Ref: 568

4) Protein and peptide hormones are lipid–soluble.

Answer: FALSE
Page Ref: 569

5) Lipid–soluble hormones diffuse into target cells, but water–soluble hormones do not.

Answer: TRUE
Page Ref: 570

6) The effect of a water–soluble hormone on a target cell depends on the type of protein kinase activated within the target cell.

Answer: TRUE
Page Ref: 571

7) A water–soluble hormone binds to adenylate cyclase on the membranes of target cells.

Answer: FALSE
Page Ref: 571

8) The hypothalamus regulates secretion of hormones from the pituitary gland.

Answer: TRUE
Page Ref: 573

9) Prolactin is an example of a tropic hormone.

Answer: FALSE
Page Ref: 575

10) Hypoglycemia stimulates increased secretion of GHIH.

Answer: FALSE
Page Ref: 576

11) The receptors in the feedback loop regulating ADH secretion are osmoreceptors in the kidneys.

Answer: FALSE
Page Ref: 580

12) The thyroid gland normally contains most of the iodide in the body.

Answer: TRUE
Page Ref: 581

13) Calcitonin and PTH act as antagonist hormones with regard to levels of serum calcium ions.

Answer: TRUE
Page Ref: 584

14) The major stimulus for release of aldosterone is angiotensin II.

Answer: TRUE
Page Ref: 589

15) Insulin is the main hormone involved in the resistance reaction of the stress response.

Answer: FALSE
Page Ref: 600

SHORT ANSWER. Write the word or phrase that best completes each statement or answers the question.

1) The signs and symptoms of Cushing's syndrome result from hypersecretion of _____.
Answer: cortisol (glucocorticoids)
Page Ref: 604

2) Harmful stress is called _____ , while "productive" stress is called _____.
Answer: distress; eustress
Page Ref: 599

3) Tumor angiogenesis factor is so-called because it stimulates the growth of new _____.
Answer: capillaries
Page Ref: 599

4) Erythropoietin is a hormone produced by the _____ to increase _____.
Answer: kidneys; red blood cell production
Page Ref: 598

5) Secretion of _____ by the pineal gland stimulates sleepiness.
Answer: melatonin
Page Ref: 596

6) The primary androgen is _____.
Answer: testosterone
Page Ref: 595

7) Low blood glucose stimulates release of _____ from the pancreas.
Answer: glucagon
Page Ref: 594

8) Acetylcholine released from parasympathetic neurons causes a(n) _____ in secretion of insulin.
Answer: increase
Page Ref: 594

9) Somatostatin is secreted by both the _____ and the _____.

Answer: hypothalamus; pancreas (delta cells)

Page Ref: 592

10) The specialized sympathetic postganglionic neurons that are the hormone–producing cells of the adrenal medulla are called _____.

Answer: chromaffin cells.

Page Ref: 591

11) The major androgen secreted by the adrenal cortex is _____.

Answer: dehydroepiandrosterone (DHEA)

Page Ref: 591

12) The most abundant glucocorticoid is _____.

Answer: cortisol (hydrocortisone)

Page Ref: 589

13) The enzyme _____ is secreted by the juxtaglomerular cells of the kidneys in response to a drop in blood pressure.

Answer: renin

Page Ref: 589

14) Aldosterone targets the kidneys to increase reabsorption of _____ into the blood and secretion of _____ into the urine.

Answer: sodium ions; potassium ions

Page Ref: 589

15) The two main targets for angiotensin II are the _____ and the _____.

Answer: adrenal cortex; smooth muscle in walls of arterioles

Page Ref: 589

16) Anti–inflammatory effects are important effects of _____ produced by the adrenal cortex.

Answer: glucocorticoids

Page Ref: 590

17) The _____ glands are located just superior to each kidney.

Answer: adrenal

Page Ref: 585

18) The major hormonal antagonist to glucagon is _____.
Answer: insulin
Page Ref: 594

19) PTH stimulates reabsorption of calcium ions by the kidneys, but excretion of _____.
Answer: phosphates
Page Ref: 585

20) Increased secretion of CRH would be stimulated by low levels of the hormone _____.
Answer: cortisol
Page Ref: 591

21) Increased secretion of CRH directly increases the secretion of _____ by the _____ gland.
Answer: ACTH; anterior pituitary
Page Ref: 591

22) Formation of calcitriol in the kidneys is promoted by the hormone _____.
Answer: PTH
Page Ref: 585

23) If levels of T_3 and T_4 are low, one would expect this to stimulate an increase in secretion of both _____ from the _____ and _____ from the _____ to correct the situation.
Answer: TRH; hypothalamus; TSH; anterior pituitary gland
Page Ref: 584

24) The amino acid that is iodinated during the formation of T_3 and T_4 is _____.
Answer: tyrosine
Page Ref: 582

25) The three target tissues/organs for ADH are the _____ , the _____ , and the _____.
Answer: kidneys; sweat glands; smooth muscle in blood vessel walls
Page Ref: 580

26) Ejection ("let-down") of milk from the mammary glands is an important effect of the hormone _____.
Answer: oxytocin
Page Ref: 580

27) _____ are cells in the _____ that secrete ACTH.
   Answer: Corticotrophs; anterior pituitary gland
   Page Ref: 578

28) Prolactin inhibiting hormone is the same molecule as the neurotransmitter _____.
   Answer: dopamine
   Page Ref: 577

29) FSH stimulates follicular cells to secrete _____.
   Answer: estrogens
   Page Ref: 577

30) LH stimulates the testes to _____.
   Answer: secrete testosterone
   Page Ref: 577

31) Somatotrophs are cells that secrete _____.
   Answer: human growth hormone
   Page Ref: 576

32) Human growth hormone acts indirectly on tissues by promoting the synthesis and secretion of small protein hormones called _____.
   Answer: insulinlike growth factors
   Page Ref: 575

33) GnRH stimulates the release of _____ and _____ from the anterior pituitary gland.
   Answer: FSH; LH
   Page Ref: 575

34) Releasing hormones and inhibiting hormones are secreted by the _____ to regulate the _____.
   Answer: hypothalamus; anterior pituitary gland
   Page Ref: 573

35) Hormone receptors on the outer surface of the plasma membranes of target cells are linked to adenylate cyclase molecules by _____.
   Answer: G proteins
   Page Ref: 572

ESSAY. Write your answer in the space provided or on a separate sheet of paper.

1) Describe the role of G proteins in hormone function.

Answer: G proteins provide the link between hormone receptors on the outer surface of the plasma membrane and adenylate cyclase on the inner surface of the membrane. When a water–soluble hormone binds to its receptor, the binding activates a G protein, which in turn activates adenylate cyclase. Adenylate cyclase catalyzes the formation of the second messenger cAMP.

Page Ref: 572

2) Describe and explain the similarities between starvation and diabetes mellitus.

Answer: A starving person is lacking energy–providing nutrient sources, and so, must use structural components of the body as energy sources. The diabetic consumes adequate nutrients, but due to the lack of insulin, is unable to move glucose into cells, and so, cannot use the nutrients. In both cases, energy generation is dependent on non–glucose sources, such as fatty acids and amino acids. Mobilization and metabolism of fats and proteins for energy production purposes leads to ketoacidosis, weight loss, and hunger.

Page Ref: 605

3) Define up–regulation and down–regulation as they relate to hormone action. Under what circumstances would you expect to see these phenomena?

Answer: These terms refer to changes in the number of receptors present on target cells depending on the concentration of a hormone. Down–regulation occurs when hormone levels are chronically high to decrease responsiveness, while up–regulation occurs in circumstances of hormone deficiency to increase sensitivity of target cells.

Page Ref: 568

4) Compare and contrast the mechanisms of action of lipid–soluble vs. water–soluble hormones.

Answer: Upon reaching their targets, lipid–soluble hormones diffuse through the phospholipid bilayer of the target cell membrane and bind to receptors in the cytosol or nucleus. The activated receptor turns a gene on or off, thus regulating synthesis of a protein. Water–soluble hormones bind to membrane receptors, activating a G protein, which activates adenylate cyclase, which converts ATP to the second messenger cAMP, which activates a protein kinase to regulate enzyme action.

Page Ref: 570–571

5) Tameekah has had a series of medical tests that show persistent hyperglycemia. Her pancreas seems to be functioning normally. What other hormone tests and general observations might be made to determine the source of her problem? Use your knowledge of feedback loops to propose an answer.

Answer: Human growth hormone might be elevated (check GHRH levels—if GHRH is low but hGH is high, then maybe tumor of somatotrophs; check for gross anatomical changes in size). Glucocorticoids might be high (check ACTH levels —if ACTH is low but cortisol is high, then problem is in adrenal cortex; if ACTH is high, then problem with corticotrophs; check for unusual fat deposition and masculinization of females).

Page Ref: 576, 578, 589

6) Thursday night is party night at Porter and Stout College, and Itzhak is taking full advantage of it. He finds that after three beers, he has made several trips to the men's room. Explain the hormonal basis for this response. Predict what will happen to Itzhak's hormone and water balance as the night progresses and more beers are consumed. Predict what his hormone balance will be like the next day.

Answer: Increased fluid intake decreases ADH secretion, so fluid output increases. Additionally, alcohol inhibits ADH secretion, so more fluid is lost via urine output than would be needed for water balance, thus leading to dehydration. Once the effects of the alcohol wane, ADH secretion and aldosterone secretion will increase to save water and increase thirst until water balance is restored.

Page Ref: 580

7) Wanda is in an abusive relationship in which she lives in constant fear of physical and verbal attack. Describe the probable effect of this relationship on Wanda's physiological systems.

Answer: The initial alarm reaction is a typical sympathetic (fight-or-flight) response of the ANS and adrenal medulla. This response would occur each time there is an imminent threat of danger and during any attack. Over time, the resistance reaction boosts activity of the adrenal cortex via ACTH, the liver via hGH, and the thyroid via TRH/TSH, leading to exhaustion of these organs.

Page Ref: 599–601

8) What is a goiter? Using the appropriate negative feedback loops in your answer, explain how goiters can develop in both hyposecretion and hypersecretion disorders. In these hyposecretion and hypersecretion disorders, would you expect the levels of other hormones involved in the loops to be high or low. Why?

Answer: A goiter is an enlarged thyroid gland. Hyposecretion goiters are usually due to insufficient iodide in the diet. Resulting low levels of thyroid hormones cause increased TRH and TSH until adequate thyroid activity is restored. Graves' disease causes hyperthyroidism by mimicking TSH. Thyroid enlargement occurs, and production of thyroid hormones increases. TRH and natural TSH remain low due to negative feedback, but false TSH pushes thyroid activity.

Page Ref: 604

9) Describe in detail the negative feedback loop involving both the adrenal gland and the kidney in the control of blood pressure.

Answer: Low blood pressure triggers release of renin from JG cells of the kidney. In blood, renin converts angiotensinogen to angiotensin I, which is converted to angiotensin II by ACE in lung capillaries. Angiotensin II stimulates secretion of aldosterone by the adrenal cortex which causes the kidneys to save sodium ions. Water is reabsorbed for osmotic balance, thus increasing blood volume and blood pressure.

Page Ref: 590

10) Many people are on long–term therapy with drugs in the glucocorticoid family. What would you expect the long–term effects of these drugs to be? Explain your answer.

Answer: Expect chronically high levels of glucose due to increased gluconeogenesis; weakening of bones and muscles due to increased protein catabolism; redistribution of fat to face, back, and abdomen; decreased resistance to stress and infection due to anti–inflammatory effects.

Page Ref: 590

11) Describe the role of the hypothalamus in the regulation of the pituitary gland.

Answer: The hypothalamus is the integrating center for much sensory input. It secretes releasing and inhibiting hormones which diffuse into the hypophyseal portal system to regulate secretion of all hormones from the anterior pituitary gland. It also contains receptors that monitor blood osmotic pressure and neural input from reproductive structures. Integration of this input leads to production of ADH and OT by neurosecretory cells. These hormones are then transported through the hypothalamohypophyseal tract to be secreted by exocytosis from the posterior pituitary in response to nerve impulses.

Page Ref: 573

CHAPTER 19   The Cardiovascular System: The Blood

MULTIPLE CHOICE. Choose the one alternative that best completes the statement or answers the question.

1) The buffy coat of centrifuged blood consists mainly of:
   A) the ejected nuclei of red blood cells.
   B) gamma globulins.
   C) ruptured red blood cells whose hemoglobin has sunk to the bottom.
   D) white blood cells and platelets.
   E) serum.

   Answer: D
   Page Ref: 611

2) The most abundant of the leukocytes are the:
   A) lymphocytes.
   B) basophils.
   C) monocytes.
   D) neutrophils.
   E) eosinophils.

   Answer: D
   Page Ref: 621

3) The function of hemoglobin is to:
   A) protect the DNA of erythrocytes.
   B) produce red blood cells.
   C) produce antibodies.
   D) carry oxygen.
   E) trigger the cascade of clotting reactions.

   Answer: D
   Page Ref: 616

4) The formed elements that are fragments of larger cells called megakaryocytes are:
   A) neutrophils.
   B) lymphocytes.
   C) erythrocytes.
   D) thrombocytes.
   E) plasma proteins.

   Answer: D
   Page Ref: 622

5) The most abundant of the plasma proteins are the:

   A) albumins.

   B) hemoglobins.

   C) gamma globulins.

   D) clotting proteins.

   E) alpha globulins.

   Answer: A
   Page Ref: 611

6) A person's ABO blood type is determined by antigens present on the:

   A) erythrocytes.

   B) platelets.

   C) leukocytes.

   D) gamma globulins.

   E) blood vessels walls.

   Answer: A
   Page Ref: 627

7) The pluripotent stem cells that are the parent cells for all formed elements are derived from:

   A) mesenchyme.

   B) ectoderm.

   C) osteoblasts in bone surrounding the marrow cavity.

   D) the endothelium that forms the lining of blood vessels.

   E) fibroblasts in the endosteum.

   Answer: A
   Page Ref: 615

8) Myeloid stem cells can develop into any of the following **EXCEPT**:

   A) neutrophils.

   B) basophils.

   C) thrombocytes.

   D) lymphocytes.

   E) erythrocytes.

   Answer: D
   Page Ref: 615

9) Agranular leukocytes that are phagocytic are the:
   A) neutrophils.
   B) monocytes.
   C) lymphocytes.
   D) eosinophils.
   E) All of the above except eosinophils.

   Answer: B
   Page Ref: 619

10) "5 million per cubic millimeter" is a value falling within the normal adult range for the number of:
   A) platelets.
   B) all leukocytes.
   C) erythrocytes.
   D) hemoglobin molecules.
   E) neutrophils.

   Answer: C
   Page Ref: 615

11) In the adult, red bone marrow would normally be found in the:
   A) sternum.
   B) diaphysis of the femur.
   C) diaphysis of the humerus.
   D) irregular bones of the face.
   E) All of the above except the bones of the face.

   Answer: A
   Page Ref: 615

12) Prothymocytes are stem cells that differentiate into:
   A) thrombocytes.
   B) monocytes.
   C) lymphocytes.
   D) erythrocytes.
   E) Both B and C are correct.

   Answer: C
   Page Ref: 615

13) Which of the following would be **TRUE** for a person with Type B blood?

    A) He could theoretically donate to a Type O person.

    B) His own plasma contains anti-B antibodies.

    C) He must be Rh positive.

    D) He could theoretically donate to a Type AB person.

    E) He could theoretically receive blood from a Type AB person.

Answer: D
Page Ref: 630

14) Which of the following would be **TRUE** for a normal person with anti-A antibodies circulating in his blood?

    A) He could be blood type A.

    B) He could be blood type B.

    C) He could be blood type AB.

    D) He could be either type B or type AB.

    E) It is impossible to know his possible blood types.

Answer: B
Page Ref: 630

15) Thrombopoietin is a hormone that is:

    A) produced by the liver to activate thrombin.

    B) produced by the liver to block the action of thrombin.

    C) produced by the liver to stimulate platelet formation.

    D) produced by the kidney to stimulate platelet formation.

    E) produced by the kidney to activate the intrinsic clotting pathway.

Answer: C
Page Ref: 615

16) A person with end-stage kidney disease may have a red blood cell count that is lower than normal because:

    A) the kidneys are an important site of erythropoiesis.

    B) red blood cells are lost into the urine.

    C) the kidneys don't synthesize enough hemoglobin.

    D) not enough erythropoietin is secreted to stimulate red blood cell formation.

    E) the damaged kidneys actively destroy red blood cells as they flow through renal vessels.

Answer: D
Page Ref: 615

17) Heparin works as an anticoagulant by:

   A) preventing clumping of platelets.

   B) acting as an antagonist to vitamin K.

   C) working with AT-III to interfere with the action of thrombin.

   D) binding calcium ions.

   E) enhancing the production of tissue plasminogen activator.

   Answer: C
   Page Ref: 627

18) When red blood cells wear out, the iron is saved and the remainder of the hemoglobin is:

   A) also save.

   B) excreted as bile pigments.

   C) rearranged into gamma globulins.

   D) broken down by plasmin.

   E) used as an anticoagulant.

   Answer: B
   Page Ref: 618

19) Formed elements that are biconcave discs about 7–8 μm in diameter are:

   A) platelets

   B) band cells.

   C) blast cells that should not be present in circulation.

   D) small lymphocytes.

   E) erythrocytes.

   Answer: E
   Page Ref: 616

20) Red blood cells do not consume any of the oxygen they transport because they:

   A) do not have the cellular machinery for aerobic ATP production.

   B) cannot remove oxygen from heme once it is attached.

   C) use carbon dioxide in the electron transport chain instead of oxygen.

   D) do not need to generate ant ATP.

   E) convert oxygen to globin during transport.

   Answer: A
   Page Ref: 616

21) The initial stimulus for the vasoconstriction that occurs in hemostasis is:

    A) prothrombinase.

    B) mechanical damage to the vessel.

    C) thromboxane A2.

    D) plasmin.

    E) thrombin.

    Answer: B
    Page Ref: 622

22) Platelets initially stick to the wall of a damaged blood vessel because:

    A) exposed collagen fibers make a rough surface to which the platelets are attracted.

    B) histamine causes vasoconstriction so that platelets can't fit through the opening.

    C) fibrin threads act like glue to hold them there.

    D) prothrombinase alters the electrical charge of the vessel wall.

    E) the intracellular fluid released by damaged cells in the blood vessel wall has a higher viscosity than plasma.

    Answer: A
    Page Ref: 614

23) The total blood volume in an average adult is about:

    A) 8 liters.

    B) one liter.

    C) 3 liters.

    D) 5 liters.

    E) 10 liters.

    Answer: D
    Page Ref: 611

24) **ALL** of the following are important functions of plasma proteins **EXCEPT**:

    A) protection against bacteria and viruses.

    B) maintenance of osmotic pressure.

    C) protection against blood loss.

    D) transportation of steroid hormones.

    E) transportation of oxygen.

    Answer: E
    Page Ref: 611

25) When carbon dioxide is carried by red blood cells it is carried in part by:

   A) attaching to the iron ion in heme.

   B) the amino acids in globin.

   C) integrins in the plasma membrane.

   D) nitric oxide.

   E) All of these are correct.

Answer: B
Page Ref: 616

26) When hemoglobin releases oxygen and super nitric oxide to tissues, the super nitric oxide causes:

   A) attachment of carbon dioxide to globin.

   B) emigration of red blood cells into interstitial fluid.

   C) vasoconstriction.

   D) vasodilation.

   E) erythropoiesis.

Answer: D
Page Ref: 617

27) The primary organs whose macrophages are responsible for phagocytizing worn-out red blood cells are the:

   A) spleen and liver.

   B) spleen and kidneys.

   C) liver and kidneys.

   D) lungs and liver.

   E) lungs and kidneys.

Answer: A
Page Ref: 617

28) The function of transferrin is to:

   A) help white blood cells emigrate from blood vessels.

   B) carry iron ions in the bloodstream.

   C) convert fibrinogen to fibrin.

   D) promote differentiation of blast cells in bone marrow.

   E) store iron in the spleen or liver.

Answer: B
Page Ref: 617

29) Erythropoietin is synthesized by the:

   A) red bone marrow.

   B) yellow bone marrow.

   C) erythrocytes.

   D) spleen.

   E) kidneys.

   Answer: E
   Page Ref: 615

30) Oxygen is transported by red blood cells by binding to:

   A) specific receptors on the plasma membrane.

   B) specific receptors within the nucleus of the red blood cell.

   C) the beta polypeptide chain of the globin portion of hemoglobin.

   D) the polypeptide chain of the heme portion of hemoglobin.

   E) the iron ion in the heme portion of hemoglobin.

   Answer: E
   Page Ref: 616

31) The function of ferritin and hemosiderin is to:

   A) transport iron via facilitated diffusion from the small intestine into the bloodstream.

   B) store iron within muscle fibers, liver, and spleen.

   C) transport iron through the bloodstream.

   D) catalyze the formation of bile pigments.

   E) stimulate the formation of hemoglobin in developing erythrocytes.

   Answer: B
   Page Ref: 617

32) Biliverdin and bilirubin are:

   A) pigments that form during the breakdown of the non-iron portion of heme.

   B) compound that transport iron in the bloodstream.

   C) storage molecules for iron in the liver and spleen.

   D) precursors to hemoglobin seen in immature red blood cells.

   E) inactive forms of clotting factors secreted by platelets.

   Answer: A
   Page Ref: 618

33) In the negative feedback loop that controls the rate of erythropoiesis, the stress is:
   A) a change in the normal percentages of each type of formed element.
   B) increased levels of carbon dioxide in the red bone marrow.
   C) increased levels of carbon dioxide in the cerebrospinal fluid.
   D) decreased levels of oxygen in the kidney.
   E) decreased solute concentration of blood circulating in the hypothalamus.

   Answer: D
   Page Ref: 618

34) In the negative feedback loop that controls the rate of erythropoiesis, the target for erythropoietin is the:
   A) kidney.
   B) spleen.
   C) proerythroblasts in red bone marrow.
   D) erythrocytes in circulation.
   E) liver.

   Answer: C
   Page Ref: 618

35) Your lab slip reporting your blood work results states, "PMNs 72%." This indicates that:
   A) your hematocrit is very high.
   B) your neutrophils are within normal range.
   C) you don't have enough granular leukocytes.
   D) you have too many immature red blood cells in circulation.
   E) your platelets are making up an abnormally high percentage of formed elements.

   Answer: B
   Page Ref: 619

36) The role of integrins on the surfaces of neutrophils is to:
   A) bind oxygen.
   B) bind carbon dioxide.
   C) attach to endothelium and facilitate emigration.
   D) poke holes in microbial membranes.
   E) stabilize the neutrophils while they undergo mitosis in the bloodstream.

   Answer: C
   Page Ref: 620

37) Production of enzymes such as histaminase that combat the effects of the mediators of inflammation is an important function of:

A) monocytes.

B) basophils.

C) plasma cells.

D) T lymphocytes.

E) eosinophils.

Answer: E
Page Ref: 621

38) So-called *natural killer cells* are a form of:

A) thrombocyte.

B) lymphocyte.

C) monocyte.

D) granular leukocyte.

E) erythrocyte.

Answer: B
Page Ref: 621

39) Contact with collagen activates clotting factor:

A) I.

B) II.

C) IV.

D) VIII.

E) XII.

Answer: E
Page Ref: 625

40) People suffering from disorders that prevent absorption of fat from the intestine may suffer uncontrolled bleeding because:

A) the fat-soluble vitamin K cannot be absorbed, so levels of prothrombin and other clotting factors drop.

B) fat droplets in the blood normally help platelets and other formed elements stick together during hemostasis.

C) vitamin B_{12} cannot be absorbed, so there are inadequate formed elements present to produce a clot.

D) fatty acids are necessary for the complete synthesis of fibrin.

E) fat prevents the complete inactivation of plasmin.

Answer: A
Page Ref: 626

41) Type O is considered the theoretical universal:

A) recipient because there are no A or B isoantigens on RBCs.

B) donor because there are no A or B isoantigens on RBCs.

C) recipient because there are no anti-A or anti-B antibodies in plasma.

D) donor because there are no anti-A or anti-B antibodies in plasma.

E) donor because there are no A or B isoantigens on RBCs, nor are there anti-A or anti-B isoantibodies in plasma.

Answer: B
Page Ref: 630

42) The symptoms of hemolytic disease of the newborn occur because:

A) the baby has a faulty gene that makes its hemoglobin unable to bind oxygen.

B) the baby begins making antibodies to its own A or B isoantigens.

C) anti-Rh antibodies produced by the mother pass the placenta into the bloodstream of the fetus.

D) the baby is premature and is unable to produce enough plasma proteins to keep osmotic pressure at the correct levels.

E) the mother took high doses of aspirin during the last trimester of development.

Answer: C
Page Ref: 629

43) The purpose for giving RhoGAM to women who have just delivered a child or who have had a miscarriage or abortion is to:

A) stimulate contraction of uterine smooth muscle to expel all uterine contents.

B) trigger the clotting cascade to prevent excessive bleeding.

C) block the stimulation of pain receptors.

D) stimulate erythropoiesis to replace red blood cells lost during delivery.

E) block recognition of any fetal red blood cells by the mother's immune system.

Answer: E
Page Ref: 629

44) A normal number of thrombocytes in circulation is:

A) about 5 million per cubic millimeter.

B) about 7000 per cubic millimeter.

C) about 300,000 per cubic millimeter.

D) about 25 percent of all formed elements.

E) about 25,000 per cubic millimeter.

Answer: C
Page Ref: 622

45) Prothrombinase is formed by:
    A) the liver.
    B) the extrinsic and intrinsic pathways.
    C) basophils.
    D) activation of plasmin.
    E) damaged endothelium.

    Answer: B
    Page Ref: 624

46) Thrombin's positive feedback effects include:
    A) acceleration of prothrombinase formation.
    B) activation of platelets.
    C) production of thromboplastin.
    D) production of fibrinogen.
    E) Both A and B are correct.

    Answer: E
    Page Ref: 625

47) A clot in an unbroken vessel is called:
    A) thrombosis.
    B) embolism.
    C) agglutination.
    D) adhesion.
    E) aggregation.

    Answer: A
    Page Ref: 627

48) MHC antigens are:
    A) the antigens that determine the ABO blood types.
    B) viral antigens whose presence indicates presence infectious disease.
    C) proteins encoded by genes present in nucleated cells that must be matched for successful tissue transplantation.
    D) the antigens that are attacked in hemolytic disease of the newborn.
    E) the molecules to which emigrating leukocytes attach before leaving the bloodstream.

    Answer: C
    Page Ref: 620

49) Which of the following indicates a normal differential count in a healthy adult?
    A) 50% neutrophils, 30% lymphocytes, 15% monocytes, 4% eosinophils, 1% basophils
    B) 65% lymphocytes, 20% neutrophils, 10% monocytes, 4% eosinophils, 1% basophils
    C) 65% neutrophils, 25% lymphocytes, 6% eosinophils, 2% monocytes, 2% basophils
    D) 65% neutrophils, 25% lymphocytes, 6% monocytes, 3% eosinophils, 1% basophils
    E) 50% lymphocytes, 30% neutrophils, 10% eosinophils, 8% monocytes, 2% basophils

Answer: D
Page Ref: 621

50) If 100 leukocyte are counted in a normal adult blood sample, how many monocytes would you expect to see?
    A) 60–70
    B) 20–25
    C) 3–8
    D) 2–4
    E) one

Answer: C
Page Ref: 621

MATCHING. Choose the item in column 2 that best matches each item in column 1.

Choose the item from column 2 that best matches each item in column 1.

1) Column 1: **a type of adhesion molecule
            on neutrophils**
   Column 2: integrin
   Answer: integrin
   Page Ref: 620

2) Column 1: enzyme that digests fibrin
   Column 2: plasmin
   Answer: plasmin
   Page Ref: 626

3) Column 1: **the end result of the extrinsic
            and intrinsic pathways**
   Column 2: prothrombinase
   Answer: prothrombinase
   Page Ref: 625

4) Column 1: enzyme that converts
fibrinogen to fibrin
Column 2: thrombin

Answer: thrombin

Page Ref: 625

5) Column 1: a mixture of lipoproteins and
phospholipids released by
damaged cells in the extrinsic
pathway
Column 2: thromboplastin

Answer: thromboplastin

Page Ref: 625

6) Column 1: forms the protein threads of a
blood clot
Column 2: fibrin

Answer: fibrin

Page Ref: 625

7) Column 1: a vasoconstricting
prostaglandin that activates
platelets
Column 2: thromboxane A2

Answer: thromboxane A2

Page Ref: 622

8) Column 1: a hormone from the kidneys
that increases red blood cell
precursor cells
Column 2: erythropoietin

Answer: erythropoietin

Page Ref: 615

9) Column 1: an iron-storage protein
Column 2: hemosiderin

Answer: hemosiderin

Page Ref: 617

10) Column 1: a prostaglandin that inhibits
           platelet adhesion and release

   Column 2: prostacyclin

   Answer: prostacyclin

   Page Ref: 627

MATCHING. Choose the item in column 2 that best matches each item in column 1.

Choose the item from column 2 that best matches each item in column 1.

   1) Column 1: transport most oxygen and
            some carbon dioxide in blood

      Column 2: erythrocytes

      Answer: erythrocytes

      Page Ref: 615

   2) Column 1: cell fragments that form a
            plug and release
            vasoconstrictors during
            hemostasis

      Column 2: thrombocytes

      Answer: thrombocytes

      Page Ref: 622

   3) Column 1: phagocytic granular
            leukocytes; most numerous
            leukocytes

      Column 2: neutrophils

      Answer: neutrophils

      Page Ref: 619

   4) Column 1: intensify inflammatory
            response via release of
            histamine and serotonin

      Column 2: basophils

      Answer: basophils

      Page Ref: 619

   5) Column 1: combat effects of histamine in
            allergic reactions

      Column 2: eosinophils

      Answer: eosinophils

      Page Ref: 619

6) Column 1: develop into plasma cells that secrete antibodies

   Column 2: B lymphocytes

   Answer: B lymphocytes
   Page Ref: 621

7) Column 1: attack viruses, cancer cells, and transplanted cells

   Column 2: T lymphocytes

   Answer: T lymphocytes
   Page Ref: 621

8) Column 1: develop into macrophages outside of circulation

   Column 2: monocytes

   Answer: monocytes
   Page Ref: 619

9) Column 1: form of red blood cell that enters circulation from the bone marrow; serve as indicators of rate of erythropoiesis

   Column 2: reticulocytes

   Answer: reticulocytes
   Page Ref: 618

10) Column 1: young neutrophils with rod-shaped nuclei

    Column 2: band cells

    Answer: band cells
    Page Ref: 619

TRUE/FALSE. Write 'T' if the statement is true and 'F' if the statement is false.

1) The hematocrit measures the amount of hemoglobin in red blood cells.

   Answer: FALSE
   Page Ref: 611

2) Most plasma proteins are synthesized by hepatocytes.

   Answer: TRUE
   Page Ref: 611

3) Erythropoietin is a hormone produced by the liver to stimulate red blood cell production.

Answer: FALSE
Page Ref: 615

4) Mature leukocytes lack a nucleus.

Answer: FALSE
Page Ref: 619

5) Bilirubin forms from the ejected DNA of developing red blood cells.

Answer: FALSE
Page Ref: 618

6) Oxygen reversibly binds to the iron ions in the heme of hemoglobin.

Answer: TRUE
Page Ref: 616

7) When hemoglobin picks up oxygen in the lungs, it also picks up super nitric oxide.

Answer: TRUE
Page Ref: 616

8) Macrophages form from lymphocytes that have migrated into tissues and differentiated.

Answer: FALSE
Page Ref: 620

9) Neutrophils are phagocytes.

Answer: TRUE
Page Ref: 620

10) A high eosinophil count may indicate a parasitic infection.

Answer: TRUE
Page Ref: 621

11) T lymphocytes develop into plasma cells that secrete antibodies.

Answer: FALSE
Page Ref: 623

12) Thromboplastin converts prothrombin to thrombin.

Answer: FALSE
Page Ref: 625

13) People who have difficulty absorbing fats from the gastrointestinal tract may suffer clotting difficulties due to vitamin K deficiency.

Answer: TRUE
Page Ref: 626

14) An increased number of band cells in circulation indicates an increased demand for neutrophils.

Answer: TRUE
Page Ref: 619

15) People who are blood type B have B antigens on the membranes of their red blood cells and anti–B antibodies circulating in their plasma.

Answer: FALSE
Page Ref: 628

SHORT ANSWER. Write the word or phrase that best completes each statement or answers the question.

1) The normal pH of blood ranges from _____ to _____.
Answer: 7.35; 7.45
Page Ref: 611

2) Blood is about _____ % formed elements and _____ % plasma.
Answer: 45; 55
Page Ref: 611

3) The most abundant of the plasma proteins are the _____.
Answer: albumins
Page Ref: 611

4) Males have a higher hematocrit range than females because testosterone stimulates synthesis of the hormone _____.
Answer: erythropoietin
Page Ref: 611

5) Immunoglobulins are produced by _____ , which develop from B lymphocytes.
Answer: plasma cells
Page Ref: 613

6) After birth, hemopoiesis takes place only in _____.
Answer: red bone marrow
Page Ref: 615

7) Thrombopoietin is produced by the _____ to stimulate formation of platelets.

Answer: liver

Page Ref: 615

8) One microliter of blood contains about _____ red blood cells in the adult male.

Answer: 5.4 million

Page Ref: 615

9) Red blood cells are highly specialized for the function of _____.

Answer: oxygen transport

Page Ref: 616

10) Each heme pigment in hemoglobin contains a(n) _____ that can combine reversibly with one oxygen molecule.

Answer: iron ion

Page Ref: 616

11) When hemoglobin passes into the lungs, it releases carbon dioxide and _____ , a gas produced by the endothelial cells lining blood vessels.

Answer: nitric oxide.

Page Ref: 616

12) Vasodilation is triggered by _____ as it is released with oxygen from hemoglobin; this triggers a(n) _____ in blood pressure.

Answer: super nitric oxide; decrease

Page Ref: 617

13) Red blood cells survive about _____ days in circulation.

Answer: 120

Page Ref: 617

14) The iron-storage proteins in muscle fibers, liver cells, and macrophages are _____ and _____ .

Answer: ferritin; hemosiderin

Page Ref: 617

15) The non-iron portion of heme is converted first to the green pigment _____ , then to the yellow-orange pigment _____ , which is transported to the liver for secretion in bile.

Answer: biliverdin; bilirubin

Page Ref: 618

16) The stimulus for release of erythropoietin is _____.

Answer: hypoxia in the kidney

Page Ref: 618

17) The target cells for erythropoietin are the _____ in the red bone marrow.

Answer: proerythroblasts

Page Ref: 618

18) A few days after donating blood at the local blood drive, a person would probably exhibit an elevated level of immature cells called _____, demonstrating an increased demand for red blood cells.

Answer: reticulocytes

Page Ref: 619

19) On a standard blood smear, cells that stain pale lilac are the _____, those that stain red-orange are the _____, and those that stain blue–purple are the _____.

Answer: neutrophils; eosinophils; basophils

Page Ref: 619

20) The largest of the leukocytes are the _____.

Answer: monocytes

Page Ref: 619

21) _____ are the unique "cell identity marker" proteins protruding from the plasma membranes of white blood cells but not red blood cells.

Answer: Major histocompatibility antigens

Page Ref: 620

22) The normal number of white blood cells per microliter ranges from _____ to _____ cells.

Answer: 5,000; 10,000

Page Ref: 620

23) Mast cells develop from _____, and intensify the inflammatory response by releasing the chemicals _____, _____, and _____.

Answer: basophils; histamine; heparin; serotonin

Page Ref: 621

24) The attraction of phagocytes to chemicals released by microbes and inflamed tissues is called _____.

Answer: chemotaxis

Page Ref: 620

25) The molecule _____ released from dense granules of platelets makes other platelets sticky during platelet aggregation.

Answer: ADP

Page Ref: 622

26) Plasma minus the clotting proteins is called _____.

Answer: serum

Page Ref: 623

27) Prothrombinase catalyzes the conversion of _____ to _____ , which then catalyzes the conversion of soluble _____ to insoluble _____.

Answer: prothrombin; thrombin; fibrinogen; fibrin

Page Ref: 624–625

28) Dissolution of a blood clot is called _____ , which occurs via the action of the enzyme _____.

Answer: fibrinolysis; plasmin

Page Ref: 626

29) Aspirin inhibits vasoconstriction and platelet aggregation by blocking synthesis of the prostaglandin _____.

Answer: thromboxane A2

Page Ref: 627

30) A person who has circulating anti–A and anti–B agglutinins is blood type _____.

Answer: O

Page Ref: 630

ESSAY. Write your answer in the space provided or on a separate sheet of paper.

1) Explain the proposed role of hemoglobin in the maintenance of blood pressure.

Answer: Hemoglobin releases carbon dioxide and nitric oxide when passing through the lungs. It then picks up oxygen and super nitric oxide, which are then circulated and released to tissues. Release of super nitric oxide causes vasodilation and so, a decrease in blood pressure. Nitric oxide causes vasoconstriction and an increase in blood pressure.

Page Ref: 616

2) A young woman with severe immune deficiency problems has been found to be lacking certain selectins. What are selectins? Predict what specific problems this woman might have. Explain your answer.

Answer: Selectins are adhesion molecules on endothelial cells displayed in response to injury and inflammation. They stick to carbohydrates on neutrophils to slow them down, so they can bind to the endothelium prior to emigration to surrounding tissues. The patient would suffer deficiencies related to loss of neutrophil function —i.e., phagocytosis in interstitial fluid surrounding damaged tissues.

Page Ref: 620

3) List and briefly describe the functions of blood.

Answer: 1) Transportation —carries oxygen, carbon dioxide, nutrients, wastes, hormones and heat
2) Regulation—helps maintain pH via buffers, body temperature via properties of water in plasma, and water balance via osmotic pressure created by plasma proteins
3) Protection—via clotting, antibodies, phagocytosis, and complement

Page Ref: 610

4) Kevin's father has been advised by his physician to take an aspirin a day "to reduce his risk of heart attack." What is the physiological basis for this advice?

Answer: Aspirin inhibits vasoconstriction and platelet aggregation by blocking synthesis of the prostaglandin thromboxane A2. This prostaglandin is present in the dense granules of platelets and is released as they begin clumping.

Page Ref: 627

5) Why does damaged endothelium present an increased risk of blood clotting?

Answer: Blood may come in contact with collagen in the surrounding basal lamina, which activates clotting factor XII, which ultimately leads to the formation of fibrin clots. Platelets are also damaged by contact with damaged endothelium and begin their release reaction.

Page Ref: 622

6) On a differential white blood cell count, Ezra is found to have 85 percent neutrophils and an elevated number of band cells. What is the most likely cause of Ezra's high neutrophil count? What benefits are being provided by all these neutrophils? What is the significance of the band cells?

Answer: High neutrophil count indicates bacterial infection (most likely), and increased band cells indicates a rapid turnover of neutrophils with an increased demand for replacements. Neutrophils are phagocytes that, upon engulfing a pathogen, release antimicrobial substances, such as lysozyme, oxidants, and defensins.

Page Ref: 621

7) Natalya is concerned because her feces are a chalky white color. Explain why this might occur. Why should Natalya consult her physician?

Answer: The lack of a normal brown color indicates lack of stercobilin. Stercobilin is produced from urobilinogen, which is produced from bilirubin by bacteria in the large intestine. The most likely scenario is a problem with delivery of bile (containing bilirubin) into the intestines (e.g., a blockage), or a problem in the liver that prevents formation of bilirubin. Natalya may need surgical intervention for a possible blockage, and if the liver is not working properly, then it would be important to find the precipitating cause.

Page Ref: 618

8) Describe the negative feedback loop that controls the rate of erythropoiesis. Under what circumstances would you expect the rate of erythropoiesis to be increased? How would it be possible to tell if the rate of erythropoiesis is elevated?

Answer: Hypoxia in the kidney leads to secretion of erythropoietin, which targets proerythroblasts in red marrow to mature into reticulocytes, which enter circulation to increase oxygen carrying capacity of blood. The rate should be increased in any form of anemia (reduced oxygen carrying capacity of blood), or when oxygen levels in the external environment are low (e.g., high altitudes). High levels of reticulocytes in circulation indicate an increase in erythropoiesis.

Page Ref: 618

9) A patient who is blood type B is inadvertently transfused with type AB blood. Explain the specific interactions, if any, that will occur between the donor's and recipient's blood.

Answer: The anti–A isoantibodies in the recipient's blood will bind to the A antigens on the donated red blood cells, causing them to undergo hemolysis. The donated blood contains neither anti–A nor anti–B antibodies, so the recipient's blood cells are not affected by the immune interaction. Ruptured RBCs release their hemoglobin, which may damage the kidneys.

Page Ref: 628

10) When malaria parasites invade red blood cells, they cause the red blood cells to become sticky, and ultimately cause them to rupture. Based on this information, what would you expect some of the symptoms of malaria to be? Explain your answers.

Answer: It is not necessary for answers to be absolutely correct, only to show appropriate thought processes. Students may suggest 1) intravascular clotting leading to ischemia, 2) hemolytic anemia leading to increased erythropoiesis and high reticulocyte count and possible kidney failure, or 3) increased activity of phagocytes in liver and spleen to handle ruptured RBCs. Other answers may be acceptable based on student reasoning.

Page Ref: 618–625

CHAPTER 20   The Cardiovascular System: The Heart

MULTIPLE CHOICE. Choose the one alternative that best completes the statement or answers the question.

1) Blood flows from the pulmonary veins into the:
   A) pulmonary arteries.
   B) right atrium.
   C) lungs.
   D) left atrium.
   E) left ventricle.

   Answer: D
   Page Ref: 641

2) The space between the parietal and visceral layers of the pericardium is normally filled with:
   A) air.
   B) blood.
   C) adipose tissue.
   D) serous fluid.
   E) serum.

   Answer: D
   Page Ref: 638

3) The bicuspid valve is located between the:
   A) right ventricle and the aorta.
   B) right ventricle and the pulmonary trunk.
   C) left atrium and the left ventricle.
   D) right and left atria.
   E) right and left ventricles.

   Answer: C
   Page Ref: 641

4) There is a semilunar valve between the:
   A) right ventricle and the aorta.
   B) right ventricle and the pulmonary trunk.
   C) left atrium and the left ventricle.
   D) right atrium and right ventricle.
   E) left ventricle and the pulmonary trunk..

   Answer: B
   Page Ref: 641

5) Blood flows from the superior vena cava into the:

    A) right atrium.

    B) inferior vena cava.

    C) left atrium.

    D) aorta.

    E) pulmonary trunk.

Answer: A
Page Ref: 639

6) The layer of the heart wall responsible for its pumping action is the:

    A) fibrous pericardium.

    B) serous pericardium.

    C) epicardium.

    D) myocardium.

    E) endocardium.

Answer: D
Page Ref: 638

7) Excess fluid filling the pericardial space interferes with the heart's pumping ability because:

    A) the fluid compresses the heart so it can't beat normally.

    B) it distorts the gradients needed for ion movements in the cardiac cycle.

    C) it causes cardiac myofibers to swell, so they pull apart from each other.

    D) the fluid dilutes the blood entering the atria.

    E) the fluid stretches the cardiac myofibers too much, and the force of contraction is reduced.

Answer: A
Page Ref: 638

8) Which of the following lists the elements of the heart's conduction system in the correct order?

    A) SA node, AV bundle, bundle branches, AV node, conduction myofibers

    B) AV node, SA node, AV bundle, bundle branches, conduction myofibers

    C) SA node, AV node, AV bundle, bundle branches, conduction myofibers

    D) conduction myofibers, AV bundle, bundle branches, AV node, SA node

    E) SA node, AV bundle, AV node, bundle branches, conduction myofibers

Answer: C
Page Ref: 648–649

9) The fossa ovalis is a prominent depression seen in the:

A) wall of the aorta.

B) interventricular septum.

C) coronary sinus.

D) semilunar valves.

E) interatrial septum.

Answer: E
Page Ref: 639

10) During the normal cardiac cycle, the atria contract when they are directly stimulated by the:

A) SA node.

B) AV node.

C) conduction myofibers.

D) baroreceptors.

E) vagus nerve.

Answer: A
Page Ref: 648

11) The atrioventricular valves close when the:

A) SA node fires.

B) atria contract.

C) vagus nerve stimulates them.

D) ventricles relax.

E) ventricles contract.

Answer: E
Page Ref: 643

12) The myocardium is made of:

A) smooth muscle.

B) cardiac muscle.

C) skeletal muscle.

D) endothelium.

E) dense connective tissue.

Answer: B
Page Ref: 638

13) The trabeculae carneae are:

   A) cords of tissue that prevent the AV valves from everting.
   B) raised bundles of cardiac muscle fibers in the walls of the ventricles that convey part of the heart's conduction system.
   C) ridges in the wall of the right atrium that are essential for conduction of nerve impulses through the atria.
   D) the fibrous rings supporting the valves.
   E) special cells making up the AV bundle.

   Answer: B
   Page Ref: 641

14) Blood flows into the coronary arteries from the:

   A) coronary sinus.
   B) superior vena cava.
   C) descending aorta.
   D) pulmonary trunk.
   E) ascending aorta.

   Answer: E
   Page Ref: 641

15) The function of the chordae tendineae is to:

   A) pull the walls of the ventricles inward during contraction.
   B) open the semilunar valves.
   C) open the AV valves.
   D) prevent eversion of the AV valves during ventricular systole.
   E) hold the heart in place within the mediastinum.

   Answer: D
   Page Ref: 643

16) The initiation of the heart beat is the responsibility of the:

   A) cardiovascular center.
   B) baroreceptors.
   C) vagus nerve.
   D) SA node.
   E) fossa ovalis.

   Answer: D
   Page Ref: 648

17) The decrease in speed of conduction from the AV node through the AV bundle results in:

A) failure of the ventricles to contract.

B) adequate time for the ventricles to fill.

C) delayed opening of the atrioventricular valves.

D) the sensation of a skipped beat.

E) a decrease in the rate of blood flow from the atria to the ventricles.

Answer: B
Page Ref: 651

18) If acetylcholine is applied to the heart, but cardiac output is to remain constant, which of the following would have to happen?

A) Stroke volume must increase.

B) Venous return must decrease.

C) Force of contraction must decrease.

D) Rate of conduction of impulses through the AV bundle must increase.

E) The oxygen content of blood in the coronary circulation must increase.

Answer: A
Page Ref: 660

19) The Frank–Starling Law of the Heart states that:

A) the heart is dependent upon the autonomic nervous system for a stimulus to contract.

B) the heart contracts to the fullest extent possible for the conditions, or not at all.

C) cardiac output equals heart rate times stroke volume.

D) the absolute refractory period for the heart must be longer that the duration of contraction for efficient heart functioning.

E) a greater force of contraction can occur if the heart muscle is stretched first.

Answer: E
Page Ref: 658

20) The role of the papillary muscles is to:

A) secrete pericardial fluid into the pericardial space.

B) hold the heart in position within the mediastinum.

C) tighten the chordae tendineae by contracting during ventricular systole.

D) transmit the action potential to the AV valves.

E) There is no known function.

Answer: C
Page Ref: 643

21) All deoxygenated blood returning from the systemic circulation flows into the:
   A) right atrium.
   B) right ventricle.
   C) coronary sinus.
   D) left atrium.
   E) left ventricle.

   Answer: A
   Page Ref: 645

22) A blockage in the marginal branch of the coronary circulation would most affect the:
   A) right atrium.
   B) right ventricle.
   C) pericardium.
   D) left atrium.
   E) left ventricle.

   Answer: B
   Page Ref: 647

23) Cardiac muscle cells have less sarcoplasmic reticulum than skeletal muscle cells. The effect of this is that cardiac muscle cells:
   A) do not depolarize as quickly.
   B) can function as a single unit.
   C) generate less ATP.
   D) have a smaller intracellular reserve of calcium ions.
   E) are autorhythmic cells.

   Answer: D
   Page Ref: 648

24) A heart beat is normally initiated when:
   A) a nerve impulse arrives from the cardiovascular center in the brain.
   B) a critical volume of blood fills the ventricles.
   C) enough sodium and calcium ions leak into the cells of the SA node to reverse their resting potentials.
   D) enough potassium ions leak out of the cells of the SA node to reverse their resting potentials.
   E) the chordae tendineae recoil after being stretched.

   Answer: C
   Page Ref: 649–650

25) The typical heart sounds are made by the:

    A) vibration of the chordae tendineae.

    B) flow of blood into the coronary arteries.

    C) opening of the valves.

    D) closing of the valves.

    E) recoil of the aorta and pulmonary trunk.

Answer: D
Page Ref: 656

26) On an ECG, depolarization of the ventricles is represented by the:

    A) P wave.

    B) T wave.

    C) QRS complex.

    D) P–Q interval.

    E) S–T segment.

Answer: C
Page Ref: 653

27) On an ECG, depolarization of the atria is represented by the:

    A) P wave.

    B) T wave.

    C) QRS complex.

    D) P–Q interval.

    E) S–T segment.

Answer: A
Page Ref: 653

28) The SA node is located:

    A) near the fossa ovalis in the interatrial septum.

    B) in the left atrial wall near the openings of the right pulmonary veins.

    C) in the right atrial wall near the opening of the superior vena cava.

    D) in the aortic wall near the openings to the coronary arteries.

    E) within the pectinate muscles of the right atrium.

Answer: C
Page Ref: 648

29) The reason that the resting heart rate is lower than the autorhythmic rate of the SA node is that:

    A) at rest, the AV node is the pacemaker, but the SA node operates only in fight-or-flight situations.

    B) norepinephrine keeps calcium ion channels closed.

    C) at rest, potassium ions are prevented from re-entering the intracellular fluid.

    D) acetylcholine from parasympathetic neurons slows the SA node's rate of initiation of action potentials.

    E) the gap junctions between cardiac muscle cells only open in response to input from skeletal muscle proprioceptors during movement.

Answer: D
Page Ref: 650

30) Opening of voltage-gated K^+ channels in cardiac myofibers allows for:

    A) rapid depolarization.

    B) a long refractory period.

    C) repolarization.

    D) rapid conduction between myofibers.

    E) the maintenance of a plateau phase.

Answer: C
Page Ref: 651

31) Increased firing of impulses by the sympathetic nervous system would cause:

    A) an increase in force of contraction of the heart.

    B) a shorter absolute refractory period in the SA node.

    C) vasoconstriction in coronary circulation.

    D) an increase in cardiac output.

    E) All of the above except vasoconstriction in coronary circulation.

Answer: E
Page Ref: 659

32) The function of intercalated discs is to:

    A) initiate the heart beat.

    B) anchor the heart in place within the mediastinum.

    C) prevent eversion of valves.

    D) provide a mechanism for rapid conduction of action potentials among myofibers.

    E) provide an anchoring point for chordae tendineae.

Answer: D
Page Ref: 648

33) Cardiac muscle fibers remain depolarized longer than skeletal muscle fibers because:

   A) voltage-gated Na^+ channels close more quickly to trap Na^+ inside longer.

   B) Ca^{2+} enters the cytosol from the extracellular fluid to contribute more positive charges slightly after Na^+ have entered.

   C) voltage-gated K^+ channels open at the same time as Na^+ channels, allowing more positively charged K^+ to enter

   D) it takes longer to reach threshold, and the duration of depolarization is directly proportional to the time is takes to reach threshold.

   E) the intercalated discs are very thick relative to the rest of the sarcolemma, it takes longer for K^+ to exit the cell to cause repolarization.

   Answer: B
   Page Ref: 651

34) The force of cardiac muscle contraction is influenced primarily by the:

   A) number of calcium ions entering the cells through slow channels.

   B) rate at which sodium ions diffuse into the cells.

   C) number of calcium ions that can be stored in the sarcoplasmic reticulum.

   D) duration of the absolute refractory period.

   E) up-and down-regulation of beta adrenergic receptors on the cells.

   Answer: A
   Page Ref: 651

35) Atrioventricular valves open when:

   A) the chordae tendineae contract.

   B) they are stimulated by the AV node.

   C) ventricular pressure falls below atrial pressure.

   D) atrial pressure falls below ventricular pressure.

   E) the papillary muscles contract.

   Answer: C
   Page Ref: 643

36) The second heart sound (dupp) is created by the:

   A) closing of the atrioventricular valves.

   B) opening of the atrioventricular valves.

   C) closing of the semilunar valves.

   D) opening of the semilunar valves.

   E) vibration of the chordae tendineae during ventricular systole.

   Answer: C
   Page Ref: 656

37) An extended P–Q interval on an ECG usually indicates:

   A) excessive K^+ in the extracellular fluid.

   B) a blockage in the conduction system.

   C) damage to the cardiac myofibers in the ventricles.

   D) enlarged ventricles.

   E) nothing unusual or abnormal.

   Answer: B
   Page Ref: 654

38) **ALL** of the following are **TRUE** regarding the ventricles **EXCEPT**:

   A) the lumen of the left ventricle is rounder than that of the right ventricle.

   B) the wall of the left ventricle is thicker than that of the right ventricle.

   C) walls of both ventricles have trabeculae carneae and papillary muscles.

   D) the left ventricle expels a greater volume of blood per beat than does the right ventricle.
   E) the left ventricle pumps blood to the systemic circulation and the right ventricle pumps blood to the pulmonary circulation.

   Answer: D
   Page Ref: 654

39) Once ventricular pressure falls below atrial pressure:

   A) AV valves open.

   B) the heart is in its relaxation period.

   C) the ventricles begin to fill.

   D) blood flows out of the ventricles.

   E) A, B, and C are all correct.

   Answer: E
   Page Ref: 656

40) All valves are closed during:

   A) atrial systole.

   B) ventricular ejection.

   C) rapid ventricular filling.

   D) diastasis.

   E) isovolumetric contraction.

   Answer: E
   Page Ref: 656

41) If heart rate increases to very high levels, then:
   A) the autonomic nervous system will release more epinephrine to the SA node to stabilize the heart rate.
   B) stroke volume increases to keep cardiac output constant.
   C) the oxygen content of blood falls to levels insufficient to maintain cardiac activity.
   D) end–diastolic volume drops because ventricular filling time is so short.
   E) end–systolic volume increases because the valves are open for only a short time.

   Answer: D
   Page Ref: 658

42) A substance that acts as a negative inotropic agent during contraction of cardiac muscle fibers will:
   A) increase stroke volume by promoting inflow of calcium ions.
   B) decrease stroke volume by preventing inflow of calcium ions.
   C) decrease stroke volume by promoting inflow of calcium ions.
   D) increase stroke volume by preventing inflow of calcium ions.
   E) decrease stroke volume by preventing outflow of calcium ions.

   Answer: B
   Page Ref: 658

43) The term *afterload* refers to:
   A) end–systolic volume.
   B) end–diastolic volume.
   C) the pressure that must be overcome before semilunar valves can open.
   D) the pressure in blood vessels necessary to cause the semilunar valves to close.
   E) the maximum possible cardiac output above resting cardiac output.

   Answer: C
   Page Ref: 658

44) Increased stimulation of the heart by the cardiac accelerator nerves causes:
   A) stimulation by acetylcholine of muscarinic receptors on the SA node and cardiac muscle fibers of the ventricles.
   B) stimulation by norepinephrine of the SA node and of the beta receptors on the cardiac muscle fibers of the ventricles.
   C) stimulation by norepinephrine of the SA node, but no effect on the cardiac muscle fibers of the ventricles.
   D) stimulation by acetylcholine of nicotinic receptors on the SA node and cardiac muscle fibers of the ventricles
   E) stimulation by norepinephrine of the SA node and of the alpha receptors on the cardiac muscle fibers of the ventricles.

   Answer: B
   Page Ref: 659

45) Stimulation of the heart by autonomic nerve fibers traveling with the vagus nerve causes:

    A) increased heart rate and increased ventricular contractility.

    B) decreased heart rate and decreased ventricular contractility.

    C) increased heart rate and no change in ventricular contractility.

    D) decreased heart rate and no change in ventricular contractility.

    E) decreased heart rate and increased ventricular contractility.

Answer: D
Page Ref: 660

46) Normal resting cardiac output for an average adult is approximately:

    A) 70 ml/min.

    B) one liter/min.

    C) 2 liters/min.

    D) 5 liters/min.

    E) 10 liters/min.

Answer: D
Page Ref: 658

47) The sound associated with the closure of the aortic semilunar valves is best heard near the:

    A) superior right point.

    B) superior left point.

    C) inferior right point.

    D) inferior left point.

    E) midpoint of all the above points.

Answer: A
Page Ref: 656

48) The ratio between a person's maximum cardiac output and resting cardiac output is called the:

    A) afterload.

    B) preload.

    C) cardiac reserve.

    D) S–T segment.

    E) stroke volume.

Answer: C
Page Ref: 658

49) An increase in afterload decreases:

A) stroke volume.

B) end–systolic volume.

C) sympathetic autonomic activity.

D) end–diastolic volume.

E) Both A and B are correct.

Answer: E
Page Ref: 659

50) Angina pectoris is:

A) an embryonic structure that develops into the aorta.

B) pain accompanying myocardial ischemia.

C) the heart's location within the mediastinum.

D) part of the cardiac conduction system.

E) the covering of the heart.

Answer: B
Page Ref: 664

MATCHING. Choose the item in column 2 that best matches each item in column 1.

Choose the item from column 2 that best matches each item in column 1.

1) Column 1: carries oxygenated blood to
the left atrium

Column 2: pulmonary vein

Answer: pulmonary vein

Page Ref: 645

2) Column 1: carries deoxygenated blood
from the upper body to the
right atrium

Column 2: superior vena cava

Answer: superior vena cava

Page Ref: 639

3) Column 1: splits into the anterior
interventricular branch and
the circumflex branch

Column 2: left coronary artery

Answer: left coronary artery

Page Ref: 647

4) Column 1: splits into the posterior
interventricular branch and
the marginal branch
Column 2: right coronary artery
Answer: right coronary artery
Page Ref: 647

5) Column 1: drains blood from the anterior
aspect of the heart
Column 2: great cardiac vein
Answer: great cardiac vein
Page Ref: 648

6) Column 1: drains blood from the
posterior aspect of the heart
Column 2: middle cardiac vein
Answer: middle cardiac vein
Page Ref: 648

7) Column 1: receives blood from the left
ventricle
Column 2: aorta
Answer: aorta
Page Ref: 644

8) Column 1: receives blood from the right
ventricle
Column 2: pulmonary trunk
Answer: pulmonary trunk
Page Ref: 645

9) Column 1: formed from the union of the
veins draining the heart
Column 2: coronary sinus
Answer: coronary sinus
Page Ref: 648

10) Column 1: supplies oxygenated blood to
the walls of the left atrium
and left ventricle
Column 2: circumflex branch
Answer: circumflex branch
Page Ref: 647

MATCHING. Choose the item in column 2 that best matches each item in column 1.

Choose the item from column 2 that best matches each item in column 1.

1) Column 1: receives blood from the
   superior vena cava, inferior
   vena cava, and coronary sinus
   Column 2: right atrium
   Answer: right atrium
   Page Ref: 639

2) Column 1: receives blood from the
   pulmonary veins
   Column 2: left atrium
   Answer: left atrium
   Page Ref: 641

3) Column 1: pumps blood into the
   pulmonary trunk
   Column 2: right ventricle
   Answer: right ventricle
   Page Ref: 641

4) Column 1: pumps blood into the aorta
   Column 2: left ventricle
   Answer: left ventricle
   Page Ref: 641

5) Column 1: located between the right
   atrium and the right ventricle
   Column 2: tricuspid valve
   Answer: tricuspid valve
   Page Ref: 639

6) Column 1: located between the left
   atrium and the left ventricle
   Column 2: bicuspid valve
   Answer: bicuspid valve
   Page Ref: 641

7) Column 1: opens when left ventricular pressure rises above 80 mm Hg.

Column 2: aortic semilunar valve

Answer: aortic semilunar valve

Page Ref: 641

8) Column 1: opens when right ventricular pressure rises above 15 mm Hg.

Column 2: pulmonary semilunar valve

Answer: pulmonary semilunar valve

Page Ref: 641

9) Column 1: located in atrial wall near opening of superior vena cava

Column 2: SA node

Answer: SA node

Page Ref: 648

10) Column 1: located in interatrial septum

Column 2: AV node

Answer: AV node

Page Ref: 650

TRUE/FALSE. Write 'T' if the statement is true and 'F' if the statement is false.

1) The apex of the heart is directed superiorly.

Answer: FALSE
Page Ref: 636

2) The visceral layer of the serous pericardium is also known as the epicardium.

Answer: TRUE
Page Ref: 638

3) The pectinate muscles anchor the chordae tendineae.

Answer: FALSE
Page Ref: 639

4) The bicuspid valve is located between the right atrium and the right ventricle.

Answer: FALSE
Page Ref: 641

5) The endocardium forms the fibrous skeleton of the heart.

Answer: FALSE
Page Ref: 642

6) Chordae tendineae prevent the eversion of AV valves.

Answer: TRUE
Page Ref: 643

7) Blood in the pulmonary veins flows into the pulmonary capillaries to pick up oxygen.

Answer: FALSE
Page Ref: 646

8) The anterior interventricular branch and the circumflex branch are branches of the right coronary artery.

Answer: FALSE
Page Ref: 647

9) The middle cardiac vein drains the anterior aspect of the heart.

Answer: FALSE
Page Ref: 648

10) The SA node is the heart's pacemaker because it initiates action potentials at a faster rate than other areas of the conduction system.

Answer: TRUE
Page Ref: 650

11) During the plateau phase of an action potential in a cardiac contractile fiber, voltage–gated slow Ca^{2+} channels open.

Answer: TRUE
Page Ref: 651

12) Increasing the concentration of calcium ions in the cytosol of a cardiac contractile fiber decreases the force of contraction.

Answer: FALSE
Page Ref: 651

13) Stroke volume equals the end–diastolic volume minus the end–systolic volume.

Answer: TRUE
Page Ref: 656

14) An increase in heart rate will increase end–diastolic volume.

Answer: FALSE
Page Ref: 658

15) The resting heart rate is usually lower than the autorhythmic rate of the SA node due to the effects of the parasympathetic nervous system.

Answer: TRUE
Page Ref: 660

SHORT ANSWER. Write the word or phrase that best completes each statement or answers the question.

1) The membrane surrounding and protecting the heart is the _____.
Answer: pericardium
Page Ref: 638

2) The epicardium is composed of _____ and delicate connective tissue; the myocardium is composed of _____; the endocardium is composed of _____ over a thin layer of connective tissue.
Answer: mesothelium; cardiac muscle; endothelium
Page Ref: 638

3) Cardiac tamponade results from compression created by the buildup of fluid in the _____.
Answer: pericardial space
Page Ref: 638

4) Pectinate muscles are present in the walls of the _____ , and papillary muscles are present in the walls of the _____.
Answer: right atrium; ventricles
Page Ref: 639

5) Valves are composed of _____ covered by _____.
Answer: dense connective tissue; endocardium
Page Ref: 639

6) Most of the base of the heart is formed by the _____ , while the apex of the heart is formed by the _____.
Answer: left atrium; left ventricle
Page Ref: 641

7) The pulmonary semilunar valve is located between the _____ and the pulmonary trunk, and the aortic semilunar valve is located between the _____ and the aorta.

Answer: right ventricle; left ventricle

Page Ref: 641

8) The _____ ventricle has a smaller workload than the _____ ventricle because it only needs to pump blood to the _____.

Answer: right; left; lungs (pulmonary circuit)

Page Ref: 642

9) As pressure in the ventricles rises, the _____ valves open, while the _____ valves close.

Answer: semilunar; AV

Page Ref: 644

10) Blood flows from the superior and inferior venae cavae into the _____.

Answer: right atrium

Page Ref: 646

11) The _____ branch of the left coronary artery distributes oxygenated blood to the walls of the left atrium and left ventricle.

Answer: circumflex

Page Ref: 647

12) Thickenings of the sarcolemmas called _____ hold cardiac muscle fibers together.

Answer: intercalated discs

Page Ref: 648

13) Normally the atria contract in response to an action potential generated by the _____.

Answer: SA node

Page Ref: 648

14) The electrical connection between the atria and ventricles is the _____.

Answer: AV bundle

Page Ref: 650

15) An action potential originating in the SA node ultimately reaches the cardiac muscle fibers of the ventricles via large-diameter cells known as _____.

Answer: conduction myofibers

Page Ref: 650

16) When a site other than the SA node becomes the pacemaker, that site is called a(n) _____ pacemaker.

Answer: ectopic

Page Ref: 650

17) In the heart's conduction system, the action potential is conducted most slowly between the _____ and the _____ , which gives the ventricles a chance to fill as completely as possible.

Answer: AV node; AV bundle

Page Ref: 651

18) The depolarization phase of a cardiac action potential occurs with the opening of voltage-gated fast _____ channels; the plateau phase involves the opening of voltage-gated slow _____ channels; repolarization results when voltage-gated _____ channels open.

Answer: sodium ion; calcium ion; potassium ion

Page Ref: 651

19) Calcium ions allow contraction of cardiac muscle fibers by binding to the regulator protein _____.

Answer: troponin

Page Ref: 651

20) An ECG can be used to determine three conditions: 1) _____; 2) _____; 3) _____.

Answer: status of the conduction pathway; enlargement of the heart; presence of myocardial damage

Page Ref: 653

21) The three upward deflections on an ECG are the _____ , the _____ , and the _____. The first represents _____ , the second represents _____ , and the third represents _____.

Answer: P wave; QRS complex; T wave; atrial depolarization; ventricular depolarization; ventricular repolarization (order doesn't matter, but answers from first sentence must be matched appropriately with answers in the second sentence)

Page Ref: 653

22) On an ECG, conduction time from the beginning of atrial excitation to the beginning of ventricular excitation is represented by the _____.

Answer: P-Q interval

Page Ref: 654

23) During the isovolumetric relaxation phase of the cardiac cycle, the AV valves are _____ and the semilunar valves are _____.

Answer: closed; closed

Page Ref: 656

24) The relaxation period of the cardiac cycle includes the three periods known as _____, _____, and _____.

Answer: isovolumetric relaxation; rapid ventricular filling; diastasis

Page Ref: 656

25) During the period of ventricular filling, the AV valves are _____ and the semilunar valves are _____.

Answer: open; closed

Page Ref: 656

26) During the period of isovolumetric contraction, the AV valves are _____ and the semilunar valves are _____.

Answer: closed; closed

Page Ref: 656

27) The end-systolic volume is the volume of blood that _____ at the end of systole.

Answer: remains in a ventricle

Page Ref: 656

28) Cardiac output equals _____ times _____.

Answer: stroke volume; heart rate

Page Ref: 658

29) The three important factors affecting stroke volume are _____, _____, and _____.

Answer: preload; contractility; afterload

Page Ref: 658

30) If preload is constant and a substance is applied to the heart that increases calcium ion inflow during a cardiac action potential, then contractility will _____.

Answer: increase

Page Ref: 658

31) Cardiac accelerator nerves extend from the _____ to the _____; these nerves contain _____ autonomic neurons.

Answer: thoracic spinal cord; SA node; sympathetic

Page Ref: 659

32) Norepinephrine enhances contractility by increasing the number of _____ entering cardiac muscle cells via voltage-gated channels.

Answer: calcium ions

Page Ref: 659

33) Parasympathetic neurons reach the heart via the _____ nerves.

Answer: vagus

Page Ref: 659

34) The heart sounds are caused by _____.

Answer: turbulence in the blood as the valves close

Page Ref: 656

35) Depolarization of cardiac muscle fibers lasts much longer than that of skeletal muscle fibers due to the influx of _____ into the cytosol from the ECF.

Answer: calcium ions

Page Ref: 651

ESSAY. Write your answer in the space provided or on a separate sheet of paper.

1) A person who is hemorrhaging has a very rapid heart rate. Using your knowledge of the formulas governing cardiac function, explain why. Do you think a rapid heart rate will improve or exacerbate the situation? Why or why not?

Answer: The decrease in blood volume means a decrease in the blood available for end-diastolic volume. If EDV decreases, then stroke volume decreases. If stroke volume decreases, then cardiac output decreases. The increase in heart rate is an attempt to maintain cardiac output (CO = HR X SV), but if the heart rate increases too much, the EDV decreases even further, since ventricular filling time is too short.

Page Ref: 655-658

2) Steve is at the starting line of his big race at the track meet. His heart rate is elevated while at the starting line, and it increases dramatically as the race begins. Explain what is happening with Steve's heart rate.

Answer: At the starting line, higher brain centers are probably increasing sympathetic fight-or-flight activity. Proprioceptors in muscles and joints send nerve impulses to the cardiovascular center in the medulla to increase heart rate as physical activity begins. Chemoreceptors and baroreceptors also provide feedback to the cardiovascular center. (note: More can be expected if Chapter 21 is included.)

Page Ref: 659

3) Explain the importance of calcium ions to cardiac physiology.

Answer: Calcium ions are responsible for the plateau phase following depolarization. As calcium ions enter the cytosol from the ECF through voltage-gated slow channels and from the sarcoplasmic reticulum, depolarization is maintained for 250 msec, thus allowing complete ventricular filling. Calcium also binds to troponin to allow sliding of actin and myosin filaments during contraction, and changes in calcium ion levels alter the force of contraction, and thus, stroke volume.

Page Ref: 651; 658

4) Coarctation of the aorta is a congenital defect in which a segment of the aorta is too narrow. Predict what the heart would need to do to compensate for this problem. Explain your answer.

Answer: Answers need not be absolutely correct —just thoughtful. Students should suggest that blocked flow leads to increased pressure proximal to the blockage. The heart must increase the force of contraction and stroke volume to push blood through the semilunar valve and into the aorta (increased afterload). Chronically high blood pressure may lead to congestive heart failure. Other answers may be acceptable depending on rationale given.

Page Ref: 658

5) Explain how regular exercise reduces the risk of heart disease.

Answer: Maximum cardiac output and maximum oxygen delivery are increased by increasing the stroke volume while decreasing the heart rate, thus increasing pumping efficiency. Accompanying weight loss reduces blood pressure. Also, HDLs are increased and triglycerides decreased, both helping to decrease the risk of plaque buildup. Increased fibrinolytic activity reduces the risk of intravascular clotting.

Page Ref: 662

6) Describe how the histological structure of the heart supports its function as a pump.

Answer: Cardiac muscle fibers form two separate networks (that of the atria and that of the ventricles). Cells within each network are branched and interconnected via intercalated discs. These discs contain desmosomes and gap junctions. The latter allow action potentials to spread among fibers so that all cells within the network contract as a single functional unit.

Page Ref: 648

7) Define *stenosis* as it relates to heart valves. If stenosis were chronic and severe, what effects would you expect to see on the heart's pumping ability? Explain your answer.

Answer: Stenosis is the narrowing of a valve, usually via scar formation or congenital defect. This leads to a need for an increased force of contraction to open the valve. Depending on which valve is involved, effects may be more or less severe—e.g., aortic stenosis leading to increased left ventricular afterload, ultimately to congestive heart failure. Student answers need not be absolutely correct, but merely thoughtful.

Page Ref: 657-659

8) State the Frank–Starling Law of the Heart, and explain its relationship to cardiac output using the appropriate formula for determining cardiac output.

Answer: A greater preload (EDV, stretch) on cardiac muscle fibers just before they contract increases the force of contraction. Because preload directly affects stroke volume, as EDV increases so does stroke volume; thus force of contraction remains appropriate for the volume in the ventricles. Because CO = HR X SV, as stroke volume increases, so does cardiac output (assuming heart rate stays constant).

Page Ref: 658

9) Describe the role of the autonomic nervous system in regulating heart rate, and explain the effect on cardiac output using the appropriate formula for determining cardiac output.

Answer: The cardiovascular center in the medulla oblongata initiates increases or decreases in heart rate by altering the rate of depolarization of the SA node. Sympathetic stimulation increases heart rate via norepinephrine and epinephrine. Parasympathetic stimulation decreases heart rate via acetylcholine. Because CO = HR X SV, as heart rate increases so does cardiac output (to a point), and as the heart rate decreases so does cardiac output (assuming stroke volume stays constant).

Page Ref: 659–660

10) Define stroke volume and discuss how stroke volume can be altered. Explain the effect of changes in stroke volume on cardiac output using the appropriate formula for determining cardiac output.

Answer: Stroke volume is the volume of blood ejected by each ventricle per contraction. Stroke volume is affected by preload (EDV) that stretches cardiac muscle, myocardial contractility (force of contraction at a given preload), and afterload (pressure needed to open the semilunar valves). Force of contraction increases if EDV increases (Frank–Starling), or if inflow of calcium ions into cardiac muscle fibers increases. Increased afterload decreases stroke volume. Because CO = HR X SV, changes in stroke volume have a direct effect (i.e., as oppposed to an inverse effect) on cardiac output.

Page Ref: 658

CHAPTER 21   The Cardiovascular System: Blood Vessels and Hemodynamics

MULTIPLE CHOICE. Choose the one alternative that best completes the statement or answers the question.

1) The basilar artery is formed by the union of the:
   A) internal jugular veins.
   B) vertebral arteries.
   C) internal carotid arteries.
   D) posterior cerebral arteries.
   E) middle cerebral arteries.

   Answer: B
   Page Ref: 697

2) The hepatic portal vein is formed by the union of the superior mesenteric vein and the:
   A) hepatic artery.
   B) inferior mesenteric vein.
   C) splenic vein.
   D) pancreatic vein.
   E) hepatic vein.

   Answer: C
   Page Ref: 726

3) The function of baroreceptors is to monitor changes in:
   A) heart rate.
   B) stroke volume.
   C) peripheral resistance.
   D) blood pressure.
   E) blood viscosity.

   Answer: D
   Page Ref: 683

4) Baroreceptors are located in the:

   A) wall of the right ventricle.

   B) medulla oblongata.

   C) SA node.

   D) walls of the aorta and carotid arteries.

   E) walls of the capillaries.

   Answer: D
   Page Ref: 683

5) The vasomotor region of the cardiovascular center directly controls:

   A) heart rate by stimulating the SA node.

   B) stroke volume by regulating total blood volume.

   C) peripheral resistance by changing the diameter of blood vessels.

   D) peripheral resistance by altering blood viscosity.

   E) total blood volume by regulating release of ADH from the posterior pituitary gland.

   Answer: C
   Page Ref: 682

6) The internal jugular veins receive blood from the:

   A) superior vena cava.

   B) brachiocephalic veins.

   C) sigmoid sinuses.

   D) internal iliac veins.

   E) subclavian veins.

   Answer: C
   Page Ref: 712

7) The first major branch off the aorta below the diaphragm is the:

   A) left subclavian artery.

   B) brachiocephalic trunk.

   C) celiac artery.

   D) superior mesenteric artery.

   E) renal artery.

   Answer: C
   Page Ref: 702

8) The primary arteries of the pelvis are the:
   A) gonadal arteries.
   B) renal arteries.
   C) femoral arteries.
   D) internal iliac arteries.
   E) external iliac arteries.

   Answer: D
   Page Ref: 707

9) The left colic, sigmoid, and superior rectal arteries are all branches of the:
   A) aorta.
   B) brachiocephalic trunk.
   C) celiac artery.
   D) superior mesenteric artery.
   E) inferior mesenteric artery.

   Answer: E
   Page Ref: 704

10) Blood in the vertebral veins flows next into the:
    A) sigmoid sinuses.
    B) brachiocephalic veins.
    C) common carotid veins.
    D) internal jugular veins.
    E) subclavian veins.

    Answer: B
    Page Ref: 713

11) Anterior to the elbows, the median cubital veins connect the:
    A) axillary and brachial veins.
    B) cephalic and brachial veins.
    C) radial and ulnar veins.
    D) cephalic and basilic veins.
    E) basilic and brachial veins.

    Answer: D
    Page Ref: 715

12) If the inferior vena cava or hepatic portal vein becomes obstructed, blood can be returned from the lower body to the superior vena cava via the:

A) azygos vein.

B) hepatic vein.

C) superior mesenteric vein.

D) brachiocephalic vein.

E) None of these—there is no way blood from the lower body can reach the superior vena cava.

Answer: A
Page Ref: 718

13) Which of the following flows directly into the inferior vena cava?

A) internal iliac vein.

B) hepatic portal vein.

C) superior vena cava.

D) hepatic vein.

E) All of these are correct.

Answer: D
Page Ref: 721

14) Blood in the great saphenous vein flows into the:

A) femoral vein.

B) popliteal vein.

C) peroneal vein.

D) inferior vena cava.

E) internal iliac vein.

Answer: A
Page Ref: 722

15) Deoxygenated blood in the fetal circulation is carried in the:

A) umbilical vein.

B) umbilical artery.

C) ductus venosus.

D) Both A and C are correct.

E) Both B and C are correct.

Answer: B
Page Ref: 728

16) The tunica interna of a blood vessel is made of:
   A) smooth muscle.
   B) cardiac muscle.
   C) skeletal muscle.
   D) endothelium.
   E) dense connective tissue.

   Answer: D
   Page Ref: 670

17) Valves are present in:
   A) arteries.
   B) arterioles.
   C) veins.
   D) capillaries.
   E) All of the above except capillaries.

   Answer: C
   Page Ref: 674

18) The layer of a blood vessel wall that determines the diameter of the lumen is the:
   A) adventitia.
   B) tunica externa.
   C) tunica interna.
   D) tunica media.
   E) vasa vasorum.

   Answer: D
   Page Ref: 670

19) A deficiency of ADH would result in:
   A) reduced venous return.
   B) a drop in systemic blood pressure.
   C) reduced stroke volume.
   D) decreased cardiac output.
   E) All of the above are correct.

   Answer: E
   Page Ref: 687

20) Increased levels of epinephrine cause:

   A) a decrease in systemic blood pressure due to net vasodilation.

   B) an increase in systemic blood pressure due to net vasoconstriction.

   C) a decrease in systemic blood pressure due to a decrease in force of contraction in cardiac muscle.

   D) an increase in systemic vascular resistance due to an increase in the rate of erythropoiesis.

   E) a decrease in systemic blood pressure due to increased movement of fluid from plasma to the interstitial fluid.

   Answer: B
   Page Ref: 685

21) An increase in venous return most directly affects:

   A) blood pressure.

   B) systemic vascular resistance.

   C) stroke volume.

   D) blood viscosity.

   E) heart rate.

   Answer: C
   Page Ref: 680

22) The viscosity of blood most directly affects:

   A) venous return.

   B) stroke volume.

   C) systemic vascular resistance.

   D) heart rate.

   E) net filtration pressure.

   Answer: C
   Page Ref: 680

23) Increased levels of aldosterone cause:

   A) an increase in venous return because more water is reabsorbed into the blood from the kidneys to increase total blood volume.

   B) increased vasodilation because of direct hormone action on the tunica media of arterioles.

   C) decreased heart rate because of the decrease in the sodium ion gradient in the SA node.

   D) a decrease in systemic blood pressure because of increased fluid loss from the kidneys.

   E) an increase in blood viscosity because of the addition of water and sodium ions to the plasma.

   Answer: A
   Page Ref: 687

24) Blood flow increases if:

   A) vasodilation increases.

   B) sympathetic stimulation to vessels with alpha adrenergic receptors increases.

   C) blood viscosity increases.

   D) net filtration pressure increases.

   E) parasympathetic stimulation to the heart increases.

   Answer: A
   Page Ref: 682

25) Starling's Law of the Capillaries states that:

   A) blood flows more slowly through capillaries than arteries or veins because of their smaller diameter.

   B) the volume of fluid reabsorbed at the venous end of a capillary is nearly equal to the volume of fluid filtered out at the arterial end.

   C) if blood pressure is low, blood is diverted around large capillary beds.

   D) if oxygen levels are low, blood is diverted into large capillary beds.

   E) blood pressure in capillaries equals cardiac output divided by resistance.

   Answer: B
   Page Ref: 676

26) Net filtration pressure equals:

   A) $($blood hydrostatic pressure $+$ blood colloid osmotic pressure$)$ $-$ $($interstitial fluid hydrostatic pressure $+$ interstitial fluid osmotic pressure$)$

   B) $($blood hydrostatic pressure $+$ interstitial fluid osmotic pressure$)$ $-$ $($blood colloid osmotic pressure $+$ interstitial fluid hydrostatic pressure$)$

   C) $($blood hydrostatic pressure $-$ blood colloid osmotic pressure$)$ $-$ $($interstitial fluid hydrostatic pressure $-$ interstitial fluid osmotic pressure$)$

   D) $($blood hydrostatic pressure $+$ interstitial fluid hydrostatic pressure$)$ $-$ $($blood colloid osmotic pressure $+$ interstitial fluid osmotic pressure$)$

   E) $($blood hydrostatic pressure $-$ interstitial fluid hydrostatic pressure$)$ $+$ $($blood colloid osmotic pressure $-$ interstitial fluid osmotic pressure$)$

   Answer: B
   Page Ref: 677

27) Of the pressure involved in determining net filtration pressure, the highest pressure at the arterial end of a capillary is usually:

   A) interstitial fluid hydrostatic pressure.

   B) interstitial fluid osmotic pressure.

   C) blood colloid osmotic pressure.

   D) blood hydrostatic pressure.

   E) blood hydrostatic pressure and blood colloid osmotic pressure are always equally high.

   Answer: D
   Page Ref: 677

28) Of the pressure involved in determining net filtration pressure, the highest pressure at the venous end of a capillary is usually:

A) interstitial fluid hydrostatic pressure.

B) interstitial fluid osmotic pressure.

C) blood colloid osmotic pressure.

D) blood hydrostatic pressure.

E) blood hydrostatic pressure and blood colloid osmotic pressure are always equally high.

Answer: C
Page Ref: 677

29) Most fluid and proteins that escape from blood vessels to the interstitial fluid are normally:

A) excreted via the urinary system.

B) reabsorbed via the urinary system.

C) returned to the blood via the hepatic portal system.

D) returned to the blood via the lymphatic system.

E) absorbed into tissue cells.

Answer: D
Page Ref: 678

30) If blood hydrostatic pressure equals 30 mm Hg, blood colloid osmotic pressure equals 26 mm Hg, interstitial fluid osmotic pressure equals 5 mm Hg, and interstitial fluid hydrostatic pressure equals 2 mm Hg, the net filtration pressure will be:

A) +7 mm Hg.

B) −7 mm Hg.

C) +1 mm Hg.

D) −1 mm Hg.

E) +49 mm Hg.

Answer: A
Page Ref: 677

31) If blood hydrostatic pressure equals 30 mm Hg, blood colloid osmotic pressure equals 26 mm Hg, interstitial fluid osmotic pressure equals 5 mm Hg, and interstitial fluid hydrostatic pressure equals 2 mm Hg, the net filtration pressure will:

A) tend to filter fluids and solutes.

B) tend to reabsorb fluids and solutes.

C) not be useful because interstitial fluid hydrostatic pressure can't be greater than 1 mm Hg.

D) indicate no net movement of fluids or solutes.

E) be impossible to calculate.

Answer: A
Page Ref: 677

32) If mean arterial blood pressure is 80 mm Hg, the blood pressure measured with the sphygmomanometer might have been:

A) recorded improperly, because there should be two numbers.

B) $\dfrac{150}{70}$.

C) $\dfrac{120}{60}$.

D) $\dfrac{120}{80}$.

E) There is no way to know.

Answer: C
Page Ref: 679

33) If plasma proteins are lost due to kidney disease, then which of the following pressure changes occur as a direct result?

A) Blood hydrostatic pressure increases.

B) Blood colloid osmotic pressure increases.

C) Interstitial fluid hydrostatic pressure decreases.

D) Blood colloid osmotic pressure decreases.

E) Interstitial fluid osmotic pressure decreases.

Answer: D
Page Ref: 677

34) If lymph channels are blocked, then in areas drained by the blocked vessels:

A) interstitial fluid hydrostatic pressure increases.

B) blood hydrostatic pressure increases.

C) blood colloid osmotic pressure increases.

D) interstitial fluid hydrostatic pressure decreases.

E) interstitial fluid osmotic pressure decreases.

Answer: A
Page Ref: 677

35) Blood flows most slowly through:

A) elastic arteries because of the elastic tissue in the walls.

B) superior and inferior venae cavae because of their large diameters and thin walls.

C) superior and inferior venae cavae because of their low pressure.

D) capillaries because of their small diameters.

E) capillaries because their total cross–sectional area is the largest.

Answer: E
Page Ref: 678

36) Blood pressure would be highest in which of the following vessels?

   A) superior sagittal sinus.

   B) brachiocephalic trunk.

   C) inferior vena cava.

   D) right subclavian vein.

   E) blood pressure is the same in all vessels.

   Answer: B
   Page Ref: 679

37) Cardiac output equals:

   A) stroke volume × resistance.

   B) mean arterial blood pressure × resistance.

   C) $\dfrac{\text{stroke volume}}{\text{resistance}}$.

   D) $\dfrac{\text{mean arterial blood pressure}}{\text{resistance}}$.

   E) mean arterial blood pressure × heart rate.

   Answer: D
   Page Ref: 679

38) The diameter of blood vessels most directly affects:

   A) venous return.

   B) blood viscosity.

   C) resistance.

   D) heart rate.

   E) stroke volume.

   Answer: C
   Page Ref: 680

39) To say that smooth muscle in arteriole walls exhibits a *myogenic response* means that:

   A) more smooth muscle cells are added as blood pressure remains chronically high.

   B) the cells possess beta adrenergic receptors for response to epinephrine.

   C) the cells respond to sympathetic cholinergic stimulation.

   D) the cells contract only in response to stimulation by vasomotor nerves.

   E) the cells contract more forcefully when stretched by increased blood flow.

   Answer: E
   Page Ref: 686

40) During compensated shock, production of **ALL** of the following hormones increases **EXCEPT**:

A) atrial natriuretic peptide.

B) angiotensin II.

C) epinephrine.

D) aldosterone.

E) ADH.

Answer: A
Page Ref: 688

41) Standing still for long periods may decrease cardiac output because:

A) too much lactic acid is produced, so blood vessels dilate and blood pressure drops.

B) heart rate falls too low to maintain cardiac output without proprioceptive input to the cardiovascular center.

C) venous return decreases due to lack of skeletal muscle pumping of veins, so stroke volume drops.

D) increased blood colloid osmotic pressure allows plasma to leak into the interstitial fluid.

E) parasympathetic activity causes vasodilation.

Answer: C
Page Ref: 681

42) The major regulator of regional blood flow in the brain is:

A) autoregulation.

B) aldosterone.

C) angiotensin.

D) the carotid sinus reflex.

E) the aortic reflex.

Answer: A
Page Ref: 686

43) Kristen is allergic to bee venom, and when she goes into anaphylactic shock, epinephrine is administered. This is, in part, because:

A) she has an abnormal parasympathetic response that causes loss of vasomotor tone.

B) the immune response to the venom clogs the vessels, and epinephrine opens them.

C) the venom binds to the cardiovascular center neurons and decreases sympathetic activity.

D) the venom itself alters capillary permeability and increases plasma loss to the interstitial fluid, so epinephrine returns capillary permeability to normal.

E) histamine, a potent vasodilator has been released, and epinephrine stimulates vasoconstriction.

Answer: E
Page Ref: 687

44) "ACE inhibitors" work as antihypertensive drugs by:

A) blocking renin release.

B) binding to the cardiovascular center to decrease sympathetic stimulation.

C) blocking release of ADH.

D) decreasing angiotensin II formation.

E) binding to aldosterone receptors in the kidney.

Answer: D
Page Ref: 733

45) Resting pulse rate in an average adult is:

A) 40–50 beats per minute.

B) 50–60 beats per minute.

C) 70–80 beats per minute.

D) 90–100 beats per minute.

E) at least 120 beats per minute.

Answer: C
Page Ref: 689

46) A superficial vein in the leg that is frequently used for prolonged administration of IV fluids is the:

A) femoral.

B) popliteal.

C) great saphenous.

D) common iliac.

E) peroneal.

Answer: C
Page Ref: 722

47) Blood flows into the left common carotid artery from the:

A) arch of the aorta.

B) brachiocephalic trunk.

C) right common carotid artery.

D) left subclavian artery.

E) left internal carotid artery.

Answer: A
Page Ref: 698

48) Vessels that are part of the cerebral arterial circle include the:
   A) superior and inferior sagittal sinuses.
   B) external carotid arteries.
   C) internal carotid arteries.
   D) vertebral arteries.
   E) All of the above except the sagittal sinuses.

   Answer: C
   Page Ref: 697

49) Blood flows directly into the superior vena cava from the:
   A) inferior vena cava.
   B) brachiocephalic veins.
   C) coronary sinus.
   D) internal jugular veins.
   E) axillary veins.

   Answer: B
   Page Ref: 713

50) Compared with systemic capillaries pulmonary capillaries have:
   A) large spaces between their endothelial cells.
   B) a much lower blood colloid osmotic pressure.
   C) thicker walls.
   D) a much higher net filtration pressure.
   E) a much lower blood hydrostatic pressure.

   Answer: E
   Page Ref: 726

MATCHING. Choose the item in column 2 that best matches each item in column 1.

Choose the item from column 2 that best matches each item in column 1.

1) Column 1: artery
   Column 2: vessel with relatively thick
            wall; blood under highest
            pressure
   Answer: vessel with relatively thick wall; blood under highest pressure
   Page Ref: 670

2) Column 1: vein
   Column 2: vessel with valves; blood
            under lowest pressure
   Answer: vessel with valves; blood under lowest pressure
   Page Ref: 674

3) Column 1: fenestrated capillary
   Column 2: special capillary in which
             plasma membranes of
             endothelial cells contain pores

   Answer: special capillary in which plasma membranes of endothelial cells contain pores

   Page Ref: 673

4) Column 1: arteriole
   Column 2: nearly microscopic vessel that
             plays key role in regulating
             flow into capillaries

   Answer: nearly microscopic vessel that plays key role in regulating flow into capillaries

   Page Ref: 672

5) Column 1: venule
   Column 2: formed by the merging of
             capillaries

   Answer: formed by the merging of capillaries

   Page Ref: 674

6) Column 1: thoroughfare channel
   Column 2: low resistance pathway
             bypassing a capillary bed; the
             distal end of a metarteriole

   Answer: low resistance pathway bypassing a capillary bed; the distal end of a metarteriole

   Page Ref: 672

7) Column 1: vasa vasorum
   Column 2: vessels providing blood flow
             to the cells in walls of large
             vessels

   Answer: vessels providing blood flow to the cells in walls of large vessels

   Page Ref: 670

8) Column 1: sinusoid
   Column 2: special capillary with spaces
             between endothelial cells and
             lacking a complete basement
             membrane

   Answer: special capillary with spaces between endothelial cells and lacking a complete
           basement membrane

   Page Ref: 673

9) Column 1: vascular sinus
   Column 2: vein whose wall lacks smooth
             muscle and is supported by
             dense connective tissue
   Answer: vein whose wall lacks smooth muscle and is supported by dense connective tissue
   Page Ref: 674

10) Column 1: anastomosis
    Column 2: union of vessels serving the
              same body region, providing
              collateral circulation
    Answer: union of vessels serving the same body region, providing collateral circulation
    Page Ref: 675

MATCHING. Choose the item in column 2 that best matches each item in column 1.

Choose the item from column 2 that best matches each item in column 1.

1) Column 1: right subclavian artery
   Column 2: brachiocephalic trunk
   Answer: brachiocephalic trunk
   Page Ref: 698

2) Column 1: left subclavian artery
   Column 2: aorta
   Answer: aorta
   Page Ref: 698

3) Column 1: brachial artery
   Column 2: axillary artery
   Answer: axillary artery
   Page Ref: 698

4) Column 1: basilar artery
   Column 2: vertebral artery
   Answer: vertebral artery
   Page Ref: 698

5) Column 1: common hepatic artery
   Column 2: celiac artery
   Answer: celiac artery
   Page Ref: 702

6) Column 1: brachiocephalic vein
   Column 2: internal jugular vein
   Answer: internal jugular vein
   Page Ref: 718

7) Column 1: azygos vein
   Column 2: superior vena cava
   Answer: superior vena cava
   Page Ref: 718

8) Column 1: femoral vein
   Column 2: great saphenous vein
   Answer: great saphenous vein
   Page Ref: 722

9) Column 1: posterior tibial vein
   Column 2: peroneal vein
   Answer: peroneal vein
   Page Ref: 722

10) Column 1: axillary vein
    Column 2: basilic vein
    Answer: basilic vein
    Page Ref: 716

TRUE/FALSE. Write 'T' if the statement is true and 'F' if the statement is false.

1) Arteries are defined as those vessels that carry oxygenated blood.

   Answer: FALSE
   Page Ref: 670

2) Parasympathetic stimulation of blood vessels causes vasodilation.

   Answer: FALSE
   Page Ref: 671

3) Normally, the only tissue that blood comes in contact with is endothelium.

   Answer: TRUE
   Page Ref: 670

4) All tissues contain capillaries.

Answer: FALSE
Page Ref: 672

5) Thoroughfare channels carry blood into capillary beds.

Answer: FALSE
Page Ref: 672

6) Sinusoids may allow large molecules and formed elements to pass in and out of the bloodstream.

Answer: TRUE
Page Ref: 673

7) The walls of veins are thinner than those of arteries.

Answer: TRUE
Page Ref: 674

8) At rest, the largest percentage of the total blood volume is in the systemic capillaries.

Answer: FALSE
Page Ref: 675

9) Blood colloid osmotic pressure promotes reabsorption of fluids into the bloodstream.

Answer: TRUE
Page Ref: 676

10) The highest pressure at the venous end of a capillary is normally the blood hydrostatic pressure.

Answer: FALSE
Page Ref: 677

11) A person whose blood pressure is measured at 140/90 has a mean arterial blood pressure of 106.7.

Answer: TRUE
Page Ref: 679

12) An increase in resistance increases cardiac output, while an increase in mean arterial blood pressure causes a decrease in cardiac output.

Answer: FALSE
Page Ref: 679

13) An obese person may develop hypertension due to an increase in the total length of the vascular circuit.

Answer: TRUE
Page Ref: 680

14) A decrease in the diameter of blood vessels increases resistance, and therefore, increases blood pressure.

Answer: TRUE
Page Ref: 681

15) Blood flows from the superior vena cava into the brachiocephalic veins.

Answer: FALSE
Page Ref: 718

SHORT ANSWER. Write the word or phrase that best completes each statement or answers the question.

1) The blood vessels that serve the blood vessel walls are called the _____.

Answer: vasa vasorum
Page Ref: 670

2) The layer of a blood vessel wall that is closest to the lumen is the tunica _____ , which is composed of _____ , a basement membrane, and elastic tissue.

Answer: interna; endothelium
Page Ref: 670

3) The tunica media of a blood vessel wall is composed of _____ fibers and _____ fibers.

Answer: elastic; smooth muscle
Page Ref: 670

4) Increased sympathetic stimulation to blood vessel walls typically causes _____.

Answer: vasoconstriction
Page Ref: 671

5) Two examples of elastic arteries include the _____ and the _____ arteries.

Answer: any two of the following: aorta, brachiocephalic, common carotid, subclavian, vertebral, pulmonary, or common iliac
Page Ref: 671

6) A vessel that emerges from an arteriole to supply a capillary bed is called a(n) _____.

Answer: metarteriole.
Page Ref: 672

7) The ring of smooth muscle fibers that regulates blood flow into a capillary bed is called a(n) _____.

Answer: precapillary sphincter

Page Ref: 673

8) Three types of capillaries include the _____ , found in skeletal and smooth muscle, the _____ , found in kidneys, and the _____ , found in the liver and red bone marrow.

Answer: continuous capillaries; fenestrated capillaries; sinusoids

Page Ref: 673

9) The most important mechanism of capillary exchange is _____.

Answer: simple diffusion

Page Ref: 676

10) Movement of large, lipid–soluble molecules across a capillary membrane via vesicles is called _____.

Answer: transcytosis

Page Ref: 676

11) Pressure–driven movement of fluid and solutes from the blood capillaries into the interstitial fluid is called _____ , while pressure–driven movement from the interstitial fluid into capillaries is called _____.

Answer: filtration; reabsorption

Page Ref: 676

12) The two pressures that promote filtration are _____ and _____ , while the main pressure that promotes reabsorption is _____.

Answer: blood hydrostatic pressure; interstitial fluid osmotic pressure; blood colloid osmotic pressure

Page Ref: 676

13) Blood colloid osmotic pressure is a force caused by the _____.

Answer: colloidal suspension of large plasma proteins

Page Ref: 677

14) Blood flows most slowly through the _____.

Answer: capillaries

Page Ref: 678

15) A person whose blood pressure measures 110/65 has a mean arterial blood pressure of _____ mm Hg.

Answer: 75

Page Ref: 679

16) An abnormal increase in formed elements, such as is seen in leukemia, increases resistance because it increases _____.

Answer: blood viscosity

Page Ref: 680

17) The primary factor affecting blood pressure under normal circumstances is _____.

Answer: blood vessel diameter/radius

Page Ref: 680

18) The part of the cardiovascular center that regulates blood vessel diameter is the _____.

Answer: vasomotor center

Page Ref: 682

19) General systemic blood pressure is regulated via the _____ reflex; nerve impulses generated by baroreceptors in this reflex are conducted via the _____ nerve to the cardiovascular center.

Answer: aortic; vagus

Page Ref: 683

20) Normal blood pressure to the brain is maintained via the _____ reflex; nerve impulses generated by baroreceptors in this reflex are conducted via the _____ nerve to the cardiovascular center.

Answer: carotid sinus; glossopharyngeal

Page Ref: 683

21) _____ is a hormone that is a potent vasoconstrictor and that stimulates secretion of aldosterone.

Answer: Angiotensin II

Page Ref: 685

22) In systemic circulation blood vessels _____ in response to a decrease in oxygen concentration, but in the pulmonary circulation, blood vessels _____ in response to a decrease in oxygen concentration.

Answer: dilate; constrict

Page Ref: 686

23) Failure of the cardiovascular system to deliver enough oxygen and nutrients to meet cellular metabolic needs is called _____.

Answer: shock

Page Ref: 686

24) Hemorrhage can lead to _____ shock, while a myocardial infarction leads to _____ shock.

Answer: hypovolemic; cardiogenic

Page Ref: 687

25) Shock stemming from the action of certain bacterial toxins on blood vessels is called _____ shock.

Answer: septic

Page Ref: 687

26) If hypovolemic shock develops, one would expect to see a(n) _____ in ADH secretion.

Answer: increase

Page Ref: 687

27) A pulse taken posterior to the knee is taken in the _____ artery.

Answer: popliteal

Page Ref: 689

28) The branches of the aorta that carry blood to the lower limbs are the _____ arteries.

Answer: common iliac

Page Ref: 692

29) The brachiocephalic trunk branches to form the _____ and the _____.

Answer: right subclavian artery; right common carotid artery

Page Ref: 696

30) Blood in the renal veins flows next into the _____.

Answer: inferior vena cava

Page Ref: 718

ESSAY. Write your answer in the space provided or on a separate sheet of paper.

1) What is the function of capillaries? How is their structure and arrangement especially suited to their function?

Answer: The function of capillaries is to permit exchange of nutrients, wastes, and gases between the blood and cells via the interstitial fluid. Walls of capillaries consist of a single layer of endothelial cells, so exchange is favored by the short distance traveled. Also, capillaries form networks that serve to increase surface area. This large cross-sectional area favors slow blood flow. Both slow flow and large surface area facilitate capillary exchange.

Page Ref: 672; 678

2) What is venoconstriction and what is its significance?

Answer: Venoconstriction is the constriction of veins in response to increased sympathetic stimulation. Systemic veins and venules contain about 60 percent of the total blood volume. When they constrict, blood in these reservoirs is decreased and flow to skeletal muscles is increased. Such a diversion of flow might occur in cases of hemorrhage, for example.

Page Ref: 676

3) Identify and describe the effects of the forces (pressures) affecting movement of fluids and solutes across a capillary membrane.

Answer: Blood hydrostatic pressure is generated by the pumping action of the heart and is the force of water in blood plasma against the inner walls of vessels. This pressure favors filtration. Blood colloid osmotic pressure is generated by the suspension of plasma proteins and is a reabsorptive force. Interstitial fluid osmotic pressure is generated by proteins that leak into the interstitial fluid. This force tends to promote filtration. Interstitial fluid hydrostatic pressure opposes blood colloid osmotic pressure, but is generally considered to be negligible under normal circumstances.

Page Ref: 677

4) Describe the arterial blood flow from the aorta to the brain. Identify all vessels and describe collateral circulation where appropriate.

Answer: See outline in Exhibit 21.3. Include discussion of the cerebral arterial circle for collateral circulation.

Page Ref: 697–698

5) Describe the mechanisms by which edema can develop.

Answer: Blood hydrostatic pressure may increase due to high blood volume created by excretion problems or due to increased venous pressure created by heart failure or intravascular clotting. Blood colloid osmotic pressure may be low if plasma protein levels are reduced by malnutrition, burns, or liver/kidney disease. Interstitial fluid osmotic pressure may be high if plasma proteins leak out of vessels and water follows in conditions of inflammation or if lymph flow is blocked preventing return of proteins and fluid to blood. (Formula for net filtration pressure is helpful in explaining answers.)

Page Ref: 678

6) Identify and discuss the factors that contribute to systemic vascular resistance.

Answer: 1) Blood viscosity—ratio of formed elements and proteins to plasma; increasing viscosity via increasing formed elements or decreasing plasma volume increases resistance
2) Total blood vessel length—directly proportional to resistance; increasing length of circuit (by adding new blood vessels to serve added tissue) increases resistance
3) Diameter/radius of blood vessels—has major effect on resistance; increased diameter decreases resistance, thus increasing flow; controlled by ANS; small vessels have greater effect because more surface area is in contact with blood

Page Ref: 680

7) Explain the mechanisms by which the autonomic nervous system regulates flow of blood to particular tissues in any given circumstance.

Answer: Control is principally via sympathetic vasomotor nerves. Small arteries and arterioles have alpha adrenergic receptors for norepinephrine, and are vasconstricted when stimulated. Most vessels in skeletal muscle and the heart have beta adrenergic receptors, and are vasodilated when stimulated. Some sympathetic fibers to skeletal muscles are cholinergic, and dilate in response to acetylcholine. Tissues with dilated arterioles receive greater blood flow.

Page Ref: 683

8) List five of the signs and symptoms of circulatory shock. Explain the physiological basis for the development of each.

Answer: Increased epinephrine and norepinephrine cause 1) clammy, cool skin due to vasoconstriction in skin vessels, 2) tachycardia, 3) sweating, and 4) nausea. Decreased cardiac output leads to hypotension and weak rapid pulse, as well as an altered mental state. Decreased urine formation results from increased ADH and aldosterone and from hypotension. Thirst is triggered by loss of ECF. Acidosis results from an increase in production of lactic acid from anaerobic respiration.

Page Ref: 687

9) Explain how the muscular system and respiratory system assist in maintaining venous return.

Answer: Both operate by alternating compression and decompression of veins. Skeletal muscles "milk" blood through the valve system, and pressure gradients change along the course of a vein to open and close valves. The respiratory system creates alternating pressure gradients in the thoracic cavity and abdominal cavity during inhalation and exhalation, again causing valves in veins to open and close as pressures change.

Page Ref: 681

10) The bacteria that cause cholera produce a toxin that alters intestinal permeability causing severe diarrhea. Without treatment, as many as 70 percent of victims die from shock. Explain in detail why fatal shock does or does not develop in these cases.

Answer: Nervous system loops start with baroreceptors sensing a drop in blood pressure as fluid volume falls. Information is transmitted to the cardiovascular center to increase sympathetic stimulation to increase heart rate, force of contraction, and net vasoconstriction. All will increase cardiac output. Endocrine loops include the renin–angiotensin–aldosterone loop, ADH loop, and the epinephrine loop, all of which will either increase fluid volume or enhance vasconstriction (or both). If these loops cannot counteract the fluid loss, total plasma volume decreases to the point that venous return and stroke volume are insufficient to maintain cardiac output. Decreased cardiac output to the heart further reduces force of contraction, and decreased flow to the brain further decreases vasomotor activity increasing net vasodilation. Death results when cardiac output falls too low to maintain vital functions.

Page Ref: 687

CHAPTER 22   The Lymphatic System, Nonspecific Resistance to Disease, and Immunity

MULTIPLE CHOICE. Choose the one alternative that best completes the statement or answers the question.

1) The composition of lymph is most similar to:

   A) plasma.

   B) serum.

   C) cytosol.

   D) interstitial fluid.

   E) intestinal juice.

   Answer: D
   Page Ref: 738

2) The cisterna chyli is:

   A) the point at which lymph is returned to venous blood.

   B) a dilation at the beginning of the thoracic duct.

   C) the embryonic thymus gland.

   D) the organ that produces the largest amount of lymph.

   E) the array of lacteals associated with the small intestine.

   Answer: B
   Page Ref: 741

3) Which of the following correctly lists the structures according to the sequence of fluid flow?
   A) lymphatic capillaries, interstitial spaces, blood capillaries, lymphatic vessels, lymphatic ducts, subclavian veins
   B) blood capillaries, lymphatic vessels, interstitial spaces, lymphatic capillaries, lymphatic ducts, subclavian veins
   C) blood capillaries, interstitial spaces, lymphatic capillaries, lymphatic ducts, lymphatic vessels, subclavian veins
   D) blood capillaries, interstitial spaces, lymphatic capillaries, lymphatic vessels, lymphatic ducts, subclavian veins
   E) blood capillaries, interstitial spaces, lymphatic vessels, lymphatic ducts, lymphatic capillaries, subclavian veins

   Answer: D
   Page Ref: 742

4) One known function of the reticular epithelial cells of the thymus is to:

   A) produce and secrete thymic hormones.

   B) produce and secrete antibodies.

   C) act as antigen-presenting cells.

   D) produce and secrete interleukin-1.

   E) differentiate into natural killer cells.

   Answer: A
   Page Ref: 742

5) B cells proliferate and differentiate into plasma cells in the:

   A) liver.

   B) bloodstream.

   C) germinal centers of lymph nodes.

   D) red pulp of the spleen.

   E) Both C and D are correct.

   Answer: C
   Page Ref: 744

6) Lysozyme is:

   A) an enzyme found in body fluids that flow over epithelial surfaces that destroys certain bacteria.

   B) a type of antibody that makes something more recognizable to a phagocyte.

   C) a cytokine produced by helper T cells.

   D) one of the self-antigens on the surface of antigen-presenting cells.

   E) an antihistamine released by eosinophils.

   Answer: A
   Page Ref: 748

7) Antibodies are:

   A) plasma cells.

   B) B lymphocytes.

   C) T lymphocytes.

   D) gamma globulin glycoproteins.

   E) cytokines released by macrophages.

   Answer: D
   Page Ref: 761

8) In cell-mediated immunity, the antigenic cell/molecule is destroyed by:

A) killer T cells.

B) mast cells.

C) opsonizing antibodies.

D) complement.

E) plasma cells.

Answer: A
Page Ref: 759

9) Antibodies are produced by:

A) macrophages.

B) killer T cells.

C) neutrophils.

D) mast cells.

E) plasma cells.

Answer: E
Page Ref: 760

10) The most common structural class of antibody molecules is:

A) IgA.

B) IgM.

C) IgG.

D) IgD.

E) IgE.

Answer: C
Page Ref: 763

11) Immunoglobulins that circulate in the interstitial spaces and bloodstream attached to mast cells and basophils are classed as:

A) IgA.

B) IgM.

C) IgG.

D) IgD.

E) IgE.

Answer: E
Page Ref: 763

12) Which of the following lists the structures in the correct order of lymph flow through a lymph node?
   A) afferent lymphatic vessels, medullary sinuses, trabecular sinus, subcapsular sinus, efferent lymphatic vessels
   B) efferent lymphatic vessels, trabecular sinus, subcapsular sinus, medullary sinuses, afferent lymphatic vessels
   C) afferent lymphatic vessels, subcapsular sinus, trabecular sinus, medullary sinuses, efferent lymphatic vessels
   D) efferent lymphatic vessels, medullary sinuses, trabecular sinus, subcapsular sinus, afferent lymphatic vessels
   E) Either C or D is correct because lymph can flow either way through a lymph node.

Answer: C
Page Ref: 743–744

13) Which of the following is **NOT** a function of the spleen?
   A) site of stem cell maturation into T and B cells
   B) destruction of blood–borne pathogens by macrophages
   C) removal of worn–out blood cells and platelets by macrophages
   D) storage of platelets
   E) hemopoiesis during fetal development

Answer: A
Page Ref: 746

14) Which of the following would most likely increase a person's risk of invasion by pathogenic microbes?
   A) increased urine flow
   B) loss of epidermal tissue
   C) increased action of cilia
   D) increased intestinal motility
   E) decreased interstitial fluid osmotic pressure

Answer: B
Page Ref: 748

15) The function of interferons is to:
   A) breakdown bacterial cell walls.
   B) fragment bacterial DNA.
   C) opsonize microbes.
   D) increase capillary permeability.
   E) prevent viral replication.

Answer: E
Page Ref: 748

16) Proteins known as CD4 and CD8 are:

   A) identifying proteins on the surfaces of helper and cytotoxic T cells.

   B) different protein chains seen in IgG and IgM antibodies.

   C) proteins on microbes that identify them as foreign.

   D) the proteins antigen-presenting cells display with foreign antigens.

   E) complement proteins that trigger inflammation.

   Answer: A
   Page Ref: 752

17) "Teaching" lymphocytes to recognize self from non-self antigens is the function of the:

   A) plasma cell.

   B) spleen.

   C) thymus.

   D) macrophage.

   E) liver.

   Answer: C
   Page Ref: 742

18) Plasma cells are a form of:

   A) helper T cell.

   B) B cell.

   C) killer T cell.

   D) macrophage.

   E) complement.

   Answer: B
   Page Ref: 752

19) The thoracic duct empties lymph into the:

   A) right lymphatic duct.

   B) cisterna chyli.

   C) left subclavian vein.

   D) ventricles of the brain.

   E) right atrium of the heart.

   Answer: C
   Page Ref: 741

20) During specific immunity, competent T cells are activated by:
    A) plasma cells.
    B) complement.
    C) antibodies.
    D) interleukin–1.
    E) histamine.

Answer: D
Page Ref: 759

21) Antibody-mediated immunity is most effective against:
    A) fungi.
    B) intracellular viruses.
    C) cancer cells.
    D) antigens in body fluids.
    E) foreign tissue transplants.

Answer: D
Page Ref: 753

22) A hapten is:
    A) a small substance that has reactivity but lacks immunogenicity.
    B) the heavy chain of an immunoglobulin molecule.
    C) the antigen binding site of an immunoglobulin molecule.
    D) the part of a lymphoid organ where antigens are processed.
    E) a self-antigen genetically encoded by the Major Histocompatibility Complex.

Answer: A
Page Ref: 754

23) The significance of haptens in immune responses is that:
    A) they must be presented to T cells along with foreign antigens to trigger T cell cloning.
    B) they can combine with larger proteins in the body to become immunogenic, but are reactive without the larger protein.
    C) they determine the immunoglobulin class to which an antibody molecule belongs.
    D) they prevent entry of viruses into cells.
    E) they are the T and B cells that have undergone negative selection.

Answer: B
Page Ref: 754

24) ALL of the following had MHC-I antigens EXCEPT:

   A) neurons in the brain.

   B) lymphocytes.

   C) macrophages.

   D) neutrophils.

   E) erythrocytes.

   Answer: E
   Page Ref: 755

25) Which of the following possess Class II MHC antigens?

   A) antigen-presenting cells

   B) erythrocytes

   C) cardiac muscle cells

   D) simple columnar epithelial cells in the gastrointestinal tract.

   E) All of the above are correct except erythrocytes.

   Answer: A
   Page Ref: 755

26) Possibly fatal constriction of the bronchioles and a rapid drop in blood pressure are typical of:

   A) anaphylactic hypersensitivity.

   B) phagocytosis when it occurs too rapidly.

   C) overproduction of memory B cells.

   D) delayed hypersensitivity.

   E) immune complex hypersensitivity.

   Answer: A
   Page Ref: 769

27) T cells and B cells are:

   A) phagocytes.

   B) antibodies.

   C) lymphocytes.

   D) complement proteins.

   E) both phagocytes and lymphocytes.

   Answer: C
   Page Ref: 743

28) The process of coating an antigenic microbe with antibodies to make it more susceptible to phagocytosis is called:

A) chemotaxis.

B) opsonization.

C) cloning.

D) anergy.

E) inflammation.

Answer: B
Page Ref: 762

29) Giving someone an intravenous injection of immunoglobulin would:

A) protect him from a specific disease by giving him passively acquired immunity.

B) cause him to produce his own antibodies to the pathogen causing the disease.

C) protect him for several years.

D) trigger formation of memory B cells that can make antibodies to protect him from this disease in the future.

E) All of the above are correct.

Answer: A
Page Ref: 765

30) The immunoglobulin important for providing passively acquired immunity to the fetus *in utero* is:

A) IgA.

B) IgM.

C) IgG.

D) IgD.

E) IgE.

Answer: C
Page Ref: 763

31) As part of the processing of exogenous antigens, an antigen–presenting cell digests an antigen into fragments and also synthesizes and packages:

A) alpha interferon.

B) MHC–II antigens.

C) histamine.

D) antibodies.

E) thymic hormones.

Answer: B
Page Ref: 755

32) Presentation of an endogenous antigen bound to an MHC–I molecule signals that:

    A) everything is normal.

    B) the cell has differentiated into a plasma cell.

    C) a helper T cell is ready to secrete interleukin–2.

    D) a phagocyte is "full" and cannot ingest more antigens.

    E) a cell has been infected.

Answer: E
Page Ref: 756

33) Cytotoxic T cells recognize antigens combined with:

    A) interleukin–1.

    B) interleukin–2.

    C) MHC–I antigens.

    D) MHC–II antigens.

    E) complement proteins.

Answer: C
Page Ref: 759

34) Which of the following occurs in delayed hypersensitivity?

    A) The complement system is activated by killer T cells.

    B) Memory B cells produce antibodies within hours of a second exposure to an antigen.

    C) Sensitized T cells migrate to the antigen site within 48 –72 hours.

    D) IgE antibodies cause histamine to be released from mast cells when they combine with an antigen.

    E) Immune complexes precipitate into joint and kidney tubules.

Answer: C
Page Ref: 769

35) Receiving an immunization with an altered form of the tetanus toxin results in:

    A) naturally acquired active immunity.

    B) naturally acquired passive immunity.

    C) artificially acquired active immunity.

    D) artificially acquired passive immunity.

    E) no response, because altered toxins cannot act as antigens.

Answer: C
Page Ref: 765

36) The term *immunological tolerance* refers to:

A) inability of the immune system to respond to a particular antigen.

B) lack of reactivity to peptide fragments from one's own proteins.

C) the maximum dosage of an antigen to which one can be exposed without initiating an immune response.

D) the actual number of microbes necessary to cause signs and symptoms of a disease.

E) the ability of memory cells to recognize an antigen from prior exposure.

Answer: B
Page Ref: 765

37) The term *anergy* refers to:

A) immobilization of a bacterium by specific antibodies.

B) making a microbe more susceptible to phagocytosis by coating it with antibodies.

C) attraction of phagocytes to an area of tissue damage by chemicals released from damaged cells.

D) the lack of reactivity to peptide fragments from one's own proteins.

E) failure of a self–reactive lymphocyte to respond to antigenic stimulation.

Answer: E
Page Ref: 765

38) You would expect anchoring filaments to open spaces between endothelial cells in lymph capillaries when:

A) blood hydrostatic pressure is low.

B) blood colloid osmotic pressure is high.

C) interstitial fluid hydrostatic pressure is high.

D) interstitial fluid osmotic pressure is low.

E) sympathetic stimulation to the filaments increases.

Answer: C
Page Ref: 740

39) People who are confined to bed for long period of time often develop edema because:

A) their blood pressure becomes elevated, forcing more fluid into interstitial spaces as blood hydrostatic pressure rises.

B) lack of motor activity leads to reduced sympathetic stimulation to lymphatic vessels, so lymph tends to pool.

C) without skeletal muscle contraction to force lymph through lymphatic vessels, fluid tends to accumulate in interstitial spaces.

D) reduced vasomotor tone allows proteins to leak from plasma, and water follows the osmotic gradient.

E) heart rate and force of contraction are reduced, so the pressure gradient is insufficient to maintain lymph flow.

Answer: C
Page Ref: 742

40) Which of the following is considered to be a primary lymphatic organ?

A) red bone marrow

B) spleen

C) any lymph node

D) pharyngeal tonsil

E) liver

Answer: A
Page Ref: 742

41) Which person most likely has the largest thymus gland?

A) third trimester fetus

B) two–year–old

C) 12–year–old

D) 25–year–old

E) 65–year–old

Answer: C
Page Ref: 742

42) A chemical that is produced by virus–infected cells and released to provide nonspecific antiviral protection to neighboring cells is:

A) transferrin.

B) interleukin–1.

C) histamine.

D) interleukin–2.

E) interferon.

Answer: E
Page Ref: 748

43) Which of the following is a nonspecific mechanism of resistance?

A) activation of the complement system via the alternative pathway

B) binding of an allergen to IgE molecules on mast cells

C) a delayed hypersensitivity response to poison ivy

D) cloning of B cells in response to a measles vaccine

E) a transfusion reaction between incompatible blood types

Answer: A
Page Ref: 748

44) Which of the following is an example of a specific immune response?
    A) release of histamine from damaged cells
    B) adherence of a macrophage to a microbe
    C) release of interferon from virus–infected cells
    D) opsonization of an antigen by IgG molecules
    E) cytolysis of microbes by complement proteins

Answer: D
Page Ref: 762

45) The swelling associated with inflammation is caused by:
    A) the large numbers of phagocytes attracted to the area.
    B) blockage of blood flow in capillaries by infecting bacteria.
    C) movement of fluid out of capillaries due to increased capillary permeability.
    D) the accumulation of intracellular fluid released by damaged cells.
    E) a larger volume of blood in dilated vessels.

Answer: C
Page Ref: 750

46) Which of the following is **TRUE** about antibodies?
    A) An IgM antibody molecule is able to react with ten different types of epitopes.
    B) Some types of antibodies provide nonspecific resistance to disease.
    C) The five different immunoglobulin classes are determined by the function of the molecules.
    D) All antibodies secreted by a particular plasma cell combine specifically with only one type of epitope.
    E) People who receive an antiserum will develop active immunity once the injected antibodies begin to reproduce.

Answer: D
Page Ref: 760

47) The immunoglobulin class of an antibody molecule is determined by the:
    A) structure of the L chains.
    B) structure of the variable region.
    C) structure of the constant region of the H chains.
    D) function of the molecule.
    E) type of antigen that stimulates production of the antibodies.

Answer: C
Page Ref: 761

48) The antigen–binding site of an antibody molecule is contained in the:

   A) hinge region.

   B) disulfide bonds.

   C) constant region of the L chains.

   D) constant region of the H chains.

   E) variable regions of the H and L chains.

   Answer: E
   Page Ref: 761

49) ALL of the following are characteristic of the secondary antibody response **EXCEPT**:

   A) proliferation of differentiation of memory cells.

   B) development of a higher antibody titter than in the primary response.

   C) production of antibodies with a higher affinity for the antigen than those in the primary response.

   D) predominant production of IgM antibodies.

   E) response occurring within hours of exposure.

   Answer: D
   Page Ref: 764

50) You had a case of chickenpox when you were six years old. When you were ten, your playmates developed chickenpox, but you did not. This was most likely due to:

   A) naturally acquired active immunity.

   B) naturally acquired passive immunity.

   C) artificially acquired active immunity.

   D) artificially acquired passive immunity.

   E) changes in the surface antigens of the chickenpox virus.

   Answer: A
   Page Ref: 765

MATCHING. Choose the item in column 2 that best matches each item in column 1.

Choose the item from column 2 that best matches each item on column 1.

   1) Column 1: helper T cells
      Column 2: display CD4 proteins; secrete cytokines to enhance lymphocyte proliferation

   Answer: display CD4 proteins; secrete cytokines to enhance lymphocyte proliferation

   Page Ref: 759

2) Column 1: cytotoxic T cells
   Column 2: display CD8 molecules;
             destroy antigens in cell-
             mediated immunity

   Answer: display CD8 molecules; destroy antigens in cell-mediated immunity
   Page Ref: 759

3) Column 1: natural killer cells
   Column 2: lymphocytes that provide
             nonspecific immunity

   Answer: lymphocytes that provide nonspecific immunity
   Page Ref: 749

4) Column 1: B cells
   Column 2: may act as antigen-presenting
             cells; differentiate into
             antibody-producing cells or
             memory cells

   Answer: may act as antigen-presenting cells; differentiate into antibody-producing cells or
           memory cells
   Page Ref: 760

5) Column 1: plasma cells
   Column 2: descendants of B cells that
             produce antibodies

   Answer: descendants of B cells that produce antibodies
   Page Ref: 760

6) Column 1: dendritic cells
   Column 2: type of antigen-presenting
             cells found in skin and
             mucous membranes

   Answer: type of antigen-presenting cells found in skin and mucous membranes
   Page Ref: 755

7) Column 1: macrophages
   Column 2: wandering or fixed phagocytic
             cells; type of antigen-
             presenting cell

   Answer: wandering or fixed phagocytic cells; type of antigen-presenting cell
   Page Ref: 749

8) Column 1: reticular epithelial cells
   Column 2: produce thymic hormones in
             thymus gland
   Answer: produce thymic hormones in thymus gland
   Page Ref: 742

9) Column 1: mast cells
   Column 2: release histamine in type I
             hypersensitivity
   Answer: release histamine in type I hypersensitivity
   Page Ref: 750

10) Column 1: memory T cells
    Column 2: remain in lymphatic tissue
              after an immune response to
              provide rapid response to
              subsequent exposure to
              antigen
    Answer: remain in lymphatic tissue after an immune response to provide rapid response to
            subsequent exposure to antigen
    Page Ref: 759

MATCHING. Choose the item in column 2 that best matches each item in column 1.

Choose the item from column 2 that best matches each item on column 1.

1) Column 1: complement
   Column 2: group of proteins in blood and
             on plasma membranes that
             react in cascade to enhance
             immune, allergic, and
             inflammatory reactions
   Answer: group of proteins in blood and on plasma membranes that react in cascade to enhance
           immune, allergic, and inflammatory reactions
   Page Ref: 752

2) Column 1: interferon
   Column 2: chemical released from virus-
             infected lymphocytes,
             macrophages, or fibroblasts to
             prevent viral replication in
             neighboring cells
   Answer: chemical released from virus-infected lymphocytes, macrophages, or fibroblasts to
           prevent viral replication in neighboring cells
   Page Ref: 756

3) Column 1: perforin

   Column 2: secreted by killer T cells to
                poke holes in target cell
                membranes

   Answer: secreted by killer T cells to poke holes in target cell membranes

   Page Ref: 757

4) Column 1: lymphotoxin

   Column 2: secreted by killer T cells to
                cause DNA fragmentation in
                target cells.

   Answer: secreted by killer T cells to cause DNA fragmentation in target cells.

   Page Ref: 757

5) Column 1: histamine

   Column 2: vasodilator released from
                mast cells and basophils that
                also increases capillary
                permeability

   Answer: vasodilator released from mast cells and basophils that also increases capillary
             permeability

   Page Ref: 750

6) Column 1: interleukin–2

   Column 2: secreted by helper T cells to
                costimulate proliferation of
                helper T cells, killer T cells,
                and B cells

   Answer: secreted by helper T cells to costimulate proliferation of helper T cells, killer T cells, and
             B cells

   Page Ref: 757

7) Column 1: interleukin–1

   Column 2: secreted by macrophages to
                costimulate T and B cell
                proliferation and to act on the
                hypothalamus to induce fever

   Answer: secreted by macrophages to costimulate T and B cell proliferation and to act on the
             hypothalamus to induce fever

   Page Ref: 757

8) Column 1: tumor necrosis factor

Column 2: produced by macrophages
and T cells to inhibit
macrophage activity and T
cell proliferation

Answer: produced by macrophages and T cells to inhibit macrophage activity and T cell
proliferation

Page Ref: 757

9) Column 1: lysozyme

Column 2: enzyme in sweat, tears, saliva,
etc., that breaks down
bacterial cell walls

Answer: enzyme in sweat, tears, saliva, etc., that breaks down bacterial cell walls

Page Ref: 752

10) Column 1: leukotriene

Column 2: chemical produced by
basophils and mast cells to
break down membrane
phospholipids and to
facilitate adherence of
phagocytes to pathogens

Answer: chemical produced by basophils and mast cells to break down membrane phospholipids
and to facilitate adherence of phagocytes to pathogens

Page Ref: 751

TRUE/FALSE. Write 'T' if the statement is true and 'F' if the statement is false.

1) Transporting lipids is an important function of the lymphatic system.

Answer: TRUE
Page Ref: 738

2) Lymph capillaries are present in all tissues, including those such as epidermis that lack blood
capillaries.

Answer: FALSE
Page Ref: 740

3) The thoracic duct drains lymph into venous blood at the junction of the left brachiocephalic
vein and the superior vena cava.

Answer: FALSE
Page Ref: 741

4) The primary lymphatic organs are the thymus and the red bone marrow.

Answer: TRUE
Page Ref: 742

5) B lymphocytes and plasma cells are tightly packed into the stroma of a lymph node.

Answer: FALSE
Page Ref: 743

6) The spleen is located on the right side between the stomach and the diaphragm.

Answer: FALSE
Page Ref: 744

7) Tonsils are examples of lymphatic nodules.

Answer: TRUE
Page Ref: 746

8) Interferons provide a mechanism of specific resistance.

Answer: FALSE
Page Ref: 748

9) Chemotaxis is the destruction of microbes inside phagocytes via oxidative bursts.

Answer: FALSE
Page Ref: 749

10) Histamine causes vasodilation and increased capillary permeability during inflammation.

Answer: TRUE
Page Ref: 750

11) Much of the pain associated with inflammation is caused by kinins.

Answer: TRUE
Page Ref: 751

12) Both T cells and B cells are involved in cell-mediated immunity.

Answer: FALSE
Page Ref: 752

13) Class I MHC antigens are only present on antigen–presenting cells, thymus cells, and activated T cells.

Answer: FALSE
Page Ref: 755

14) Interleukin–2 is the prime trigger for T cell proliferation in an immune response.

Answer: TRUE
Page Ref: 759

15) The antigen–binding site of an immunoglobulin molecule is located at the tips of the variable regions of the H and L chains.

Answer: TRUE
Page Ref: 761

SHORT ANSWER. Write the word or phrase that best completes each statement or answers the question.

1) The structure of the _____ region of the _____ chain of an antibody molecule determines its immunoglobulin class.

Answer: constant; H

Page Ref: 761

2) The first antibody to appear in an infection belong to the immunoglobulin class _____.

Answer: IgM

Page Ref: 761

3) The process by which a microbe is coated with antibodies that make it more susceptible to phagocytosis is called _____.

Answer: opsonization

Page Ref: 762

4) The only antibodies that can cross the placenta belong to the immunoglobulin class _____.

Answer: IgG

Page Ref: 763

5) Antibodies that circulate bound to basophils and mast cells belong to the immunoglobulin class _____.

Answer: IgE

Page Ref: 763

6) The amount of antibody in serum is called the antibody _____.

Answer: titer

Page Ref: 764

7) The process of negative selection weeds out self-reactive T cells via _____ , in which self-reactive T cells undergo apoptosis, or via _____ , in which they remain alive, but unresponsive to antigenic stimulation.

Answer: deletion; anergy

Page Ref: 765

8) The three types of antigen-presenting cells includes the _____ , the _____ , and the _____ .

Answer: macrophage; B cell; dendritic cell

Page Ref: 767

9) Specialized lymph capillaries in the small intestine are called _____ , and the lipid-rich lymph they transport is called _____ .

Answer: lacteals; chyle

Page Ref: 740

10) The largest lymphatic vessel is the _____ , which begins as a dilation called the _____ .

Answer: thoracic duct; cisterna chyli

Page Ref: 741

11) The thymus gland is located posterior to the _____ .

Answer: sternum

Page Ref: 742

12) The reticular cells of the germinal centers of lymph nodes are antigen-presenting cells known as _____ .

Answer: dendritic cells

Page Ref: 743

13) The spleen consists of two tissue types —white pulp, which is _____ , and red pulp, which is _____ .

Answer: lymphatic tissue; venous sinuses (and splenic cords)

Page Ref: 745

14) _____ are chemicals produced by lymphocytes, macrophages, and fibroblasts to stop viral replication in neighboring cells.

Answer: Interferons

Page Ref: 748

15) Transferrins inhibit the growth of certain bacteria by reducing the amount of available
_____.

Answer: iron

Page Ref: 748

16) Histiocytes in the skin and microglia in the brain are examples of a group of cells called
_____.

Answer: fixed macrophages

Page Ref: 749

17) The four characteristic (cardinal) signs of inflammation are _____ , _____ ,
_____ , and _____.

Answer: heat; redness; swelling; pain

Page Ref: 750

18) _____ are substances that are recognized as foreign and provoke an immune response.

Answer: Antigens

Page Ref: 752

19) In cell–mediated immunity, the invading antigen is destroyed by _____.

Answer: cytotoxic T cells

Page Ref: 752

20) Cell–mediated immunity is especially effective against _____ , _____ , and
_____.

Answer: intracellular pathogens; certain cancer cells; foreign tissue transplants

Page Ref: 752

21) Antibody–mediated immunity is especially effective against _____ and _____.

Answer: antigens in body fluids; extracellular pathogens

Page Ref: 753

22) Antigens have two important characteristics —_____ , which is the ability to provoke an
immune response, and _____ , which is the ability to react specifically with the
antibodies or cells provoked.

Answer: immunogenicity; reactivity

Page Ref: 753

23) The specific portion of an antigen that triggers an immune response is called a(n) _____.

Answer: epitope (antigenic determinant)

Page Ref: 754

24) The three main types of differentiated T cells are _____ T cells that display CD4 proteins, _____ T cells that display CD8 proteins, and _____ T cells that are members of a clone that remain after an immune response.

Answer: helper; cytotoxic; memory

Page Ref: 759

25) Killer T cells destroy antigens via _____ , which forms holes in target cell membranes, and _____ , which activates DNA fragmenting enzymes in target cells.

Answer: perforin; lymphotoxin

Page Ref: 759

26) Differentiated B cells that secrete antibodies are _____ .

Answer: plasma cells

Page Ref: 760

27) The Human Immunodeficiency Virus (HIV) contains the enzyme _____ that allows DNA to be made from a viral RNA template.

Answer: reverse transcriptase

Page Ref: 768

28) The reactions of type I hypersensitivity are collectively called _____ .

Answer: anaphylaxis

Page Ref: 769

29) Lymph nodes are considered organs, while lymphatic nodules are not, because lymph nodes have _____ .

Answer: a capsule

Page Ref: 742

30) The spread of cancer cells from one organ to another not directly connected to it is called _____ .

Answer: metastasis

Page Ref: 744

ESSAY. Write your answer in the space provided or on a separate sheet of paper.

1) Identify the components of the lymphatic system, and describe the functions of the lymphatic system.

Answer: Components include lymph, lymphatic vessels, and lymphatic tissue (nodes, spleen, thymus, red bone marrow, MALT). Functions include returning lost fluid and proteins to blood plasma to maintain BHP and BCOP, transport of dietary fats and lipid–soluble vitamins from the GI tract to the blood, and protection via specific and nonspecific immunity.

Page Ref: 738–739

2) What is the difference between fever and the heat that is one of the characteristic signs of inflammation?

Answer: The heat of inflammation is a local event related to vasodilation induced by histamine. Greater blood flow means more heat is distributed to affected areas. Fever is a systemic increase in body temperature triggered by bacterial products and endogenous cytokines that reset the hypothalamic thermostat.

Page Ref: 750–751

3) Compare and contrast active and passive immunity.

Answer: In active immunity antibodies are made by self cells in response to exposure to antigens —either naturally or artificially (via immunization with treated antigens). In passive immunity, antibodies are made by someone else—either by the mother to protect the fetus via placental passage of antibodies or mother to newborn via ingestion of breast milk or by intravenous injection of immunoglobulins collected from other individuals.

Page Ref: 764–765

4) Describe the complement system and describe its role in the immune response.

Answer: Complement is about 20 different plasma proteins activated in a cascade either by an Ag–Ab complex or by microbial polysaccharides. Activated proteins enhance the immune response in several ways—activation of inflammation, opsonization of microbes, and cytolysis of microbes (via MAC).

Page Ref: 762–763

5) Describe the immunological mechanism by which anaphylactic shock occurs. Why is epinephrine useful in reversing the effects on the cardiovascular system?

Answer: IgE made in a primary response to an allergen binds to the surface of mast cells and basophils. In the secondary response, the allergen binds to the IgE and causes release of histamine (etc.) from mast cells and basophils. The result is increased vasodilation, increased capillary permeability, increased smooth muscle contraction in the bronchioles, and increased mucus secretion. Loss of fluid volume to the interstitial spaces leads to shock. Epinephrine increases the force of contraction of the heart to increase cardiac output and blood pressure and counteracts the vasodilation.

Page Ref: 769

6) Identify and briefly describe the functions of the various types of lymphocytes in the immune response.

Answer: Natural killer (NK) cells nonspecifically attack and destroy microbes and tumor cells via perforin and direct cytolysis. Helper T cells (CD4 cells) recognize antigens with MHC-II molecules. They are costimulated by IL-1 to secrete cytokines needed for all immune responses. Cytotoxic T cells (CD8 cells) recognize foreign antigens with MHC-I molecules. They are cytolytic when costimulated by IL-2 or other cytokines. B cells can act as antigen-presenting cells and are the cells that differentiate into plasma cells that secrete antibodies. Memory cells (T and B) stay after the immune response for rapid secondary responses.

Page Ref: 749; 758–760

7) Describe the process of phagocytosis, and identify the cell types involved.

Answer: Macrophages and neutrophils are the major phagocytes. The process involves chemotaxis (attraction of phagocytes to chemicals released at the site of damage), adherence (attachment of phagocyte to foreign material), ingestion (formation of phagocytic vesicle around foreign material), and digestion (via lysosomal enzymes and oxidative bursts).

Page Ref: 749–750

8) List the four cardinal signs of inflammation, and describe how each develops. What benefit is derived from the development of each sign?

Answer: Pain is stimulated mainly by kinins and makes a person aware of damage. Swelling results when histamine increases capillary permeability and water follows escaping proteins. This allows protective proteins and cells to reach the site. Redness and heat result as histamine increases vasodilation, which increases blood flow to the area. Increased blood flow brings needed oxygen and nutrients to cells and removes wastes. Increased temperature increases the rate of reactions and the activity of phagocytes.

Page Ref: 750–751

9) Describe the process by which antigen–presenting cells process and present an exogenous antigen.

Answer: Steps include: 1) phagocytosis or endocytosis of antigen; 2) digestion of antigen into fragments within vesicles; 3) vesicles containing fragments and MHC–II molecules merge and fuse; 4) antigen fragments bind to MHC–II molecules; 5) vesicle undergoes exocytosis, and Ag–MHC–II complexes are inserted into the membrane of the antigen-presenting cell.

Page Ref: 755

10) Every cell in the body possesses molecules that could act as antigens in others. How does your own immune system "learn" not to attack your own antigens?

Answer: Some immature T cells in the thymus undergo positive selection when they become able to recognize self–MHC molecules. Those that cannot recognize MHC molecules die. Those that survive undergo negative selection, in which those cells that recognize frgaments of self antigens are eliminated (deletion) or inactivated (anergy) by failure of costimulation. Similar selection of B cells occurs in red bone marrow and peripheral tissues.

Page Ref: 765

CHAPTER 23   The Respiratory System

MULTIPLE CHOICE. Choose the one alternative that best completes the statement or answers the question.

1) Which of the following is **NOT** considered a function of the respiratory system?
   A) regulation of acid–base balance
   B) production of sound
   C) filtering inspired air
   D) transport of oxygen and carbon dioxide to tissue cells
   E) intake of oxygen and elimination of carbon dioxide

   Answer: D
   Page Ref: 775

2) Which of the following is **NOT** considered part of the lower respiratory system?
   A) trachea
   B) larynx
   C) pharynx
   D) bronchi
   E) alveoli

   Answer: C
   Page Ref: 775

3) Which of the following is **NOT** a function of the nose?
   A) warming of incoming air
   B) acting as a resonating chamber for speech
   C) filtering incoming air
   D) detecting olfactory stimuli
   E) gas exchange

   Answer: E
   Page Ref: 777

4) Air pressure in the middle ear is equalized via the auditory tube, which opens into the:
   A) nasal cavity.
   B) maxillary sinus.
   C) nasopharynx.
   D) oropharynx.
   E) laryngopharynx.

   Answer: C
   Page Ref: 779

5) The cough reflex is triggered by irritation of an important medical landmark called the:

A) carina.

B) fauces.

C) cardiac notch.

D) cricoid cartilage.

E) internal choanae.

Answer: A
Page Ref: 784

6) The respiratory membrane through which gases diffuse includes ALL of the following **EXCEPT:**

A) type I alveolar cells.

B) type II alveolar cells.

C) capillary endothelium.

D) an epithelial basement membrane.

E) a layer of smooth muscle.

Answer: E
Page Ref: 788

7) During normal resting pulmonary ventilation, **ALL** of the following are **TRUE EXCEPT:**

A) the phrenic nerve stimulates contraction of the diaphragm.

B) intrapleural pressure increases above atmospheric pressure during exhalation.

C) air comes in during inspiration because alveolar pressure falls below atmospheric pressure.

D) thoracic volume increases as the diaphragm contracts during inspiration.

E) the diaphragm forms a dome as it relaxes.

Answer: B
Page Ref: 790

8) Which of the following muscles helps increase the size of the thoracic cavity during forced inspiration?

A) external oblique

B) external intercostals

C) internal oblique

D) internal intercostals

E) pectoralis major

Answer: B
Page Ref: 791

9) Surface tension exists in alveoli because:

   A) surfactant is very sticky.

   B) elastic fibers in the basement membrane form linkages that collapse alveoli.

   C) movement of gas molecules within alveoli creates electrical charges that attract each other.

   D) polar water molecules are more strongly attracted to each other than to gas molecules in the air.

   E) polar water molecules are more strongly attracted to gas molecules in the air than to each other.

   Answer: D
   Page Ref: 793

10) The normal resting minute volume is:

    A) 6 liters/minute.

    B) 500 mL/minute.

    C) 4.5 liters/minute.

    D) 1200 mL/minute.

    E) 3.6 liters/minute.

    Answer: A
    Page Ref: 795

11) On a very humid day, people with chronic respiratory diseases may experience greater difficulty breathing because:

    A) they are dehydrated.

    B) atmospheric pressure is much lower, so respiratory gradients are decreased.

    C) water vapor contributes a greater partial pressure to inhaled air, thus interfering with normal gradients of other respiratory gases.

    D) the water vapor condenses within the alveoli.

    E) the water vapor decreases the solubility of oxygen.

    Answer: C
    Page Ref: 796

12) The reason the gradients for carbon dioxide can be smaller that those for oxygen and still meet the body's gas exchange needs is that:

    A) carbon dioxide is a smaller molecule than oxygen.

    B) carbon dioxide is more water–soluble than oxygen.

    C) carbon dioxide receives assistance crossing membranes from a carrier molecule.

    D) much of the oxygen, but not the carbon dioxide, is consumed by red blood cells during transport.

    E) oxygen forms ions once it enters the alveoli, and the electrical charges slow its movement across membranes.

    Answer: B
    Page Ref: 798

13) Expired air has a greater oxygen content than alveolar air because:

   A) more oxygen diffuses in across the mucosa of the bronchioles and bronchi.

   B) newly inspired air is entering as expired as it is leaving.

   C) oxygen is being generated by microbes in the upper respiratory tract.

   D) alveolar air mixes with air in the anatomic dead space on its way out.

   E) some carbon dioxide is converted to oxygen in respiratory passages.

   Answer: D
   Page Ref: 799

14) To say that hemoglobin is *fully saturated* means that:

   A) the red blood cells contain as many hemoglobin molecules as possible.

   B) oxygen is attached to both the heme and the globin portions of the molecule.

   C) it is carrying both oxygen and carbon dioxide simultaneously.

   D) some molecule other than oxygen is attached to the oxygen binding sites on hemoglobin.

   E) there is an oxygen molecule attached to each of the four heme groups.

   Answer: E
   Page Ref: 800

15) Which of the following would be **TRUE** if the oxygen–hemoglobin dissociation curve is shifted to the right?

   A) Partial pressure of carbon dioxide is increased.

   B) pH is increased.

   C) Temperature is decreased.

   D) Levels of BPG are decreased.

   E) Partial pressure of oxygen is decreased.

   Answer: A
   Page Ref: 800

16) BPG is a substance that:

   A) is responsible for the detergent activity of surfactant.

   B) catalyzes the conversion of carbon dioxide to bicarbonate ion.

   C) is produced during glycolysis in erythrocytes and increases the dissociation of oxygen from hemoglobin.

   D) inhibits the activity of the central chemoreceptors to prolong inspiration.

   E) binds extra oxygen onto fetal hemoglobin.

   Answer: C
   Page Ref: 801

17) High partial pressure of carbon dioxide favors the formation of:

    A) BPG.

    B) carbaminohemoglobin.

    C) chloride ions.

    D) oxyhemoglobin.

    E) carbon monoxide.

Answer: B
Page Ref: 802

18) Which of the following lists the structures in the correct order of air flow?

    A) trachea, laryngopharynx, nasopharynx, oropharynx, larynx

    B) nasopharynx, oropharynx, laryngopharynx, trachea, larynx

    C) nasopharynx, oropharynx, laryngopharynx, larynx, trachea

    D) oropharynx, laryngopharynx, nasopharynx, larynx, trachea

    E) nasopharynx, laryngopharynx, oropharynx, larynx, trachea

Answer: C
Page Ref: 778

19) The trachea extends from the:

    A) larynx to vertebra T5.

    B) soft palate to the hyoid bone.

    C) atlas to vertebra C7.

    D) epiglottis to the thyroid cartilage.

    E) foramen magnum to vertebra C5.

Answer: A
Page Ref: 783

20) The vocal folds are part of the:

    A) nasal cavity.

    B) laryngopharynx.

    C) trachea.

    D) larynx.

    E) lungs.

Answer: D
Page Ref: 780

21) The function of the epiglottis is to:

   A) hold the pharynx open during speech.

   B) produce surfactant.

   C) close off the nasal cavity during swallowing.

   D) close off the larynx during swallowing.

   E) vibrate to produce sound as air passes over it.

   Answer: D
   Page Ref: 780

22) What is normally found between the visceral and parietal layers of the pleura?

   A) the lungs

   B) venous blood

   C) serous fluid

   D) air

   E) lymph

   Answer: C
   Page Ref: 785

23) A function of type II alveolar cells is to:

   A) help control what passes between squamous epithelial cells of the alveoli.

   B) produce surfactant.

   C) act as phagocytes.

   D) produce mucus in the upper respiratory tract.

   E) store oxygen until it can be transported into the blood.

   Answer: B
   Page Ref: 786

24) Airway resistance is affected primarily by the:

   A) amount of surfactant.

   B) thickness of the cartilage in the bronchial wall.

   C) amount of elastic tissue in the lungs.

   D) diameter of the bronchioles.

   E) partial pressure of each type of gas in inspired air.

   Answer: D
   Page Ref: 794

25) Dalton's Law states that:

A) at a constant temperature, the volume of a gas varies inversely with the pressure.

B) at a constant pressure, the volume of a gas is directly proportional to the temperature.

C) the rate of diffusion is directly proportional to the surface area of the membrane.

D) in a mixture of gases each gas exerts its own partial pressure.

E) at a constant temperature, the volume of a gas is directly proportional to the pressure.

Answer: D
Page Ref: 796

26) Boyle's law states that:

A) at a constant temperature, the volume of a gas varies inversely with the pressure.

B) at a constant pressure, the volume of a gas is directly proportional to the temperature.

C) the rate of diffusion is directly proportional to the surface area of the membrane.

D) in a mixture of gases each gas exerts its own partial pressure.

E) at a constant temperature, the volume of a gas is directly proportional to the pressure.

Answer: A
Page Ref: 790

27) During external respiration, gases are exchanged between the:

A) outside air and the alveoli.

B) alveoli and the blood.

C) blood and cells.

D) outside air and blood in the dermis.

E) cytosol and mitochondria.

Answer: B
Page Ref: 797

28) Compliance is affected primarily by the amount of elastic tissue in the lungs and the:

A) amount of surfactant.

B) thickness of the cartilage in the bronchial wall.

C) partial pressure of oxygen in inspired air.

D) diameter of the bronchioles.

E) temperature of inspired air.

Answer: A
Page Ref: 794

29) During internal respiration, oxygen moves:

    A) into cells by primary active transport.

    B) out of cells by primary active transport.

    C) into cells by diffusion.

    D) out of cells by diffusion.

    E) into cells by secondary active transport.

Answer: C
Page Ref: 798

30) Most oxygen is transported in blood by:

    A) the heme portion of hemoglobin.

    B) the globin portion of hemoglobin.

    C) simply dissolving in plasma.

    D) conversion to bicarbonate ion.

    E) any type of plasma protein.

Answer: A
Page Ref: 799

31) If the partial pressure of carbon dioxide rises within homeostatic range, then:

    A) more oxygen can attach to hemoglobin.

    B) the pH of blood increases.

    C) more bicarbonate ions are produced from carbonic acid.

    D) respiratory rate decreases.

    E) chemoreceptors in the walls of the carotid sinus and aortic arch fire fewer action potentials.

Answer: C
Page Ref: 802

32) If the pH of blood and interstitial fluid rises within homeostatic range, then:

    A) more oxygen can combine with hemoglobin.

    B) less oxygen can stay attached to hemoglobin.

    C) the level of hydrogen ions in these fluids has increased.

    D) the increase was caused by an elevated partial pressure of carbon dioxide.

    E) respiratory rate will increase to compensate.

Answer: A
Page Ref: 800

33) Carbonic acid is produced when:

    A) oxygen combines with bicarbonate ion.

    B) carbon dioxide combines with bicarbonate ion.

    C) carbon dioxide combines with water.

    D) oxygen and carbon dioxide combine.

    E) carbon dioxide attached to hemoglobin.

Answer: C
Page Ref: 802

34) Most carbon dioxide is transported in blood by:

    A) the heme portion of hemoglobin.

    B) the globin portion of hemoglobin.

    C) simply dissolving in plasma.

    D) conversion to bicarbonate ion.

    E) any plasma protein.

Answer: D
Page Ref: 802

35) If the partial pressure of oxygen increases, then:

    A) more oxygen can attach to hemoglobin.

    B) less oxygen can stay attached to hemoglobin.

    C) more bicarbonate ions are produced from carbonic acid.

    D) the pH of blood decreases.

    E) respiratory rate increases.

Answer: A
Page Ref: 800

36) Based on your knowledge of the gas laws and molecular activity, which of the following would you expect to result from an increase in temperature?

    A) More of a particular gas can be dissolved in a liquid.

    B) A particular gas will diffuse across membranes at a faster rate.

    C) The volume of a particular gas will decrease.

    D) The solubility coefficient of a particular gas will increase.

    E) The partial pressure of the gas will increase.

Answer: B
Page Ref: 797

37) Where would you expect to find the highest partial pressure of carbon dioxide?
    A) in the atmosphere
    B) in pulmonary arteries
    C) in pulmonary veins
    D) in alveolar air
    E) in the intracellular fluid

Answer: E
Page Ref: 797

38) The basic pattern of breathing is set by nuclei of neurons located in the:
    A) pons.
    B) diaphragm.
    C) medulla oblongata.
    D) lungs.
    E) thoracic region of the spinal cord.

Answer: C
Page Ref: 804

39) The apneustic and pneumotaxic areas are located in the:
    A) pons.
    B) diaphragm.
    C) medulla oblongata.
    D) lungs.
    E) thoracic region of the spinal cord.

Answer: A
Page Ref: 805

40) In metabolically active tissues you would expect:
    A) the percent saturation of hemoglobin will be less than it is near the lungs.
    B) the partial pressure of oxygen will be higher than in the alveoli.
    C) the pH will be slightly higher than it is in the fluid close to the lungs.
    D) the partial pressure of carbon dioxide will be at its lowest point.
    E) All of these are correct.

Answer: A
Page Ref: 800

41) Hemoglobin will tend to bind more oxygen at a given partial pressure of oxygen if:

    A) the partial pressure of carbon dioxide is increased.

    B) the temperature is increased.

    C) the pH is increased.

    D) BPG concentration increases.

    E) the concentration of hydrogen ions increases.

Answer: C
Page Ref: 801

42) The residual volume is the amount of air:

    A) remaining in the lungs after the lungs collapse.

    B) that can be inhaled above tidal volume.

    C) remaining in the lungs after forced expiration.

    D) contained in air spaces above the alveoli.

    E) that can be exhaled above tidal volume.

Answer: C
Page Ref: 796

43) The tidal volume is the:

    A) volume of air the lungs can hold when maximally inflated.

    B) volume of air moved in and out of the lungs in a single quiet breath.

    C) percentage of alveolar air that is water vapor.

    D) sum of the inspiratory and expiratory reserve volumes.

    E) volume of air left in the lungs after a forced expiration.

Answer: B
Page Ref: 796

44) You would expect the partial pressure of oxygen to be highest in the:

    A) pulmonary arteries.

    B) pulmonary veins.

    C) hepatic portal vein.

    D) intracellular fluid.

    E) interstitial fluid.

Answer: B
Page Ref: 800

45) Several small alveoli merge to form one single, larger air space. This results in a(n):
   A) increased rate of gas exchange due to an increased volume of air within the alveolus.
   B) increased rate of gas exchange due to increased partial pressure of oxygen and decreased partial pressure of carbon dioxide within the alveolus.
   C) decreased rate of gas exchange due to decreased partial pressure of oxygen and decreased partial pressure of carbon dioxide within the alveolus
   D) decreased rate of gas exchange due to a decrease in surface area.
   E) decreased rate of gas exchange due to an increase in the thickness of the respiratory membrane.

Answer: D
Page Ref: 788

46) The Haldane effect refers to the decreased:
   A) affinity of hemoglobin for oxygen in the presence of a high partial pressure of carbon dioxide.
   B) affinity of hemoglobin for oxygen as pH falls.
   C) affinity of hemoglobin for carbon dioxide as temperature increases.
   D) affinity of hemoglobin for carbon dioxide as the partial pressure of oxygen increases.
   E) rate of external respiration as surface area decreases.

Answer: D
Page Ref: 803

47) If the partial pressure of carbon dioxide is decreasing, then:
   A) the partial pressure of oxygen must be increasing.
   B) the pH will also be decreasing.
   C) the affinity of hemoglobin for oxygen is decreasing.
   D) there is an increase in the rate of the reaction converting carbonic acid into water and carbon dioxide.
   E) there is an increase in the rate of the reaction converting carbonic acid into hydrogen ion and bicarbonate ion.

Answer: D
Page Ref: 801

48) If a person is hypoventilating, then:
   A) the partial pressure of carbon dioxide is decreasing.
   B) the rate at which carbonic acid is dissociating into hydrogen ions and bicarbonate ions is increasing.
   C) the rate at which carbonic acid is dissociating into hydrogen ions and bicarbonate ions is decreasing.
   D) the pH of cerebrospinal fluid is increasing.
   E) more oxygen will be able to bind to hemoglobin.

Answer: B
Page Ref: 806

49) C-shaped cartilage rings support the:

    A) laryngopharynx.

    B) larynx.

    C) trachea.

    D) tertiary bronchi.

    E) All of these are supported by C-shaped rings.

Answer: C
Page Ref: 783

50) The alveolar ventilation rate for someone whose tidal volume = 450 mL, whose dead space air = 150 mL, and whose respiratory rate is 15 respirations per minute is:

    A) 2250 mL/min.

    B) 4500 mL/min.

    C) 6750 mL/min.

    D) 9000 mL/min.

    E) There is not enough information to calculate the alveolar ventilation rate.

Answer: B
Page Ref: 796

MATCHING. Choose the item in column 2 that best matches each item in column 1.

Choose the item from column 2 that best matches each item on column 1.

1) Column 1: total lung capacity
Column 2: 6000 mL

Answer: 6000 mL
Page Ref: 796

2) Column 1: vital capacity
Column 2: 4800 mL

Answer: 4800 mL
Page Ref: 796

3) Column 1: expiratory reserve volume
Column 2: 1200 mL

Answer: 1200 mL
Page Ref: 796

4) Column 1: inspiratory reserve volume
Column 2: 3100 mL

Answer: 3100 mL
Page Ref: 796

5) Column 1: inspiratory capacity
   Column 2: 3600 mL
   Answer: 3600 mL
   Page Ref: 796

6) Column 1: functional residual capacity
   Column 2: 2400 mL
   Answer: 2400 mL
   Page Ref: 796

7) Column 1: tidal volume
   Column 2: 500 mL
   Answer: 500 mL
   Page Ref: 795

8) Column 1: residual volume
   Column 2: 1200 mL
   Answer: 1200 mL
   Page Ref: 796

9) Column 1: tidal volume reaching the respiratory portion of the respiratory system
   Column 2: 350 mL
   Answer: 350 mL
   Page Ref: 795

10) Column 1: tidal volume remaining as dead space air
    Column 2: 150 mL
    Answer: 150 mL
    Page Ref: 795

MATCHING. Choose the item in column 2 that best matches each item in column 1.

Choose the item from column 2 that best matches each item on column 1.

1) Column 1: tidal volume
   Column 2: volume of air moved in and out of the lungs during normal quiet breathing
   Answer: volume of air moved in and out of the lungs during normal quiet breathing
   Page Ref: 795

2) Column 1: inspiratory reserve volume
   Column 2: volume of air that can be
   inhaled beyond tidal volume

   Answer: volume of air that can be inhaled beyond tidal volume
   Page Ref: 796

3) Column 1: expiratory reserve volume
   Column 2: volume of air that can be
   exhaled beyond tidal volume

   Answer: volume of air that can be exhaled beyond tidal volume
   Page Ref: 796

4) Column 1: minimal volume
   Column 2: volume of air remaining in the
   lungs after the lungs collapse

   Answer: volume of air remaining in the lungs after the lungs collapse
   Page Ref: 796

5) Column 1: residual volume
   Column 2: volume of air remaining in the
   lungs after forced expiration

   Answer: volume of air remaining in the lungs after forced expiration
   Page Ref: 796

6) Column 1: inspiratory reserve capacity
   Column 2: tidal volume + inspiratory
   reserve volume

   Answer: tidal volume + inspiratory reserve volume
   Page Ref: 796

7) Column 1: functional residual capacity
   Column 2: residual volume + expiratory
   reserve volume

   Answer: residual volume + expiratory reserve volume
   Page Ref: 796

8) Column 1: vital capacity
   Column 2: tidal volume + inspiratory
   reserve volume + expiratory
   reserve volume

   Answer: tidal volume + inspiratory reserve volume + expiratory reserve volume
   Page Ref: 796

9) Column 1: minute ventilation
   Column 2: tidal volume × respirations
            per minute

   Answer: tidal volume × respirations per minute
   Page Ref: 795

10) Column 1: alveolar ventilation rate

    Column 2: (tidal volume − dead space
             air) × respirations per minute

    Answer: (tidal volume − dead space air) × respirations per minute
    Page Ref: 796

TRUE/FALSE. Write 'T' if the statement is true and 'F' if the statement is false.

1) Internal respiration is the exchange of gases between the alveoli and the blood.

   Answer: FALSE
   Page Ref: 775

2) Both food and air normally pass through the laryngopharynx.

   Answer: TRUE
   Page Ref: 780

3) The trachea is anterior to the esophagus.

   Answer: TRUE
   Page Ref: 781

4) The carina is the part of the trachea where a tracheostomy is normally done.

   Answer: FALSE
   Page Ref: 783

5) The left lung has three lobes, and the right lung has two lobes.

   Answer: FALSE
   Page Ref: 786

6) The alveoli are composed of simple columnar epithelium.

   Answer: FALSE
   Page Ref: 786

7) The thinness of the respiratory membrane is an important factor favoring the rapid diffusion of gases.

   Answer: TRUE
   Page Ref: 788

8) When the diaphragm contracts, thoracic volume increases and alveolar pressure decreases.

Answer: TRUE
Page Ref: 790

9) The higher the surface tension, the less likely the alveoli are to collapse.

Answer: FALSE
Page Ref: 793

10) Increased sympathetic stimulation to the bronchioles increases airway resistance.

Answer: FALSE
Page Ref: 794

11) The higher the partial pressure of a gas, the more gas can be dissolved in solution.

Answer: TRUE
Page Ref: 797

12) At rest, the partial pressure of oxygen in deoxygenated blood is about 40 mm Hg and the partial pressure of carbon dioxide is about 45 mm Hg.

Answer: TRUE
Page Ref: 797

13) As the concentration of hydrogen ions rises, oxygen will dissociate from hemoglobin more readily.

Answer: TRUE
Page Ref: 800

14) The chloride shift occurs to make more room for oxygen on hemoglobin molecules.

Answer: FALSE
Page Ref: 802

15) The rate of oxygen exchange during external respiration increases if the partial pressure of oxygen in the alveoli is closer to the partial pressure of oxygen in the blood.

Answer: FALSE
Page Ref: 798

SHORT ANSWER. Write the word or phrase that best completes each statement or answers the question.

1) Proteins that bind carbon dioxide form _____ compounds.
Answer: carbamino
Page Ref: 802

2) The enzyme that catalyzes the conversion of carbon dioxide and water to carbonic acid is
_____.

Answer: carbonic anhydrase

Page Ref: 802

3) The Bohr effect occurs when the oxygen saturation of hemoglobin decreases in response to
_____.

Answer: decreased pH

Page Ref: 800

4) The areas of the brain stem that make up the respiratory center are the _____ , the
_____ , and the _____.

Answer: medullary rhythmicity center; apneustic center; pneumotaxic center

Page Ref: 804

5) Central chemoreceptors are located in the _____ , and peripheral chemoreceptors are
located in the _____ and the _____.

Answer: medulla oblongata; aortic bodies; carotid bodies

Page Ref: 806

6) If hypercapnia occurs, chemoreceptors trigger a(n) _____ in the rate and depth of
breathing, which is called _____.

Answer: increase; hyperventilation

Page Ref: 806

7) Deficiency of hemoglobin leads to _____ hypoxia, while reduction in blood flow leads to
_____ hypoxia.

Answer: anemic; ischemic

Page Ref: 807

8) The _____ is a tube extending from the internal nares to the level of the cricoid cartilage.

Answer: pharynx

Page Ref: 777

9) The single opening to the oropharynx is the _____.

Answer: fauces

Page Ref: 779

10) The space between the vocal folds is called the _____.

Answer: rima glottidis

Page Ref: 780

11) The _____ cartilage of the larynx is the landmark for making an emergency airway.
Answer: cricoid
Page Ref: 780

12) The pitch of a sound generated by the larynx is controlled by the _____.
Answer: tension on the vocal cords
Page Ref: 782

13) The epithelial portion of the mucosa of the trachea is _____ epithelium.
Answer: pseudostratified ciliated columnar
Page Ref: 783

14) An aspirated object is more likely to lodge in the _____ primary bronchus due to its structure.
Answer: right
Page Ref: 784

15) Tertiary bronchi branch to form _____.
Answer: bronchioles
Page Ref: 784

16) Binding of an antigen to IgE antibodies could result in _____ of bronchioles due to release of _____.
Answer: constriction; histamine
Page Ref: 785

17) The concavity on the medial surface of the left lung is called the _____.
Answer: cardiac notch
Page Ref: 785

18) The function of type I alveolar cells is _____ ; the function of type II alveolar cells is _____.
Answer: gas exchange; secretion of alveolar fluid
Page Ref: 786

19) The detergent component of alveolar fluid is called _____ , the function of which is to _____.
Answer: surfactant; lower surface tension of alveolar fluid
Page Ref: 786

20) The components of the respiratory membrane include the _____ , the _____ , the _____ , and the _____ .

Answer: alveolar wall (Type I and II cells); epithelial basement membrane of the alveolar wall; basement membrane of the capillary; endothelium of the capillary

Page Ref: 788

21) Pulmonary capillaries _____ in response to hypoxia.

Answer: constrict

Page Ref: 789

22) Thoracic volume decreases when the diaphragm _____ , causing alveolar pressure to _____ according to _____ Law.

Answer: relaxes; increase; Boyle's

Page Ref: 792

23) Entry of air into the intrapleural space is called _____ .

Answer: pneumothorax

Page Ref: 793

24) Forced expiration against a closed rima glottidis is called _____ .

Answer: the Valsalva maneuver

Page Ref: 794

25) Increased mucus production by the mucosa of the bronchial tree interferes with ventilation because it increases _____ .

Answer: airway resistance

Page Ref: 794

26) The two principal factors affecting compliance are _____ and _____ .

Answer: elasticity; surface tension

Page Ref: 794

27) The gas contributing the highest partial pressure to inspired air is _____ .

Answer: nitrogen

Page Ref: 796

28) At rest, the partial pressure of oxygen in fully oxygenated blood is _____ mm Hg, and in in deoxygenated blood it is about _____ mm Hg.

Answer: 105; 40

Page Ref: 797

29) Elevation of body temperature will cause hemoglobin to _____ oxygen.

Answer: release

Page Ref: 801

30) Fetal hemoglobin binds oxygen _____ strongly than adult hemoglobin because it binds _____ less strongly.

Answer: more; BPG

Page Ref: 802

ESSAY. Write your answer in the space provided or on a separate sheet of paper.

1) Describe the inward forces of elastic recoil, and explain why the lungs do not normally collapse during expiration.

Answer: Elastic recoil is the recoil of elastic fibers stretched during inspiration and the pull of the surface tension of alveolar fluid. Intrapleural pressure is always subatmospheric during normal breathing, which tends to pull lungs outward and to keep alveolar pressure from equalizing with atmospheric pressure. Surfactant in alveolar fluid decreases surface tension to help prevent collapse.

Page Ref: 790-794

2) Why is epinephrine injected as a treatment for the respiratory signs and symptoms of anaphylaxis?

Answer: Epinephrine enhances sympathetic activity to dilate airways and decrease airway resistance, which had been elevated by the effects of histamine on the bronchioles. It also raises blood pressure, which enhances oxygen delivery to tissues by increasing flow.

Page Ref: 794

3) Describe and explain the effects of smoking on the functioning of the respiratory system.

Answer: Nicotine constricts terminal bronchioles to increase airway resistance, as does the increased mucus secretion and swelling of the mucosa. Smoke inhibits the movement of cilia, which allows buildup of substances and microbes normally removed. Over time, smoking leads to destruction of elastic tissue, which decreases compliance, and ultimately to the effects of emphysema.

Page Ref: 809

4) Describe the neural, chemical, and physical changes that increase the rate and depth of ventilation during exercise.

Answer: Anticipation of exercise generates neural input to the limbic system. Sensory input is provided from proprioceptors and motor input is provided from the primary motor cortex. As the partial pressure of oxygen falls due to increased consumption, the partial pressure of carbon dioxide and the temperature increase due to metabolic activity in muscle fibers. Also, carbon dioxide is added via the buffering of the hydrogen ions produced as a result of lactic acid production. Chemoreceptors sense the changes in partial pressure and notify the medullary rhythmicity center to increase the rate and depth of breathing.

Page Ref: 809

5) State Boyle's Law and explain how it relates to the process of pulmonary ventilation.

Answer: Boyle's Law says that at a constant temperature, the pressure of a gas in a closed container is inversely proportional to the volume of the container. During inspiration, as the diaphragm contracts and flattens, the volume of the thoracic cavity is increased, thus decreasing the alveolar pressure. As the pressure falls below atmospheric pressure, air can flow into the lungs until equilibriun is reached. During expiration, the diaphragm relaxes, reducing the size of the thoracic cavity, increasing alveolar pressure above atmospheric pressure, and forcing air out of the lungs.

Page Ref: 790

6) Identify and briefly discuss the factors that affect the rate of external respiration.

Answer: 1) Partial pressure of gases —as gradients across the respiratory membrane change, rate of external respiration changes proportionally;
2) Total surface area for gas exchange —rate of external respiration is directly proportional to the surface area of the respiratory membrane;
3) Diffusion distance —rate of external respiration is inversely proportional to the thickness of the respiratory membrane;
4) Solubility combines with molecular weight of gases —rate of external respiration is directly proportional to solubility, but inversely proportional to molecular weight.

Page Ref: 797-798

7) Write out the chemical formula that describes the conversion of carbon dioxide to bicarbonate ion, and use the formula to explain why hyperventilation and hypoventilation affect acid-base balance.

Answer: $CO_2 + H_2O \longleftrightarrow H_2CO_3 \longleftrightarrow H^+ + HCO_3^-$

During hyperventilation, the partial pressure of carbon dioxide decreases, driving the reaction the the left, thus reducing the hydrogen ion concentration and raising pH. During hypoventilation, partial pressure of carbon dioxide increases, driving the reaction the to right, increasing the concentration of hydrogen ions and lowering pH.

Page Ref: 802; 806-807

8) Define the term *percent saturation of hemoglobin*, and identify the factors that affect the percent saturation of hemoglobin. What is the significance of these factors in the delivery of oxygen to tissues?

Answer: Percent saturation of hemoglobin refers to the ratio of oxyhemoglobin to total hemoglobin. As the partial pressure of oxygen increases, so does percent saturation. Conditions present in and around metabolically active tissues, such as increased partial pressure of carbon dioxide, lower pH, higher temperature, and higher BPG levels, all decrease affinity of hemoglobin for oxygen, so that oxygen is released where it is most needed. When these conditions are reversed, as they would be in the pulmonary capillaries, more oxygen can be picked up.

Page Ref: 797-798

9) In chronic emphysema, some alveoli merge together and some are replaced with fibrous connective tissue. In addition, the bronchioles are often inflamed, and expiratory volume is reduced. Using proper respiratory system terminology, explain at least four reasons why affected individuals will have problems with ventilation and external respiration.

Answer: Answers could include: reduced compliance (reduces ability to increase thoracic volume); increased airway resistance (decreases tidal volume); decreased diffusion due to increased diffusion distance, decreased surface area, and changes in partial pressures of gases (altering gradients). Other answers may be acceptable.

Page Ref: 790–793; 798

10) You have just moved from your home on the Atlantic coast to a small town high in the Rocky Mountains. Explain the effects of this move on your respiratory system. What are the short-term and long-term compensations you might expect your body to make to this new environment?

Answer: [note: This question is intended to cover multiple chapters.] Reduced partial pressure of oxygen is sensed by peripheral chemoreceptors, which trigger an increase in respiratory rate and depth. Blood pressure may be increased to maintain oxygen delivery. Over time, one might see an increase in the red blood cell count to optimize pick-up of available oxygen. (Other answers may be acceptable.)

Page Ref: 806

CHAPTER 24   The Digestive System

MULTIPLE CHOICE. Choose the one alternative that best completes the statement or answers the question.

1) The gastroileal reflex forces chyme from the:
   A) stomach to the duodenum.
   B) stomach to the ileum.
   C) ileum to the cecum.
   D) sigmoid colon to the rectum.
   E) jejunum to the ileum.

   Answer: C
   Page Ref: 859

2) The primary chemical digestion in the large intestine results from the action of:
   A) the continued action of pancreatic juice.
   B) bacterial enzymes.
   C) bilirubin.
   D) hydrochloric acid.
   E) fat–soluble vitamins.

   Answer: B
   Page Ref: 859

3) The appendix is attached to the:
   A) left lobe of the liver.
   B) gallbladder.
   C) cecum.
   D) rectum.
   E) splenic flexure.

   Answer: C
   Page Ref: 857

4) The migrating motility complex is:

   A) a plexus of the enteric nervous system that regulates contractions of the muscularis.

   B) a group of enteroendocrine cells that extends the length of the small intestine.

   C) a bolus of food that is moving from the mouth to the stomach.

   D) a wavelike type of peristalsis that migrates down the small intestine from stomach to ileum.

   E) a type of bacterial infection that causes diarrhea.

   Answer: D
   Page Ref: 857

5) Monosaccharides enter the capillaries of the villi from epithelial cells by:

   A) primary active transport.

   B) facilitated diffusion.

   C) simple diffusion.

   D) secondary active transport linked to sodium ion transport.

   E) emulsification.

   Answer: B
   Page Ref: 855

6) The folds of the gastric mucosa are called:

   A) microvilli.

   B) circular folds.

   C) gastric pits.

   D) villi.

   E) rugae.

   Answer: E
   Page Ref: 833

7) The products of the hydrolysis reaction catalyzed by carboxypeptidase are:

   A) amino acids.

   B) glucose and fructose.

   C) dextrins.

   D) nitrogenous bases.

   E) fatty acids and monoglycerides.

   Answer: A
   Page Ref: 853

8) The major stimulus for secretion of secretin is:

   A) the sight and aroma of food.

   B) entry of a bolus into the esophagus.

   C) CCK.

   D) distention of the stomach.

   E) entry of acid chyme into the small intestine.

   Answer: E
   Page Ref: 847

9) Gallstones are usually made of crystallized:

   A) glucose.

   B) bilirubin.

   C) cholesterol.

   D) chyme.

   E) fat-soluble vitamins.

   Answer: C
   Page Ref: 846

10) Without functioning hepatocytes, protein catabolism is a toxic process due to:

   A) production of ammonia.

   B) excessive HCl production.

   C) buildup of the parts of amino acids remaining after deamination.

   D) clogging of bile canaliculi with denatured proteins.

   E) increased fluid volume.

   Answer: A
   Page Ref: 845

11) Which of the following is NOT produced by the acini of the pancreas?

   A) amylase

   B) lipase

   C) carboxypeptidase

   D) somatostatin

   E) elastase

   Answer: D
   Page Ref: 840

12) Bicarbonate ions diffuse into blood capillaries of the stomach after a meal because:

A) they are being generated from amino acids absorbed by the gastric mucosa.

B) they are being exchanged for hydrogen ions that enter the stomach lumen.

C) they are being exchanged for chloride ions that enter the stomach lumen.

D) they are being exchanged for potassium ions that enter the stomach lumen.

E) carbon dioxide is generated as pepsin hydrolyzes proteins, and it is converted to bicarbonate ion.

Answer: C
Page Ref: 836

13) Intrinsic factor secreted by parietal cells of the stomach is required for:

A) activation of pepsin.

B) buffering of HCl.

C) complete gastric emptying.

D) absorption of vitamin B_{12}.

E) stimulation of mixing waves.

Answer: D
Page Ref: 833

14) Peristalsis occurs during:

A) the voluntary stage of deglutition.

B) the pharyngeal stage of deglutition.

C) the esophageal stage of deglutition.

D) mastication.

E) Both B and C are correct.

Answer: C
Page Ref: 831

15) The type of chemical reaction catalyzed by the digestive enzymes in the digestive juices of the alimentary canal is:

A) oxidation.

B) reduction.

C) hydrolysis.

D) dehydration.

E) phosphorylation.

Answer: C
Page Ref: 819

16) In areas of the gastrointestinal tract specialized for absorption of nutrients, the type of epithelium seen in the mucosa is:

   A) simple squamous.

   B) stratified squamous.

   C) transitional.

   D) simple columnar.

   E) pseudostratified ciliated columnar.

   Answer: D
   Page Ref: 821

17) The small intestine is attached to the posterior abdominal wall by a fold of the peritoneum called the:

   A) mesocolon.

   B) mesentery.

   C) falciform ligament.

   D) taeniae coli.

   E) greater omentum.

   Answer: B
   Page Ref: 822

18) The major digestive enzyme in saliva is:

   A) amylase.

   B) pepsin.

   C) carboxypeptidase.

   D) lipase.

   E) maltase.

   Answer: A
   Page Ref: 829

19) Which of the following is an example of mechanical digestion?

   A) glycolysis

   B) defecation

   C) oxidation–reduction

   D) mastication

   E) hydrolysis

   Answer: D
   Page Ref: 828

20) The pyloric sphincter is located at the junction of the:

A) esophagus and stomach.

B) stomach and duodenum.

C) ileum and cecum.

D) esophagus and larynx.

E) sigmoid colon and rectum.

Answer: B
Page Ref: 833

21) The major chemical digestion that occurs in the adult stomach is:

A) hydrolysis of fats by gastric lipase.

B) formation of chylomicrons.

C) conversion of ammonia to urea.

D) hydrolysis of sucrose by sucrase.

E) hydrolysis of proteins by pepsin.

Answer: E
Page Ref: 836

22) Increased activity of the sympathetic nervous system will:

A) increase production of all hydrolytic enzymes by abdominal organs.

B) increase only production of those digestive juices rich in buffers.

C) have no effect on the digestive system.

D) decrease production of digestive juices.

E) increase movement of food through the alimentary canal.

Answer: D
Page Ref: 840

23) Fold in the mucosa of the small intestine that increase the surface area for diffusion are called:

A) microvilli.

B) villi.

C) rugae.

D) taeniae coli.

E) haustra.

Answer: B
Page Ref: 848

24) The common bile duct is formed by the union of the:

A) right and left hepatic ducts.

B) cystic and pancreatic ducts.

C) common hepatic and cystic ducts.

D) all bile capillaries.

E) pancreatic and accessory ducts.

Answer: C
Page Ref: 843

25) Most absorption of nutrients occurs in the:

A) mouth.

B) transverse colon.

C) stomach.

D) small intestine.

E) rectum

Answer: D
Page Ref: 854

26) The function of bile is to:

A) emulsify fats.

B) transport fats through the blood.

C) hydrolyze fats.

D) actively transport fats through epithelial membranes.

E) All of these are correct.

Answer: A
Page Ref: 843

27) Specific disaccharides are hydrolyzed by enzymes found in:

A) gastric juice.

B) intestinal juice.

C) saliva.

D) pancreatic juice.

E) bile.

Answer: B
Page Ref: 853

28) The hydrolytic reactions catalyzed by trypsin and chymotrypsin would result in the production of:

A) fatty acids and glycerol.

B) monosaccharides.

C) peptides.

D) nucleotides.

E) dextrin.

Answer: C
Page Ref: 853

29) Which of the following would be considered an accessory organ of the digestive system?

A) pancreas.

B) stomach.

C) esophagus.

D) large intestine.

E) small intestine.

Answer: A
Page Ref: 818

30) Which of the following lists the tubing in the correct order of food movement?

A) nasopharynx, oropharynx, laryngopharynx, larynx, esophagus

B) oropharynx, laryngopharynx, esophagus, stomach, pyloric valve

C) laryngopharynx, oropharynx, esophagus, stomach, pyloric valve

D) oropharynx, laryngopharynx, esophagus, pyloric valve, stomach

E) nasopharynx, oropharynx, larynx, esophagus, stomach

Answer: B
Page Ref: 830

31) Which of the following lists the tubing in the correct order of food movement?

A) descending colon, splenic flexure, transverse colon, hepatic flexure, ascending colon, sigmoid colon

B) ascending colon, hepatic flexure, transverse colon, splenic flexure, descending colon, sigmoid colon

C) sigmoid colon, ascending colon, hepatic flexure, transverse colon, splenic flexure, descending colon

D) ascending colon, splenic flexure, transverse colon, hepatic flexure, descending colon, sigmoid colon

E) sigmoid colon, descending colon, splenic flexure, transverse colon, hepatic flexure, ascending colon

Answer: B
Page Ref: 858

32) Which of the following lists the tubing in the correct order of food movement?

   A) pyloric valve, duodenum, ileum, jejunum, ileocecal valve
   B) pyloric valve, jejunum, duodenum, ileum, ileocecal valve
   C) ileocecal valve, ileum, jejunum, duodenum, pyloric valve
   D) ileocecal valve, ileum, jejunum, duodenum, pyloric valve
   E) pyloric valve, duodenum, jejunum, ileum, ileocecal valve

   Answer: E
   Page Ref: 848

33) During swallowing, the nasal cavity is closed off by the soft palate and the:

   A) epiglottis.
   B) uvula.
   C) palatine tonsils.
   D) fauces.
   E) tongue.

   Answer: B
   Page Ref: 824

34) Which of the following best describes the location of the esophagus?

   A) from the fauces to the stomach
   B) posterior to the vertebral column from the laryngopharynx to the stomach.
   C) retroperitoneal
   D) posterior to the trachea, anterior to the vertebral column from laryngopharynx to stomach
   E) anterior to the trachea and heart, just under the sternum

   Answer: D
   Page Ref: 830

35) The regular contractions of the muscularis that push food through the entire gastrointestinal tract are known as:

   A) segmentations.
   B) haustral churning.
   C) peristalsis.
   D) pendular movements.
   E) migratory motility complex.

   Answer: C
   Page Ref: 831

36) The greenish color of bile is the result of the presence of breakdown products of:

A) hemoglobin.

B) urea.

C) starch.

D) the B vitamins.

E) fats.

Answer: A
Page Ref: 843

37) The large intestine absorbs mostly:

A) amino acids.

B) monosaccharides.

C) bile pigments.

D) water.

E) triglycerides.

Answer: D
Page Ref: 859

38) Partially digested food is usually passed from the stomach to the small intestine about how long after consumption?

A) an hour or less

B) 2–4 hours

C) 6–8 hours

D) 10–12 hours

E) 24 hours

Answer: B
Page Ref: 840

39) Gastric emptying is stimulated by **ALL** of the following **EXCEPT**:

A) distention of the stomach.

B) gastrin.

C) CCK.

D) partially digested proteins.

E) the vagus nerve.

Answer: C
Page Ref: 839

40) The functions of the gallbladder include:

   A) production of bile.

   B) storage and concentration of bile.

   C) formation of urea.

   D) secretin of cholecystokinin.

   E) Both A and B are correct.

   Answer: B
   Page Ref: 843

41) The difference between the effects of secretin and the effects of CCK on the pancreas is that:
   A) secretin stimulates secretion of pancreatic juice, while CCK inhibits secretion of pancreatic juice.

   B) secretin stimulates the acini of the pancreas, while CCK stimulates the pancreatic islets.

   C) secretin stimulates alpha cells, while CCK stimulates beta cells.

   D) secretin causes dilation of the pancreatic duct, while CCK causes constriction of the duct.

   E) secretin stimulates secretion of pancreatic juice rich in bicarbonate, while CCK inhibits secretion of pancreatic juice rich in digestive enzymes.

   Answer: E
   Page Ref: 847

42) The liver produces urea to:

   A) detoxify ammonia produced via deamination of proteins.

   B) keep bile in an inactive form until it reaches the small intestine.

   C) convert into glucose when blood glucose is low.

   D) store iron.

   E) bind to ingested poisons to detoxify them.

   Answer: A
   Page Ref: 845

43) Glucose is transported into epithelial cells of the villi via:

   A) secondary active transport coupled to active transport of sodium ions.

   B) secondary active transport coupled to active transport of galactose.

   C) facilitated diffusion.

   D) primary active transport.

   E) pinocytosis.

   Answer: A
   Page Ref: 854

44) The role of micelles in absorption of triglycerides is to:

   A) transport triglycerides through the lymph.

   B) make triglycerides more soluble in the water of intestinal fluid.

   C) actively transport triglycerides into intestinal cells.

   D) hydrolyze triglycerides to fatty acids and glycerol.

   E) protect triglycerides from premature hydrolysis in the stomach.

Answer: B
Page Ref: 856

45) The normal color of feces is due primarily to the:

   A) pigments in the bacteria present.

   B) breakdown products of hemoglobin.

   C) pigments in foods consumed.

   D) pigments in epithelial cells sloughed off from the mucosa.

   E) chemical interactions of undigested foods.

Answer: B
Page Ref: 859

46) The muscularis of most organs of the gastrointestinal tract consists of two layers of smooth muscle except in the:

   A) duodenum.

   B) ileum.

   C) sigmoid colon.

   D) stomach.

   E) ascending colon.

Answer: D
Page Ref: 833

47) Which of the following has the lowest pH?

   A) saliva.

   B) gastric juice.

   C) pancreatic juice.

   D) bile.

   E) intestinal juice.

Answer: B
Page Ref: 836

48) Which of the following occurs during the cephalic phase of gastric digestion?

A) Chemoreceptors detect as change in the pH of gastric juice.

B) Stretch receptors detect distention of the stomach.

C) Chemoreceptors detect fatty acids in the duodenum.

D) Sight, smell, thought, or taste of food trigger parasympathetic impulses.

E) CCK is secreted by enteroendocrine cells.

Answer: D
Page Ref: 838

49) In the neural negative feedback loop controlling secretion of gastric juice, the output in response to entry of food into the stomach would include:

A) decreased parasympathetic impulses.

B) increased secretory activity by parietal cells.

C) increased distention of the stomach wall.

D) increased sympathetic impulses.

E) decreased secretory activity of chief cells.

Answer: B
Page Ref: 838

50) The process of mastication results is:

A) passage of food from the oral cavity into the esophagus.

B) removal of pathogens from partially digested food by MALT tissues.

C) mechanical mixing of food with saliva and shaping of food into a bolus.

D) sudden movement of colonic contents into the rectum.

E) passage of feces from the anus.

Answer: C
Page Ref: 828

MATCHING. Choose the item in column 2 that best matches each item in column 1.

Choose the item from column 2 that best matches each item in column 2.

1) Column 1: parotid glands

Column 2: secrete saliva

Answer: secrete saliva

Page Ref: 825

2) Column 1: parietal cells of stomach

Column 2: secrete hydrogen ions and chloride ions

Answer: secrete hydrogen ions and chloride ions

Page Ref: 833

3) Column 1: chief cells of stomach
   Column 2: secrete pepsinogen
   Answer: secrete pepsinogen
   Page Ref: 833

4) Column 1: G cells of stomach
   Column 2: secrete gastrin
   Answer: secrete gastrin
   Page Ref: 833

5) Column 1: hepatocytes
   Column 2: secrete bile
   Answer: secrete bile
   Page Ref: 843

6) Column 1: Paneth cells of small intestine
   Column 2: secrete lysozyme
   Answer: secrete lysozyme
   Page Ref: 850

7) Column 1: duodenal glands of small
                intestine
   Column 2: secrete alkaline mucus
   Answer: secrete alkaline mucus
   Page Ref: 850

8) Column 1: intestinal glands of small
                intestine
   Column 2: secrete maltase, lactase, and
                sucrase
   Answer: secrete maltase, lactase, and sucrase
   Page Ref: 850

9) Column 1: acini of pancreas
   Column 2: secrete trypsinogen
   Answer: secrete trypsinogen
   Page Ref: 840

10) Column 1: pancreatic islets

   Column 2: secrete insulin and glucagon

   Answer: secrete insulin and glucagon

   Page Ref: 840

MATCHING. Choose the item in column 2 that best matches each item in column 1.

Choose the item from column 2 that best matches each item in column 2.

1) Column 1: stomach

   Column 2: fundus

   Answer: fundus

   Page Ref: 833

2) Column 1: small intestine

   Column 2: jejunun

   Answer: jejunun

   Page Ref: 848

3) Column 1: large intestine

   Column 2: cecum

   Answer: cecum

   Page Ref: 857

4) Column 1: liver

   Column 2: caudate lobe

   Answer: caudate lobe

   Page Ref: 843

5) Column 1: gallbladder

   Column 2: cystic duct

   Answer: cystic duct

   Page Ref: 843

6) Column 1: pancreas

   Column 2: acini

   Answer: acini

   Page Ref: 840

7) Column 1: peritoneum
   Column 2: mesentery
   Answer: mesentery
   Page Ref: 822

8) Column 1: tongue
   Column 2: fungiform papillae
   Answer: fungiform papillae
   Page Ref: 827

9) Column 1: teeth
   Column 2: cementum
   Answer: cementum
   Page Ref: 827

10) Column 1: oral cavity
    Column 2: hard palate
    Answer: hard palate
    Page Ref: 825

TRUE/FALSE. Write 'T' if the statement is true and 'F' if the statement is false.

1) The stomach is considered an accessory digestive organ.

   Answer: FALSE
   Page Ref: 818

2) Motility of the gastrointestinal tract is controlled primarily by the myenteric plexus.

   Answer: TRUE
   Page Ref: 821

3) The substrate for salivary amylase is starch.

   Answer: TRUE
   Page Ref: 825

4) Cuspids are teeth specialized for grinding food.

   Answer: FALSE
   Page Ref: 828

5) Peristalsis begins in the esophagus.

   Answer: TRUE
   Page Ref: 831

6) Bicarbonate ions are secreted into the lumen of the stomach along with hydrogen ions to buffer them.

Answer: FALSE
Page Ref: 836

7) Secretion of gastrin is stimulated by norepinephrine released by sympathetic neurons.

Answer: FALSE
Page Ref: 837

8) Enterokinase activates pepsin.

Answer: FALSE
Page Ref: 842

9) Stellate reticuloendothelial cells in the liver are phagocytes.

Answer: TRUE
Page Ref: 843

10) Oxygenated and deoxygenated blood mix in liver sinusoids.

Answer: TRUE
Page Ref: 845

11) CCK stimulates ejection of bile from the gallbladder.

Answer: TRUE
Page Ref: 847

12) The jejunum is the longest region of the small intestine.

Answer: FALSE
Page Ref: 848

13) Most monosaccharides are absorbed from the lumen of the small intestine by simple diffusion.

Answer: FALSE
Page Ref: 854

14) The gastrocolic reflex triggers mass peristalsis.

Answer: TRUE
Page Ref: 859

15) The brush border of the small intestine is formed by the microvilli of epithelial cells.

Answer: TRUE
Page Ref: 848

SHORT ANSWER. Write the word or phrase that best completes each statement or answers the question.

1) The epithelium in the mouth, pharynx, and esophagus is _____ epithelium.
   Answer: nonkeratinized stratified squamous
   Page Ref: 821

2) The part of the enteric nervous system located in the muscularis of the wall of the gastrointestinal tract is the _____.
   Answer: myenteric plexus
   Page Ref: 821

3) The condition in which fluid accumulates in the peritoneal cavity is called _____.
   Answer: ascites
   Page Ref: 822

4) The largest peritoneal fold is called the _____.
   Answer: greater omentum
   Page Ref: 822

5) The antibodies seen in saliva belong to the immunoglobulin class _____.
   Answer: IgA
   Page Ref: 825

6) The role of chloride ions in saliva is to _____ ; the role of bicarbonate and phosphate ions is to _____.
   Answer: activate salivary amylase; act as buffers
   Page Ref: 825

7) Teeth are composed primarily of _____.
   Answer: dentin
   Page Ref: 827

8) The root of a tooth is held to the periodontal ligament by _____.
   Answer: cementum
   Page Ref: 827

9) The process of mechanical digestion in the mouth is called _____.
   Answer: mastication (chewing)
   Page Ref: 828

10) The opening in the diaphragm through which the esophagus passes is called the _____.
    Answer: esophageal hiatus
    Page Ref: 830

11) Chief cells of the stomach produce _____ and _____.

Answer: pepsinogen; gastric lipase

Page Ref: 833

12) Parietal cells of the stomach secrete _____ and _____.

Answer: hydrochloric acid; intrinsic factor

Page Ref: 833

13) Mixing waves of the stomach convert solid food to a liquid called _____.

Answer: chyme

Page Ref: 836

14) During the gastric phase of gastric digestion, acetylcholine from parasympathetic neurons stimulates secretion of the hormone _____.

Answer: gastrin

Page Ref: 837

15) Once food enters the duodenum, enteroendocrine cells in the small intestine secrete _____ and _____.

Answer: CCK; secretin

Page Ref: 839

16) Gastric emptying is slowest after a meal rich in _____.

Answer: lipids (triglycerides)

Page Ref: 840

17) The principal triglyceride–digesting enzyme in adults is _____.

Answer: pancreatic lipase

Page Ref: 842

18) Bile is secreted by hepatocytes into vessels called _____.

Answer: bile canaliculi

Page Ref: 843

19) _____ is an important phospholipid in bile that helps make cholesterol more water-soluble.

Answer: Lecithin

Page Ref: 843

20) The principal bile pigment is _____.

Answer: conjugated bilirubin

Page Ref: 844

21) The phagocytic cells of the liver are called _____.

Answer: stellate reticuloendothelial cells

Page Ref: 845

22) All of the microvilli of the epithelial cells of the small intestine collectively form a fuzzy line called the _____.

Answer: brush border

Page Ref: 848

23) Aggregated lymphatic follicles (Peyer's Patches) are located in the mucosa of the _____ of the small intestine.

Answer: ileum

Page Ref: 850

24) Chyme and digestive juices are mixed by localized contractions of the muscularis of the small intestine called _____.

Answer: segmentations

Page Ref: 850

25) Chyme normally remains in the small intestine for about _____ hours.

Answer: 3–5
Page Ref: 850

26) The end-products of the hydrolysis reactions catalyzed by sucrase are _____ and _____.

Answer: glucose; fructose

Page Ref: 852

27) About 90 percent of all absorption of nutrients occurs in the _____ ; the other 10 percent occurs in the _____ and the _____.

Answer: small intestine; stomach; large intestine

Page Ref: 854

28) All dietary lipids are absorbed by the process of _____.

Answer: simple diffusion

Page Ref: 855

29) Globules of triglycerides, phospholipids, and cholesterol that are coated with protein for transport in lacteals are called _____.

Answer: chylomicrons

Page Ref: 856

30) Thickened portions of the longitudinal muscles of the large intestine are called _____ that gather the colon into pouches called _____.

Answer: taeniae coli; haustra

Page Ref: 859

ESSAY. Write your answer in the space provided or on a separate sheet of paper.

1) People with cystic fibrosis produce abnormally thick mucus that clogs ducts. One of the major organs affected is the pancreas. Predict the effects on the digestive system from this disorder.

Answer: Lack of hydrolytic enzymes in pancreatic juice affects digestion of carbohydrates, fats, and proteins, leading to malnutrition. As enzymes back up into the ducts, proteolytic enzymes self–digest pancreatic tissue (despite trypsin inhibitor). Endocrine derangements involving insulin and glucagon may also occur.

Page Ref: 842

2) Explain why food does not normally go up into your nasal cavity or down into your lungs when you swallow —even if you are standing on your head when you swallow.

Answer: Presence of food in the oropharynx stimulates the deglutition center in the medulla and pons to move the soft palate and uvula upward to close off the nasopharynx, thus keeping food out of the nasal cavity. At the same time, the larynx rises and the epiglottis moves down and back to seal off the larynx, which is further closed by the vocal cords, thus keeping food from entering the lower respiratory tract.

Page Ref: 830

3) Describe the structural characteristics of the small intestine that enhance its function as the major absorber of nutrients.

Answer: All structures increase surface area to increase the rate of reabsorption: great length (10' in living humans), microvilli on plasma membrane of each epithelial cell, villi (fingerlike projections of mucosa), and circular folds (permanent ridges in the mucosa).

Page Ref: 848

4) Describe the role of the liver in protein metabolism.

Answer: Hepatocytes deaminate amino acids. The amine group is converted to toxic ammonia. Hepatocytes convert the toxic ammonia to less toxic urea for excretion in urine. The liver also synthesizes many proteins, including most plasma proteins.

Page Ref: 845

5) Describe the structures and functions of the enteric nervous system.

Answer: The ENS consists of the submucosal plexus in the submucosa and the myenteric plexus in the musclaris. Both contain sensory and motor neurons, as well as ANS postganglionic fibers of both divisions. The myenteric plexus also contains parasympathetic ganglia. The submucosal plexus regulates movements of the mucosa, secretion from glands in the gastrointestinal tract, and vasoconstriction of blood vessels in the gastrointestinal tract. The myenteric plexus regulates gastric motility.

Page Ref: 821

6) Describe the location, gross anatomy, and microscopic anatomy of the pancreas. What are the functions of the different types of cells in the pancreas?

Answer: The pancreas lies posterior to the greater curvature of the stomach, and is connected by the pancreatic and accessory ducts to the duodenum. It is retroperitoneal and about 6" long and 1" thick. The head fits into the duodenum; the body and tail extend away from the head. Acini produce digestive enzymes, and make up about 99 percent of pancreatic cells. The pancreatic islets produce glucagon (from alpha cells), insulin (from beta cells), and somatostain (from delta cells), as well as pancreatic polypeptide.

Page Ref: 840

7) Identify the protein–hydrolyzing enzymes in the digestive tract, and name their sources. Why are these enzymes released in an inactive form?

Answer: Pepsin from the stomach, trypsin, chymotrypsin, carboxypeptidase, and elastin from the pancreas, and aminopeptidase and dipeptidase from the small intestine are the proteases in the GI tract. The enzymes are not activated until they are in the lumen of the stomach or small intestine because they would otherwise digest the proteins in the cells that produce them.

Page Ref: 853

8) Describe the flow of blood into, through, and out of the liver. What is the functional significance of this arrangement?

Answer: Oxygenated blood comes from the hepatic artery. Deoxygenated blood containing newly absorbed nutrients comes from the hepatic portal vein. Blood from each mixes in sinusoids, where oxygen, nutrients, and poisons are extracted, and other nutrients are added. Blood then passes into the central vein, then to the hepatic vein. Nutrients newly absorbed are processed quickly, without having to make the full vascular circuit.

Page Ref: 843

9) A patient is passing feces that are chalky white in color. What problems might this indicate? Explain your answer.

Answer: Lack of brown coloration indicates lack of bile pigment derivatives in the feces. Since these come from the action of the liver, the problem could be with the liver itself or with the route the bile takes to get to the small intestine.

Page Ref: 843

10) This morning you drank your coffee black with one teaspoon of sugar and you had a donut with powdered sugar on it. Describe the fates of the table sugar, grain sugar, and fats from this meal in the digestive tract.

Answer: Sucrose (table sugar) is broken down by sucrase in the small intestine into glucose and fructose. Maltose (grain sugar) is broken down by maltase in the small intestine into two molecules of glucose. The sugars are absorbed by secondary active transport (glucose) or facilitated diffusion (fructose). The fats are digested by lipases (lingual, pancreatic), emulsified by bile, and absorbed directly by simple diffusion into either epithelial cells, blood, or the lymph.

Page Ref: 853

CHAPTER 25   Metabolism

MULTIPLE CHOICE. Choose the one alternative that best completes the statement or answers the question.

1) Which of the following is **NOT** one of the possible fates of glucose 6-phosphate?
   A) synthesis of glycogen for glucose storage
   B) conversion to pyruvic acid
   C) conversion to cholesterol
   D) synthesis of nucleic acids
   E) conversion to glucose for release into the bloodstream

   Answer: C
   Page Ref: 891

2) The process of transamination results in:
   A) synthesis of nonessential amino acids.
   B) conversion of amino acids to glucose.
   C) phosphorylation of glucose.
   D) conversion of a hexose to a pentose.
   E) production of ammonia.

   Answer: A
   Page Ref: 891

3) Conversion of amino acids to oxaloacetic acid to glucose 6-phosphate is an example of:
   A) ketogenesis.
   B) beta oxidation.
   C) glycolysis.
   D) deamination.
   E) gluconeogenesis.

   Answer: E
   Page Ref: 892

4) Dietary lipids are transported in lymph and blood by:
   A) high-density lipoproteins.
   B) low-density lipoproteins.
   C) very low-density lipoproteins.
   D) chylomicrons.
   E) ketone bodies.

   Answer: D
   Page Ref: 886

5) Endogenous triglycerides synthesized in hepatocytes are transported to adipocytes for storage by:

   A) High-density lipoproteins.

   B) low-density lipoproteins.

   C) very low-density lipoproteins.

   D) chylomicrons.

   E) ketone bodies.

   Answer: C
   Page Ref: 886

6) Cholesterol is carried to cells for repair of membranes and synthesis of steroid hormones and bile salts by:

   A) high-density lipoproteins.

   B) low-density lipoproteins.

   C) very low-density lipoproteins.

   D) chylomicrons.

   E) ketone bodies.

   Answer: B
   Page Ref: 886

7) Excess cholesterol is transported to the liver for elimination by:

   A) high-density lipoproteins.

   B) low-density lipoproteins.

   C) very low-density lipoproteins.

   D) chylomicrons.

   E) ketone bodies.

   Answer: A
   Page Ref: 886

8) The apoprotein *apo C-2* of chylomicrons and VLDLs activates the enzyme:

   A) phosphatase.

   B) phosphofructokinase.

   C) ATP synthase.

   D) pancreatic lipase.

   E) endothelial lipoprotein lipase.

   Answer: E
   Page Ref: 886

9) The apoprotein *apo B100* on LDLs activates:

   A) phosphofructokinase.

   B) receptor–mediated endocytosis of an LDL.

   C) emulsification of dietary fats.

   D) ATP synthase.

   E) endothelial lipoprotein lipase.

   Answer: B
   Page Ref: 886

10) If total cholesterol = 220 mg/dL, HDL = 45 mg/dL, and triglycerides = 120 mg/dL, what can you tell from this information?

   A) All values are within the desirable range.

   B) The HDL value is acceptable, but the others are high.

   C) Total cholesterol is border–line high.

   D) The LDL value is 151 mg/dL.

   E) Both C and D are correct.

   Answer: E
   Page Ref: 887

11) If total cholesterol = 220 mg/dL, HDL = 45 mg/dL, and triglycerides = 120 mg/dL, what can you tell about LDLs from this information?

   A) LDLs are border–line high.

   B) LDLs are normal.

   C) LDLs are high.

   D) LDLs are low.

   E) There is not enough information to know anything about LDLs.

   Answer: A
   Page Ref: 887

12) Most triglycerides are stored in adipocytes in the:

   A) areas between the muscles.

   B) areas around the kidneys.

   C) subcutaneous tissue.

   D) greater omentum.

   E) large intestine.

   Answer: C
   Page Ref: 887

13) Dietary fat is required for the absorption of ALL of the following EXCEPT:

    A) vitamin A.

    B) tocopherols.

    C) vitamin K.

    D) vitamin D.

    E) thiamine.

Answer: E
Page Ref: 906

14) Beta–carotene is the provitamin form of:

    A) vitamin A.

    B) biotin.

    C) vitamin B_{12}.

    D) ascorbic acid.

    E) tocopherols.

Answer: A
Page Ref: 906

15) Sunlight converts 7–dehydrocholesterol in the skin to cholecalciferol, which is a form of:

    A) vitamin A.

    B) niacin.

    C) vitamin C.

    D) vitamin D.

    E) folic acid.

Answer: D
Page Ref: 906

16) The reactions of the Krebs cycle and the electron transport chain occur in the:

    A) cytosol.

    B) mitochondria.

    C) nucleus.

    D) interstitial fluid.

    E) ribosomes.

Answer: B
Page Ref: 878

17) Lactic acid is produced as a result of the chemical reduction of:

A) acetyl CoA.

B) oxaloacetic acid.

C) pyruvic acid

D) cytochromes.

E) NAD.

Answer: C
Page Ref: 878

18) The end–products of the complete aerobic oxidation of glucose are:

A) fatty acids and glycerol.

B) ATP and oxygen.

C) amino acids.

D) carbon dioxide and water.

E) pyruvic acid and lactic acid.

Answer: D
Page Ref: 882

19) Beta oxidation is the process by which:

A) hydrogen ions are removed from compounds in the Krebs cycle.

B) carbon dioxide is removed from compounds in the Krebs cycle.

C) amine groups are removed from proteins.

D) fatty acids are broken down for use in the Krebs cycle.

E) ADP is converted to ATP.

Answer: D
Page Ref: 888

20) Urea is produced in the process of detoxifying:

A) ammonia.

B) lactic acid.

C) carbon dioxide.

D) pyruvic acid.

E) ketone bodies.

Answer: A
Page Ref: 890

21) The compound that is converted into urea by the liver is formed from the:

   A) acetyl units formed during lipolysis.

   B) amine groups removed during deamination.

   C) reactions of the electron transport chain.

   D) reactions of glycogenolysis.

   E) lactic acid formed during anaerobic respiration.

   Answer: B
   Page Ref: 890

22) The conversion of glycerol into glyceraldehyde 3–phosphate for use in glycolysis is an example of:

   A) glycogenolysis.

   B) deamination.

   C) beta oxidation.

   D) oxidative phosphorylation.

   E) gluconeogenesis.

   Answer: E
   Page Ref: 888

23) The complete hydrolysis of proteins yields:

   A) amino acids.

   B) fatty acids and glycerol.

   C) nucleic acids.

   D) monosaccharides.

   E) carbon dioxide and water.

   Answer: A
   Page Ref: 889

24) **ALL** of the following hormones raise blood glucose **EXCEPT**:

   A) human growth hormone.

   B) glucagon.

   C) cortisol.

   D) insulin.

   E) epinephrine.

   Answer: D
   Page Ref: 895

25) The processes of lipogenesis, protein synthesis, and glycogenesis, are all promoted by the hormone:

A) human growth hormone.

B) glucagon.

C) cortisol.

D) insulin.

E) epinephrine.

Answer: D
Page Ref: 895

26) The function of the satiety center is to:

A) regulate the rate of lipogenesis.

B) stimulate consumption of food.

C) regulate the release of insulin.

D) stimulate cessation of feeding.

E) regulate body temperature.

Answer: D
Page Ref: 901

27) The hormones primarily responsible for daily regulation of production of body heat are produced by the:

A) pancreas.

B) thyroid gland.

C) adrenal cortex.

D) adrenal medulla.

E) hypothalamus.

Answer: B
Page Ref: 898

28) Most biological oxidations are:

A) dehydrogenation reactions.

B) dehydration reactions.

C) hydrolysis reactions.

D) phosphorylation reactions.

E) decarboxylation reactions.

Answer: A
Page Ref: 873

29) Conversion of NAD^+ to NADH and H^+ is an example of:

    A) oxidation.

    B) reduction.

    C) phosphorylation.

    D) hydrolysis.

    E) dehydration.

Answer: B
Page Ref: 873

30) The role of insulin in the body's utilization of glucose is to:

    A) catalyze the conversion of glucose 6-phosphate into glycogen.

    B) carry acetyl units into the Krebs cycle.

    C) increase the rate of facilitated diffusion of glucose into cells.

    D) transport hydrogen ions between compounds of the Krebs cycle and compounds of the electron transport chain.

    E) increase the rate of glycolysis.

Answer: C
Page Ref: 874

31) The function of coenzyme A in glucose metabolism is to:

    A) reduce pyruvic acid to lactic acid.

    B) convert glucose 6-phosphate into glycogen.

    C) transport glucose from the blood across cell membranes.

    D) carry hydrogen ions between compounds in the Krebs cycle and compounds in the electron transport chain.

    E) carry two-carbon units into the Krebs cycle.

Answer: E
Page Ref: 878

32) The primary significance of the Krebs cycle in terms of ATP production is:

    A) production of large amounts of GTP that can be converted to ATP.

    B) transfer of energy into NADH and $FADH_2$.

    C) generation of carbon dioxide for use in the electron transport chain.

    D) transfer of energy into ATP between each step of the cycle.

    E) production of acetyl units.

Answer: B
Page Ref: 879

33) The enzyme found in the hydrogen ion channels between the inner and outer mitochondrial membrane is:

A) cytochrome oxidase.

B) ATP synthase.

C) NADH dehydrogenase.

D) citric synthetase.

E) succinyl kinase.

Answer: B
Page Ref: 882

34) A person who is excreting large amounts of ketone bodies is probably:

A) using mostly fatty acids for energy production.

B) producing large amounts of new protein.

C) just starting to exercise after a long period of inactivity.

D) not taking in enough oxygen.

E) in renal failure.

Answer: A
Page Ref: 889

35) For glycerol to be used in carbohydrate metabolism, it is first converted into:

A) fatty acids.

B) oxaloacetic acid.

C) glyceraldehyde 3–phosphate.

D) glucose 6–phosphate.

E) citric acid.

Answer: C
Page Ref: 888

36) For glycogen to be used for energy production, it must first be converted into:

A) glycerol.

B) glucose 6–phosphate.

C) carbon dioxide.

D) lactic acid.

E) an acetyl unit.

Answer: B
Page Ref: 885

37) Vasoconstriction is considered to be a heat–saving mechanism because:

A) the energy released by vascular smooth muscle contraction warms you up.

B) sweat glands don't receive enough blood supply to produce sweat.

C) less heat can be conducted to the surface and radiated away.

D) more heat is generated by friction as a larger volume of blood is forced through a smaller space.

E) All of these are correct.

Answer: C
Page Ref: 901

38) Before amino acids can enter the Krebs cycle, they must be:

A) oxidized.

B) reduced.

C) decarboxylated.

D) deaminated.

E) dehydrated.

Answer: D
Page Ref: 889

39) A compound that is a product of ketogenesis is:

A) oxaloacetic acid.

B) cholesterol.

C) pyruvic acid.

D) glucose 6–phosphate.

E) beta–hydroxybutyric acid.

Answer: E
Page Ref: 888

40) In chemiosmosis, ATP is produced when:

A) a high energy phosphate group is passed from glucose 6–phosphate to ADP.

B) hydrogen ions are bound to NAD and FAD.

C) pyruvic acid is converted to an acetyl unit.

D) hydrogen ions diffuse into the mitochondrial matrix.

E) glucose is transported across the cell membrane.

Answer: D
Page Ref: 881

41) Each molecule of acetyl CoA that enters the Krebs cycle produces how many molecules of carbon dioxide?

   A) one.

   B) two.

   C) four.

   D) six.

   E) 36.

   Answer: B
   Page Ref: 879

42) During the complete oxidation of one glucose molecule, the electron transport chain yields how many molecules of water?

   A) one.

   B) two.

   C) four.

   D) six.

   E) 32.

   Answer: D
   Page Ref: 882

43) Most ATP generated by the complete oxidation of glucose results from the reactions of:

   A) glycogenolysis.

   B) glycolysis

   C) the Krebs cycle.

   D) the electron transport chain.

   E) gluconeogenesis.

   Answer: D
   Page Ref: 882

44) Gluconeogenesis occurs primarily in hepatocytes and:

   A) adipocytes.

   B) neurons.

   C) skeletal muscle fibers.

   D) kidney cortex cells.

   E) cardiac muscle cells.

   Answer: D
   Page Ref: 885

45) During a prolonged fast or in starvation, most tissues will:

   A) oxidize glucose at a faster rate.

   B) break down the coenzymes NAD and FAD to make ATP.

   C) switch from glucose to fatty acids as the primary energy source.

   D) increase the storage of glycogen in skeletal muscle fibers.

   E) convert more glucose to triglycerides.

   Answer: C
   Page Ref: 888

46) Which of the following is **NOT** characteristic of the absorptive state?

   A) production of ATP by oxidizing glucose to carbon dioxide and water by most body cells

   B) storage of dietary lipids in adipose tissue

   C) gluconeogenesis using amino acids in the liver

   D) packaging of fatty acids and triglycerides into VLDLs

   E) transport of amino acids into body cells

   Answer: C
   Page Ref: 896

47) Which of the following is **NOT** characteristic of the postabsorptive state?

   A) glycogenolysis of liver glycogen

   B) gluconeogenesis using lactic acid in skeletal muscle fibers

   C) beta oxidation of fatty acids by most body cells

   D) oxidation of ketone bodies by heart and kidneys

   E) lipogenesis by hepatocytes

   Answer: E
   Page Ref: 895

48) The primary hormone regulating the metabolic reactions and membrane transport activities of the absorptive state is:

   A) glucagon.

   B) thyroxine.

   C) epinephrine.

   D) insulin.

   E) cortisol.

   Answer: D
   Page Ref: 895

49) Decarboxylation reactions occur in:
   A) the electron transport chain.
   B) the Krebs cycle.
   C) chemiosmosis.
   D) glycogenolysis.
   E) ketogenesis.

   Answer: B
   Page Ref: 879

50) The function of oxygen in aerobic respiration is to:
   A) carry hydrogen ions from the Krebs cycle to the electron transport chain.
   B) bind electrons and hydrogen ions at the end of the electron transport chain.
   C) attach a high energy phosphate group to ADP.
   D) form carbon dioxide in the Krebs cycle.
   E) donate electrons to NADH to make it release a hydrogen ion.

   Answer: B
   Page Ref: 882

MATCHING. Choose the item in column 2 that best matches each item in column 1.

Choose the item from column 2 that best matches each item in column 1.

1) Column 1: calcium
   Column 2: 99% stored in bones and teeth;
             required for release of
             neurotransmitters
   Answer: 99% stored in bones and teeth; required for release of neurotransmitters
   Page Ref: 904

2) Column 1: phosphorus
   Column 2: involved in major buffer
             system and energy transfer;
             component of DNA and RNA
   Answer: involved in major buffer system and energy transfer; component of DNA and RNA
   Page Ref: 904

3) Column 1: potassium
   Column 2: principal cation in
             intracellular fluid
   Answer: principal cation in intracellular fluid
   Page Ref: 904

4) Column 1: selenium
   Column 2: antioxidant; prevents
              chromosome breakage
   Answer: antioxidant; prevents chromosome breakage
   Page Ref: 905

5) Column 1: sodium
   Column 2: most abundant cation in
              extracellular fluid
   Answer: most abundant cation in extracellular fluid
   Page Ref: 904

6) Column 1: chloride
   Column 2: principal anion in
              extracellular fluid
   Answer: principal anion in extracellular fluid
   Page Ref: 904

7) Column 1: cobalt
   Column 2: part of vitamin B_{12}; required
              for erythropoiesis
   Answer: part of vitamin B_{12}; required for erythropoiesis
   Page Ref: 905

8) Column 1: iron
   Column 2: binds oxygen in hemoglobin
   Answer: binds oxygen in hemoglobin
   Page Ref: 905

9) Column 1: copper
   Column 2: component of enzymes in
              electron transport chain;
              needed for melanin formation
   Answer: component of enzymes in electron transport chain; needed for melanin formation
   Page Ref: 905

10) Column 1: zinc
    Column 2: component of carbonic
               anhydrase
    Answer: component of carbonic anhydrase
    Page Ref: 905

MATCHING. Choose the item in column 2 that best matches each item in column 1.

Choose the item from column 2 that best matches each item in column 1.

1) Column 1: vitamin A
   Column 2: essential for formation of
   photopigments
   Answer: essential for formation of photopigments
   Page Ref: 906

2) Column 1: vitamin D
   Column 2: essential for absorption and
   utilization of calcium from the
   GI tract
   Answer: essential for absorption and utilization of calcium from the GI tract
   Page Ref: 906

3) Column 1: vitamin E
   Column 2: antioxidant thought to inhibit
   catabolism of fatty acids in
   cell membranes
   Answer: antioxidant thought to inhibit catabolism of fatty acids in cell membranes
   Page Ref: 906

4) Column 1: vitamin K
   Column 2: essential for synthesis of
   prothrombin by the liver
   Answer: essential for synthesis of prothrombin by the liver
   Page Ref: 906

5) Column 1: vitamin C
   Column 2: antioxidant important for
   collagen production and
   wound healing
   Answer: antioxidant important for collagen production and wound healing
   Page Ref: 907

6) Column 1: vitamin B_1
   Column 2: important for the synthesis of
   acetylcholine
   Answer: important for the synthesis of acetylcholine
   Page Ref: 907

7) Column 1: vitamin B_2
   Column 2: component of coenzymes FAD
   and FMN

   Answer: component of coenzymes FAD and FMN

   Page Ref: 907

8) Column 1: niacin
   Column 2: component of coenzymes
   NAD and NADP

   Answer: component of coenzymes NAD and NADP

   Page Ref: 907

9) Column 1: vitamin B_6
   Column 2: coenzyme for amino acid
   metabolism and production of
   antibodies

   Answer: coenzyme for amino acid metabolism and production of antibodies

   Page Ref: 907

10) Column 1: vitamin B_{12}
    Column 2: necessary for red blood cell
    formation and synthesis of
    methionine

    Answer: necessary for red blood cell formation and synthesis of methionine

    Page Ref: 907

11) Column 1: pantothenic acid
    Column 2: part of coenzyme A

    Answer: part of coenzyme A

    Page Ref: 907

12) Column 1: folic acid
    Column 2: necessary for purine and
    pyrimidine synthesis and
    blood cell production

    Answer: necessary for purine and pyrimidine synthesis and blood cell production

    Page Ref: 907

TRUE/FALSE. Write 'T' if the statement is true and 'F' if the statement is false.

1) Oxidation reactions increase the potential energy of a molecule.

   Answer: FALSE
   Page Ref: 872

2) FAD is chemically reduced by the addition of a hydrogen ion and a hydride ion.

Answer: TRUE
Page Ref: 873

3) Substrate–level phosphorylation occurs in the cytosol of human cells.

Answer: TRUE
Page Ref: 873

4) Glycogenesis is the synthesis of new glucose molecules.

Answer: FALSE
Page Ref: 874

5) The Krebs cycle and electron transport chain both require oxygen to produce ATP.

Answer: TRUE
Page Ref: 874

6) Pyruvic acid undergoes a reduction reaction to form lactic acid.

Answer: TRUE
Page Ref: 878

7) When acetylCoA enters the Krebs cycle it combines with citric acid.

Answer: FALSE
Page Ref: 879

8) Chemiosomosis is the movement of pyruvic acid into mitochondria.

Answer: FALSE
Page Ref: 881

9) Oxygen is the final electron acceptor in the electron transport chain.

Answer: TRUE
Page Ref: 881

10) Most ATP produced during cellular respiration comes from the reactions of glycolysis.

Answer: FALSE
Page Ref: 883

11) Copper atoms are part of the cytochrome oxidase pump of the electron transport chain.

Answer: TRUE
Page Ref: 882

12) The proton motive force is the potential energy contained in the electrochemical gradient created by hydrogen ions within mitochondria.

Answer: TRUE
Page Ref: 882

13) Oxaloacetic acid is a ketone body.

Answer: FALSE
Page Ref: 888

14) During the absorptive state, most glucose that enters hepatocytes is converted to triglycerides or glycogen.

Answer: TRUE
Page Ref: 895

SHORT ANSWER. Write the word or phrase that best completes each statement or answers the question.

1) Joining a fatty acid to glycerol in an ester linkage is an example of a(n) _____ (endergonic) reaction.

Answer: anabolic
Page Ref: 872

2) About 40% of the energy released in catabolism is used for cellular functions, and the rest is _____.

Answer: given off as heat
Page Ref: 872

3) The conversion of lactic acid to pyruvic acid is a(n) _____ reaction because it is a dehydrogenation reaction.

Answer: oxidation
Page Ref: 873

4) In redox reactions, the _____ reaction is usually an exergonic reaction.

Answer: oxidation
Page Ref: 873

5) The enzyme that is the key regulator of the rate of glycolysis is _____.

Answer: phosphofructokinase
Page Ref: 875

6) The fate of pyruvic acid depends on the availability of _____.

Answer: oxygen
Page Ref: 878

7) When acetylCoA enters the Krebs cycle, it combines with _____ to form _____.

Answer: oxaloacetic acid; citric acid

Page Ref: 879

8) In the final step of the Krebs cycle, a hydrogen atom removed from malic acid is transferred to _____.

Answer: NAD^+

Page Ref: 879

9) The most important outcome of the Krebs cycle are the reduced coenzymes _____ and _____.

Answer: NADH; $FADH_2$

Page Ref: 879

10) The three proton pumps of the electron transport chain are the _____ complex, the _____ complex, and the _____ complex.

Answer: NADH dehydrogenase; cytochrome b–c; cytochrome oxidase

Page Ref: 882

11) Glycogenesis is stimulated by the hormone _____.

Answer: insulin

Page Ref: 884

12) Hepatocytes can release glucose into the blood, but skeletal muscles cannot because hepatocytes contain the enzyme _____ that converts glucose 6–phosphate to glucose.

Answer: phosphatase

Page Ref: 885

13) Gluconeogenesis is stimulated by the hormones _____ and _____.

Answer: cortisol; glucagon

Page Ref: 886

14) If _____ are present in excessive numbers, they deposit cholesterol in and around smooth muscle fibers in arteries to form plaques.

Answer: low–density lipoproteins.

Page Ref: 886

15) The polar proteins making up the outer shell of a lipoprotein are called _____.

Answer: apoproteins

Page Ref: 886

16) The apoprotein *apo C-2* of chylomicrons and VLDLs activates the enzyme _____ , which triggers uptake of fatty acids by adipocytes.

Answer: endothelial lipoprotein lipase

Page Ref: 886

17) A person is considered to have high blood cholesterol if total blood cholesterol is greater than _____ mg/dL.

Answer: 239

Page Ref: 887

18) Rickets and osteomalacia are skeletal disorders resulting from deficiency of _____ .

Answer: vitamin D

Page Ref: 906

19) Macrocytic anemia and increased risk of neural tube defects are associated with deficiency of _____ .

Answer: folic acid

Page Ref: 907

20) A decrease in body temperature triggers a(n) _____ in the levels of thyroid hormones.

Answer: increase

Page Ref: 900

21) Nonessential amino acids can be synthesized by the process of _____ , in which an amine group is added to pyruvic acid or other acids.

Answer: transamination

Page Ref: 891

22) The rate at which the resting, fasting body breaks down nutrients to liberate energy is called the _____ .

Answer: basal metabolic rate

Page Ref: 898

23) Transfer of heat between objects without physical contact is called _____ .

Answer: radiation

Page Ref: 899

24) Formation of ATP by transfer of a high-energy phosphate group from an intermediate phosphorylated compound to ADP is called _____ phosphorylation.

Answer: substrate-level

Page Ref: 873

25) Formation of ATP via energy released during the reactions of the electron transport chain is called _____ phosphorylation.

Answer: oxidative

Page Ref: 874

26) Glycolysis is the oxidation of glucose to _____.

Answer: pyruvic acid

Page Ref: 874

27) During the Krebs cycle, two molecules of _____ are generated by substrate-level phosphorylation.

Answer: GTP

Page Ref: 879

28) Iron-containing proteins involved in the reactions of the electron transport chain are called _____.

Answer: cytochromes

Page Ref: 881

29) The theoretical maximum number of ATP molecules produced as a result of the aerobic respiration of one glucose molecule is _____.

Answer: 38

Page Ref: 882

30) The process by which new glucose is formed from non-carbohydrate sources is called _____.

Answer: gluconeogenesis

Page Ref: 885

ESSAY. Write your answer in the space provided or on a separate sheet of paper.

1) Which vitamins are considered "antioxidant vitamins?" Why is this role so important?

Answer: Vitamins C, E, and beta-carotene (a provitamin) are antioxidants that inactivate oxygen free radicals. Free radicals damage cell membranes, DNA, and other cell structures. They also contribute to the formation of atherosclerotic plaque. Antioxidant vitamins may also decrease cancer risk, delay aging, and decrease the risk of cataract formation.

Page Ref: 905

2) Describe the role of the hypothalamus in regulation of food intake.

Answer: The hypothalamus contains the neurons of the feeding center that stimulate eating and of the satiety center that signal fullness. It is thought that changes in blood chemistry (in terms of nutrients and hormone balance), as well as distention of the gastrointestinal tract, initiate appropriate hypothalamic activity.

Page Ref: 901

3) Describe the mechanisms by which heat can be transferred from the body to its surroundings.

Answer: Conduction is heat exchange between objects in direct contact. Convection is heat exchange via fluid movement (e.g., skin to moving air). Radiation is heat exchange without physical contact. Evaporation is heat transfer in the change of state of water from liquid to gas (sweat, insensible perspiration).

Page Ref: 899

4) Identify the different types of lipoproteins and describe the function of each.

Answer: Chylomicrons transport dietary lipids in the lymph and blood. Very low-density lipoproteins transport endogenous triglycerides from hepatocytes to adipocytes for storage. Low-density lipoproteins transport cholesterol through the body for use in repair of membranes and synthesis of steroid hormones and bile salts. High-density lipoproteins transport excess cholesterol to the liver for elimination.

Page Ref: 886

5) Briefly outline the possible fates of glucose in the body.

Answer: 1) immediate oxidation for ATP production
2) synthesis of amino acids for protein synthesis
3) synthesis of glycogen for storage in liver and skeletal muscle
4) formation of triglycerides via lipogenesis for long-term storage after glycogen stores are full
5) excretion in urine if blood glucose is very high

Page Ref: 874

6) What are the possible fates of pyruvic acid in the body? What is the primary determinant of the fate of pyruvic acid? What is the fate of compounds to which pyruvic acid may be converted?

Answer: Pyruvic acid in the presence of low oxygen is reduced to lactic acid, which is converted to either glycogen or carbon dioxide. In the presence of high oxygen levels, pyruvic acid is converted to an acetyl unit, which may be carried into the Krebs cycle by coenzyme A or converted into fatty acids, ketone bodies, or cholesterol.

Page Ref: 878

7) Describe the process of ketogenesis. Under what circumstances would you expect to see elevated levels of the end-products of this process?

Answer: The liver converts the acetyl units of acetyCoA to acetoacetic acid, which is converted to acetone and beta-hydroxybutyric acid. These reactions are increased during periods of fasting and starvation, and also in cases of uncontrolled diabetes mellitus. In these situations, lipolysis reactions are increased, which leads to ketogenesis.

Page Ref: 888

8) Describe the chemiosmotic mechanism of ATP generation.

Answer: The proton pump in the inner mitochondrial membrane expels hydrogen ions from the mitochondrial matrix to create an electrochemical gradient of hydrogen ions. The inner mitochondrial membrane is nearly impermeable to hydrogen ions, which results in a gradient that creates the proton motive force. In regions where specific channels exist, hydrogen ions diffuse back across the membrane, triggering ATP production via action of ATP synthase in the channels.

Page Ref: 881

9) Summarize the Krebs cycle. What defines this process as a "cycle?"

Answer: Acetyl units (2C) enter via coenzyme A to combine with oxaloacetic acid (4C) to form citric acid (6C). Two decarboxylations remove two carbon dioxides, returning the process to the 4C compound (hence the "cycle"). Two GTP are formed by substrate-level phosphorylation. Six NADH, six hydrogen ions, and two FADH$_2$ are formed by the redox reactions that occur in the cycle, all of which enter the electron transport chain to yields 22 ATP. All reactions occur in the matrix of the mitochondria.

Page Ref: 879

10) Your lab partner had the flu, but came to school anyway. Now it's two days later, and you feel chills. Explain this reaction using your knowledge of nonspecific resistance and thermoregulatory mechanisms.

Answer: [note: This question is designed to integrate material from multiple chapters.] A macrophage phagocytizes the pathogen and secretes IL-1, which acts as a pyrogen on the hypothalamus. The hypothalamus secretes PGEs to rest the hypothalamic thermostat to a higher level. Heat-promoting responses, including vasoconstriction, increased metabolism, and shivering, help raise the body temperature to the new level. The increased temperature increases T cell production, macrophage activity, heart rate, etc.

Page Ref: 908

CHAPTER 26   The Urinary System

MULTIPLE CHOICE. Choose the one alternative that best completes the statement or answers the question.

1) In the myogenic mechanism of renal autoregulation:
    A) renin causes contraction of macula densa cells to increase GFR.
    B) smooth muscle in afferent arterioles triggers vasoconstriction to decrease GFR.
    C) norepinephrine causes vasoconstriction of afferent arterioles to decrease GFR.
    D) atrial natriuretic peptide causes relaxation of mesangial cells to increase GFR.
    E) angiotensin II causes dilation of the proximal and distal convoluted tubules.

    Answer: B
    Page Ref: 928

2) The function of atrial natriuretic peptide in renal autoregulation of GFR is to stimulate:
    A) renin secretion.
    B) conversion of angiotensin I to angiotensin II.
    C) relaxation of glomerular mesangial cells.
    D) constriction in afferent and efferent arterioles.
    E) reabsorption of sodium ions.

    Answer: C
    Page Ref: 929

3) **ALL** of the following are mechanisms of renal autoregulation of GFR **EXCEPT**:
    A) sympathetic stimulation of afferent arterioles.
    B) the action of angiotensin on afferent and efferent arterioles.
    C) the action of ANP on mesangial cells.
    D) vasoconstriction in response to stretching of afferent arteriole walls.
    E) secretion of ADH in response to increased osmolarity of blood.

    Answer: E
    Page Ref: 928

4) The surface of glomerular capillaries available for filtration is regulated by:
    A) mesangial cells.
    B) macula densa cells.
    C) juxtaglomerular cells.
    D) renin.
    E) ADH.

    Answer: A
    Page Ref: 925

5) **ALL** of the following are factors in the glomerular filter **EXCEPT:**

   A) slit membranes.

   B) basal laminae.

   C) endothelial cells.

   D) fenestrations.

   E) microvilli.

   Answer: E
   Page Ref: 925

6) If sympathetic stimulation to afferent and efferent arterioles decreases, then GFR:

   A) doesn't change because the arterioles each have the same diameter.

   B) increases because the afferent arterioles dilate, but the efferent arterioles don't change.

   C) increases because both vessels are less constricted.

   D) decreases because both vessels constrict.

   E) doesn't change because the vessels do not have receptors for sympathetic neurotransmitters.

   Answer: C
   Page Ref: 929

7) Passive reabsorption of fluid between tubule cells is called:

   A) transcytosis.

   B) transcellular reabsorption.

   C) facultative reabsorption.

   D) paracellular reabsorption.

   E) obligatory reabsorption.

   Answer: D
   Page Ref: 931

8) Obligatory reabsorption of water occurs in the:

   A) proximal convoluted tubule.

   B) distal convoluted tubule.

   C) ascending limb of the loop of Henle.

   D) descending limb of the loop of Henle.

   E) both A and D are correct.

   Answer: E
   Page Ref: 931

9) Facultative reabsorption of water is regulated by:

   A) angiotensin II.
   B) epinephrine.
   C) ADH.
   D) mesangial cells.
   E) calcitriol.

   Answer: C
   Page Ref: 931

10) Facultative reabsorption of water occurs mainly in the:

   A) glomerulus.
   B) proximal convoluted tubule.
   C) descending limb of the loop of Henle.
   D) ascending limb of the loop of Henle.
   E) collecting ducts.

   Answer: E
   Page Ref: 931

11) Sodium ion transporters in the proximal convoluted tubule promote the reabsorption of **ALL** of the following **EXCEPT:**

   A) ammonium ions.
   B) bicarbonate ions.
   C) chloride ions.
   D) glucose.
   E) amino acids.

   Answer: A
   Page Ref: 932

12) Which of the following is **TRUE** about tubular fluid that has just reached the distal convoluted tubule?

   A) It has a relatively high osmolarity because ions have been added to the fluid, while water has been reabsorbed.
   B) It is identical to glomerular filtrate because nothing has been reabsorbed yet.
   C) It has a relatively low osmolarity because it has just left the ascending limb of the loop of Henle where ions were reabsorbed by water was not.
   D) It is as concentrated as tubular fluid can get.
   E) Both A and D are correct.

   Answer: C
   Page Ref: 939

13) The amount of potassium secreted by principal cells is increased by which of the following?
   A) high levels of sodium ions in tubular fluid
   B) low levels of potassium in plasma
   C) the action of mesangial cells
   D) increased ADH
   E) Both A and D are correct.

   Answer: A
   Page Ref: 935

14) A role of intercalated cells is to:
   A) secrete renin.
   B) secrete erythropoietin.
   C) reabsorb water in response to ADH.
   D) reabsorb sodium ions in response to aldosterone.
   E) excrete hydrogen ions when pH is too low.

   Answer: E
   Page Ref: 936

15) The action of ADH on principal cells is to:
   A) increase production of sodium ion pumps.
   B) increase insertion of aquaporin-2 vesicles into apical membranes.
   C) increase the number of microvilli in their membranes.
   D) decrease the number of aquaporin-1 vesicles in basolateral membranes.
   E) do nothing because principal cells do not have ADH receptors.

   Answer: B
   Page Ref: 937

16) The part of a juxtamedullary nephron that is in the renal medulla is the:
   A) glomerulus only.
   B) glomerular (Bowman's) capsule only.
   C) renal corpuscle.
   D) loop of Henle.
   E) entire nephron.

   Answer: D
   Page Ref: 920

17) Which of the following lists the vessels in the correct order of blood flow?

    A) efferent arteriole, glomerulus, afferent arteriole, peritubular capillaries

    B) peritubular capillaries, efferent arteriole, glomerulus, afferent arteriole

    C) afferent arteriole, efferent arteriole, peritubular capillaries, glomerulus

    D) afferent arteriole, glomerulus, efferent arteriole, peritubular capillaries

    E) efferent arteriole, afferent arteriole, glomerulus, peritubular capillaries

Answer: D
Page Ref: 919

18) Which of the following lists the nephron regions in the correct order of fluid flow?

    A) glomerular capsule, distal convoluted tubule, loop of Henle, proximal convoluted tubule

    B) proximal convoluted tubule, loop of Henle, distal convoluted tubule, glomerular capsule

    C) glomerular capsule, proximal convoluted tubule, loop of Henle, distal convoluted tubule

    D) loop of Henle, glomerular capsule, proximal convoluted tubule, distal convoluted tubule

    E) distal convoluted tubule, loop of Henle, proximal convoluted tubule, glomerular capsule

Answer: C
Page Ref: 918

19) The most important function of the juxtaglomerular (JG) apparatus is to:

    A) secrete water and sodium into the tubular fluid.

    B) release renin in response to a drop in renal blood pressure or blood flow.

    C) make sure that the diameter of the efferent arteriole is kept larger then that of the afferent arteriole.

    D) produce antidiuretic hormone in response to increased glomerular filtration rate (GFR).

    E) produce chemicals that change the diameter of the loop of Henle.

Answer: B
Page Ref: 929

20) If there were an obstruction in the renal artery, one might expect to see:

    A) a decrease in glomerular filtration rate (GFR).

    B) an increase in the release of renin.

    C) an increase in glomerular filtration rate (GFR).

    D) Both B and C are correct.

    E) Both A and B are correct.

Answer: E
Page Ref: 929

21) The **transport maximum** is the:

A) highest the glomerular filtration rate can increase without inhibiting kidney function.

B) greatest percentage of plasma entering the glomerulus that can become filtrate.

C) upper limit of reabsorption due to saturation of carrier systems.

D) steepest any concentration gradient can become.

E) fastest rate at which fluid can flow through the renal tubules.

Answer: C
Page Ref: 931

22) Most water is reabsorbed in the proximal convoluted tubule by **obligatory reabsorption**, which means that:

A) water is moving up its own gradient.

B) water is "following" sodium and other ions/molecules to maintain osmotic balance.

C) the carrier that transports sodium cannot do so without binding water first.

D) the proximal convoluted tubule cannot physically hold the volume of water that enters from the glomerular capsule, so water is reabsorbed because of hydrostatic pressure.

E) the rate of water reabsorption never changes, regardless of water intake.

Answer: B
Page Ref: 931

23) If the level of aldosterone in the blood increases, then:

A) more potassium is excreted in the urine.

B) more sodium is excreted in the urine.

C) blood pressure will drop.

D) glomerular filtration rate will drop.

E) First B, then C, then D.

Answer: A
Page Ref: 935

24) The significance of secretion of ammonium (NH_4^+) ions by the tubule cells is:

A) it triggers the release of renin.

B) it results from generation of new bicarbonate ions that can be reabsorbed to help maintain pH.

C) it keeps the ascending limb of Henle's loop from reabsorbing water.

D) it carries urea across the endothelium of the vasa recta.

E) there is no apparent function for this type of secretion.

Answer: B
Page Ref: 933

25) Podocytes are cells specialized for filtration that are found in the:
    A) walls of the vasa recta.
    B) ascending limb of the loop of Henle.
    C) urinary bladder.
    D) visceral layer of the glomerular capsule.
    E) collecting duct.

Answer: D
Page Ref: 923

26) The function of the macula densa cells is to:
    A) prevent water reabsorption in the ascending limb of the loop of Henle.
    B) prevent over–distension of the urinary bladder.
    C) add bicarbonate ions to the tubular fluid in the proximal convoluted tubule.
    D) monitor NaCl concentration in the tubular fluid.
    E) produce the carrier molecules used to actively transport ions into the peritubular space.

Answer: D
Page Ref: 928

27) If the diameter of the efferent arteriole is smaller than the diameter of the afferent arteriole, then:
    A) blood pressure in the glomerulus stays low.
    B) blood pressure in the glomerulus stays high.
    C) there must be an abnormal blockage in the peritubular capillaries.
    D) the endothelial–capsular membrane filters less blood than normal.
    E) capsular hydrostatic pressure increases to levels higher than glomerular blood hydrostatic pressure.

Answer: B
Page Ref: 925

28) Glomerular filtrate contains:
    A) everything in blood.
    B) everything in blood except cells and proteins.
    C) water and electrolytes only.
    D) water and waste only.
    E) water only.

Answer: B
Page Ref: 925

29) An obstruction in the proximal convoluted tubule decreases glomerular filtration rate because:
   A) blood hydrostatic pressure in the glomerulus decreases when blood can't flow through the tubule.
   B) osmotic pressure in the glomerular capsule increases due to leakage of more proteins into the filtrate.
   C) hydrostatic pressure in the glomerular capsule increases, which decreases net filtration pressure.
   D) hydrostatic pressure in the glomerular capsule decreases due to leakage of more filtrate into the peritubular space.
   E) release of renin decreases as fluid flow to the macula densa decreases.

   Answer: C
   Page Ref: 927

30) As substances are reabsorbed in the proximal convoluted tubules of the kidneys, they move from:
   A) filtered fluid to epithelial cells, to intersitial fluid to peritubular capillaries.
   B) filtered fluid to interstitial fluid, to epithelial cells, to peritubular capillaries.
   C) peritubular capillaries to interstitial fluid, to epithelial cells, to filtered fluid.
   D) vasa recta to epithelial cells, to interstitial fluid, to filtered fluid.
   E) peritubular capillaries to epithelial cells, to interstitial fluid, to filtered fluid.

   Answer: A
   Page Ref: 929

31) The renal clearance of a large protein such as albumin would be closest to which of the following values?
   A) the rate of renal blood flow
   B) the total blood volume entering both kidneys each minute
   C) the average glomerular filtration rate
   D) the transport maximum for glucose
   E) zero

   Answer: E
   Page Ref: 944

32) The permeability of the collecting ducts to water is regulated by:
   A) aldosterone.
   B) renin.
   C) antidiuretic hormone.
   D) atrial natriuretic peptide.
   E) angiotensinogen.

   Answer: C
   Page Ref: 942

33) The countercurrent mechanism in the loop of Henle builds and maintains an osmotic gradient in the renal medulla. Which of the following is **NOT** a contributing factor.?

A) Fluid flows in opposite directions in the ascending and descending limbs of the loop of Henle.

B) Chloride ions passively diffuse from the interstitial fluid into the thick portion of the ascending limb.

C) The thick portion of the ascending limb is impermeable to water.

D) The descending limb is permeable to water.

E) Fluid in the descending limb is in osmotic equilibrium with the surrounding interstitial fluid.

Answer: B
Page Ref: 941

34) Cells that have receptors for aldosterone include:

A) podocytes.

B) intercalated cells in the collecting ducts.

C) cells in the thick ascending limb of the loop of Henle.

D) cells in the proximal convoluted tubules.

E) principal cells in the collecting ducts.

Answer: E
Page Ref: 924

35) An increase in blood pressure in the afferent arterioles of the kidney will result in **ALL** of the following **EXCEPT**:

A) a decrease in the release of atrial natriuretic peptide.

B) an increase in glomerular filtration rate.

C) an increase in glomerular hydrostatic pressure.

D) a somewhat greater output of urine.

E) a decrease in release of renin by juxtaglomerular cells.

Answer: A
Page Ref: 929

36) Filtration of blood in the glomeruli is promoted by:

A) blood colloid osmotic pressure.

B) blood hydrostatic pressure.

C) capsular hydrostatic pressure.

D) both blood hydrostatic pressure and capsular hydrostatic pressure.

E) both blood colloid osmotic pressure and capsular hydrostatic pressure.

Answer: B
Page Ref: 926

37) Sympathetic nerves from the renal plexus are distributed to the:
    A) renal blood vessels.
    B) convoluted tubules.
    C) renal pyramids.
    D) collecting ducts.
    E) both renal blood vessels and convoluted tubules.

    Answer: A
    Page Ref: 918

38) The cells making up the proximal and distal convoluted tubules are:
    A) stratified squamous epithelial cells.
    B) simple squamous epithelial cells.
    C) simple cuboidal epithelial cells.
    D) transitional epithelial cells.
    E) smooth muscle cells.

    Answer: C
    Page Ref: 923

39) The renal corpuscle consists of:
    A) the proximal and distal convoluted tubules.
    B) the glomerulus and the glomerular (Bowman's) capsule.
    C) the descending and ascending limbs of the loop of Henle.
    D) all the renal pyramids.
    E) the glomerulus and the vase recta.

    Answer: B
    Page Ref: 918

40) Which of the following pressures is highest in the renal corpuscle under normal circumstances?
    A) blood colloid osmotic pressure
    B) capsular hydrostatic pressure
    C) capsular colloid osmotic pressure
    D) glomerular blood hydrostatic pressure
    E) None is higher than the others; all pressures are equal under normal circumstances.

    Answer: D
    Page Ref: 927

41) Although angiotensin II has several target tissues, all of its actions are directed toward:
   A) decreasing glomerular filtration rate.
   B) increasing glomerular filtration rate.
   C) increasing the surface area of the nephron.
   D) decreasing the concentration of urine.
   E) decreasing the secretion of aldosterone.

   Answer: B
   Page Ref: 929

42) If a substance has exceeded its transport maximum in the kidney tubules, it is likely that:
   A) urine volume will increase.
   B) urine volume will decrease.
   C) the concentration of the substance in the blood is unusually high.
   D) the concentration of the substance in the blood cannot increase further.
   E) Both A and C are correct.

   Answer: E
   Page Ref: 931

43) The effect of aldosterone on the principal cells of the distal convoluted tubule is to:
   A) increase the synthesis of sodium pumps.
   B) increase the cells' permeability to water.
   C) increase retention of potassium ions.
   D) increase the cells' secretion of antidiuretic hormone.
   E) trigger the release of renin.

   Answer: A
   Page Ref: 937

44) Blood in the renal vein may have a higher concentration of bicarbonate ions than blood in the renal artery because:
   A) bicarbonate ions cannot pass the glomerular filter, so blood becomes more concentrated as water enters the nephrons and bicarbonate ions stay behind.
   B) the rate of cellular respiration is higher in the endothelium of the renal venules than in the endothelium of the renal arterioles.
   C) newly produced bicarbonate ions (as opposed to filtered bicarbonate ions) are added to the blood by the intercalated cells of the collecting ducts as they secrete hydrogen ions into the tubular fluid.
   D) hydrogen ions must be added to venous blood to maintain pH balance, so bicarbonate ions are reabsorbed at the same time to maintain electrical balance.
   E) large ions like bicarbonate ions are necessary in the venous blood to help maintain blood colloid osmotic pressure.

   Answer: C
   Page Ref: 936

45) Urine that is hypotonic to blood plasma is produced when:

   A) levels of aldosterone are high.

   B) levels of antidiuretic hormone are high.

   C) levels of antidiuretic hormone are low.

   D) plasma concentration of sodium ions is high.

   E) levels of both aldosterone and antidiuretic hormone are high.

   Answer: C
   Page Ref: 938

46) The concentration of solutes in tubular fluid is greatest in the:

   A) glomerular (Bowman's) capsule.

   B) proximal convoluted tubule.

   C) hairpin turn of the loop of Henle.

   D) ascending limb of the loop of Henle.

   E) distal convoluted tubule.

   Answer: C
   Page Ref: 939

47) The normal daily volume of urine produced is:

   A) under 200 ml.

   B) 200–400 ml.

   C) 1000–2000 ml.

   D) 3 liters.

   E) 180 liters.

   Answer: C
   Page Ref: 943

48) **Urea recycling** in the renal medulla refers to the:

   A) conversion of urea to ammonia by the tubule cells.

   B) conversion of ammonia to ammonium ions by the tubule cells.

   C) conversion of urea into amino acids in the vasa recta.

   D) mechanism by which urea leaves the collecting duct and re-enters the loop of Henle, thus helping to maintain the hypertonic conditions of the interstitial spaces.

   E) mechanism by which urea leaves the collecting ducts and enters the vasa recta, thus helping to maintain the correct blood volume in the vasa recta.

   Answer: D
   Page Ref: 940

49) Principal cells in the distal convoluted tubules:

    A) secrete renin.

    B) monitor sodium and chloride ion concentrations in tubular fluid.

    C) secrete hydrogen ions when pH in the extracellular fluid is low.

    D) filter large proteins.

    E) respond to ADH and aldosterone.

Answer: E
Page Ref: 924

50) Which of the following would be in the highest concentration in normal urine?

    A) albumin.

    B) bilirubin.

    C) creatinine.

    D) acetoacetic acid.

    E) urobilinogen.

Answer: C
Page Ref: 943

MATCHING. Choose the item in column 2 that best matches each item in column 1.

Choose the item from column 2 that best matches each item in column 1.

1) Column 1: renal clearance
    Column 2: a measure of how effectively
            the kidneys remove a
            substance from the plasma

Answer: a measure of how effectively the kidneys remove a substance from the plasma
Page Ref: 944

2) Column 1: transport maximum
    Column 2: the upper limit of
            reabsorption of a substance
            determined by the number of
            available carrier molecules

Answer: the upper limit of reabsorption of a substance determined by the number of available carrier molecules
Page Ref: 931

3) Column 1: obligatory reabsorption
   Column 2: reabsorption of water with
             solutes in the proximal
             convoluted tubule and
             descending limb of the loop of
             Henle

   Answer: reabsorption of water with solutes in the proximal convoluted tubule and descending
            limb of the loop of Henle

   Page Ref: 931

4) Column 1: tubular secretion
   Column 2: movement of substances from
             the blood or tubule cells into
             the tubular fluid

   Answer: movement of substances from the blood or tubule cells into the tubular fluid

   Page Ref: 930

5) Column 1: tubular reabsorption
   Column 2: movement of substances from
             the tubular fluid into the
             blood

   Answer: movement of substances from the tubular fluid into the blood

   Page Ref: 929

6) Column 1: countercurrent mechanism
   Column 2: the arrangement of
             juxtamedullary nephrons and
             vasa recta that functions to
             generate and maintain the
             osmotic gradient in the renal
             medulla

   Answer: the arrangement of juxtamedullary nephrons and vasa recta that functions to generate
            and maintain the osmotic gradient in the renal medulla

   Page Ref: 941

7) Column 1: glomerular filtration rate
   Column 2: the amount of filtrate formed
             in all the renal corpuscles of
             both kidneys every minute

   Answer: the amount of filtrate formed in all the renal corpuscles of both kidneys every minute

   Page Ref: 927

8) Column 1: net filtration pressure

Column 2: the forces favoring filtration minus the forces opposing filtration

Answer: the forces favoring filtration minus the forces opposing filtration

Page Ref: 927

9) Column 1: renal autoregulation

Column 2: the ability of the kidneys to maintain a constant blood pressure and GFR

Answer: the ability of the kidneys to maintain a constant blood pressure and GFR

Page Ref: 928

10) Column 1: filtration fraction

Column 2: the percentage of plasma entering the nephrons that becomes glomerular filtrate.

Answer: the percentage of plasma entering the nephrons that becomes glomerular filtrate.

Page Ref: 925

MATCHING. Choose the item in column 2 that best matches each item in column 1.

Choose the item from column 2 that best matches each item in column 1.

1) Column 1: renal cortex

Column 2: location of all glomeruli

Answer: location of all glomeruli

Page Ref: 916

2) Column 1: renal medulla

Column 2: made up of renal pyramids

Answer: made up of renal pyramids

Page Ref: 916

3) Column 1: renal papilla

Column 2: apex of a renal pyramid

Answer: apex of a renal pyramid

Page Ref: 916

598

4) Column 1: renal capsule
   Column 2: fibrous membrane
            surrounding and maintaining
            the shape of the kidney
   Answer: fibrous membrane surrounding and maintaining the shape of the kidney
   Page Ref: 916

5) Column 1: renal fascia
   Column 2: anchors kidney to abdominal
            wall and neighboring
            structures.
   Answer: anchors kidney to abdominal wall and neighboring structures.
   Page Ref: 916

6) Column 1: renal pelvis
   Column 2: receives urine from major
            calyces
   Answer: receives urine from major calyces
   Page Ref: 917

7) Column 1: ureter
   Column 2: carries urine from kidney to
            bladder
   Answer: carries urine from kidney to bladder
   Page Ref: 945

8) Column 1: urethra
   Column 2: carries urine from bladder to
            exterior
   Answer: carries urine from bladder to exterior
   Page Ref: 947

9) Column 1: minor calyces
   Column 2: receive urine from papillary
            ducts
   Answer: receive urine from papillary ducts
   Page Ref: 917

10) Column 1: major calyces
    Column 2: pass urine into renal pelvis
    Answer: pass urine into renal pelvis
    Page Ref: 917

TRUE/FALSE. Write 'T' if the statement is true and 'F' if the statement is false.

1) Urine in a major calyx flows into a minor calyx.

Answer: FALSE
Page Ref: 917

2) Blood flows from arcuate arteries into interlobar arteries.

Answer: FALSE
Page Ref: 917

3) The kidneys help regulate blood glucose via the deamination of the amino acid glutamine.

Answer: TRUE
Page Ref: 915

4) The proximal convoluted tubule is part of the renal corpuscle.

Answer: FALSE
Page Ref: 918

5) The kidneys are retroperitoneal organs.

Answer: TRUE
Page Ref: 916

6) Principal cells of the collecting ducts have receptors for both ADH and aldosterone.

Answer: TRUE
Page Ref: 924

7) Tubular secretion removes substances from the blood.

Answer: FALSE
Page Ref: 925

8) Mesangial cells are the cells of the juxtaglomerular apparatus that secrete renin.

Answer: FALSE
Page Ref: 925

9) The fenestrations of glomerular endothelial cells allow filtration of all solutes in plasma.

Answer: TRUE
Page Ref: 925

10) The main force promoting filtration in the glomerulus is glomerular blood hydrostatic pressure.

Answer: TRUE
Page Ref: 925

11) GFR averages 125 mL/min in adult males.

Answer: TRUE
Page Ref: 927

12) Angiotensin II causes vasodilation of the afferent arteriole to increase GFR.

Answer: FALSE
Page Ref: 929

13) Passive movement of fluid between tubule cells is called paracellular reabsorption.

Answer: TRUE
Page Ref: 931

14) Facultative reabsorption of water is regulated mainly by ADH.

Answer: TRUE
Page Ref: 931

15) In the process of producing and secreting ammonium ions, tubule cells also produce bicarbonate ions that diffuse into the blood.

Answer: TRUE
Page Ref: 933

SHORT ANSWER. Write the word or phrase that best completes each statement or answers the question.

1) The measure of the total number of dissolved particles per liter of solution is _____.
Answer: osmolarity
Page Ref: 914

2) The kidneys help regulate blood pressure by secretion of the enzyme _____ and by adjusting _____.
Answer: renin; renal resistance
Page Ref: 914

3) The kidneys release two hormones: _____ , which helps regulate calcium homeostasis, and _____ , which increases red blood cell production.
Answer: calcitriol; erythropoietin
Page Ref: 915

4) The functional units of the kidneys are the _____.
Answer: nephrons
Page Ref: 916

5) Blood flows into afferent arterioles from _____.
   Answer: interlobular arteries
   Page Ref: 917

6) The tubules of the juxtamedullary nephrons are served by special capillaries called _____.
   Answer: vasa recta
   Page Ref: 918

7) Most renal nerves originate in the _____ ganglion, and their function is to regulate _____.
   Answer: celiac; renal resistance and blood flow
   Page Ref: 918

8) Fluid flows from the ascending limb of the loop of Henle into the _____.
   Answer: distal convoluted tubule
   Page Ref: 921

9) The juxtaglomerular apparatus consists of two parts: the _____ that detects the concentration of tubular fluid, and the _____ that secrete renin.
   Answer: macula densa; juxtaglomerular cells
   Page Ref: 923, 928

10) The last portion of the distal convoluted tubule and the collecting duct are made up of _____ cells, which are the target cells for ADH and aldosterone, and _____ cells that have microvilli and help regulate acid–base balance.
    Answer: principal; intercalated
    Page Ref: 924

11) In tubular reabsorption, substances move from _____ to _____.
    Answer: tubular fluid; blood
    Page Ref: 925

12) The footlike processes of podocytes are called _____ and the spaces between the processes are called _____.
    Answer: pedicels; filtration slits
    Page Ref: 925

13) Glomerular endothelial cells are leaky because they have large pores called _____.
    Answer: fenestrations
    Page Ref: 925

14) Norepinephrine causes _____ of afferent arterioles, which causes GFR to _____.

Answer: vasoconstriction; decrease

Page Ref: 928

15) Angiotensin II causes _____ of the afferent arteriole and _____ of the efferent arteriole, which causes GFR to _____.

Answer: vasoconstriction; vasoconstriction; decrease

Page Ref: 929

16) The hormone _____ increases capillary surface area available for filtration by causing relaxation of _____.

Answer: ANP; mesangial cells

Page Ref: 929

17) If there is a decrease in the delivery of sodium and chloride ions to macula densa cells, tubuloglomerular feedback causes GFR to _____.

Answer: increase

Page Ref: 928

18) The 10"–12" tubes carrying urine from the kidneys to the urinary bladder are the _____.

Answer: ureters

Page Ref: 945

19) The mucosa of the urinary bladder includes _____ epithelium.

Answer: transitional

Page Ref: 945

20) The smooth muscle layers surrounding the mucosa of the urinary bladder are collectively known as the _____.

Answer: detrusor muscle

Page Ref: 946

21) The normal component of urine that is derived from the detoxification of ammonia produced as a result of deamination of proteins is _____.

Answer: urea

Page Ref: 943

22) The enzyme secreted by the juxtaglomerular cells in response to impulses from renal sympathetic nerves is _____.

Answer: renin

Page Ref: 936

23) The substrate for the enzyme secreted by juxtaglomerular cells is _____.

Answer: angiotensinogen

Page Ref: 936

24) The blood vessels of surrounding the loop of Henle that help maintain the hypertonic conditions in the peritubular spaces of the renal medulla are called the _____.

Answer: vasa recta

Page Ref: 918

25) The percentage of plasma in afferent arterioles that becomes glomerular filtrate is called the _____.

Answer: filtration fraction

Page Ref: 925

26) In the formula for calculating net filtration pressure, those forces opposing glomerular filtration are _____ and _____ .

Answer: capsular hydrostatic pressure; blood colloid osmotic pressure

Page Ref: 926

27) Fluid flowing in opposite directions in parallel tubes is called _____ flow.

Answer: countercurrent

Page Ref: 940

28) The product of catabolism of nucleic acids that is normally present in urine and that may crystallized into kidney stones is _____.

Answer: uric acid

Page Ref: 943

29) Most tubular reabsorption of water, sodium ions, and potassium ions occurs in the _____.

Answer: proximal convoluted tubule

Page Ref: 929

30) The renal tubules are least permeable to water in the region known as the _____.

Answer: thick ascending limb (of the loop of Henle)

Page Ref: 939

ESSAY. Write your answer in the space provided or on a separate sheet of paper.

1) Describe the role of the kidney in acid–base balance.

Answer: The kidney can secrete hydrogen ions (via Na^+/H^+ antiporter). It can also reabsorb bicarbonate ions generated from carbon dioxide (from various sources) and generate new bicarbonate ions via deamination of glutamine.

Page Ref: 933

2) Describe the flow of blood through the kidneys.

Answer: Kidneys receive 20–25% of the resting cardiac output via the renal arteries. The renal arteries branch to form segmental arteries, which branch to form interlobar arteries (through renal columns) to arcuate arteries (over bases of pyramids) to interlobular arteries. The interlobular arteries branch to form afferent arterioles to each nephron. Afferent arterioles branch to form glomerular capillaries where filtration occurs. Glomerular capillaries merge to form efferent arterioles, which then branch to form peritubular capillaries. Juxtamedullary nephrons also have vasa recta capillaries around them. Peritubular capillaries merge to form peritubular veins and with the vasa recta to form interlobular veins to arcuate veins to interlobar veins to segmental veins. Blood exits the kidney via renal veins.

Page Ref: 917–919

3) What is the difference between obligatory and facultative reabsorption of water. How is reabsorption regulated?

Answer: Obligatory reabsorption of water is that which occurs with solutes for osmotic balance. This accounts for 90% of water reabsorption and is regulated by the GFR. Facultative reabsorption is the water that is reabsorbed or excreted depending of the body's needs. It is regulated by ADH.

Page Ref: 931

4) Janice has done a dipstick urine test. The glucose square indicates that glucose is present in her urine sample. Should she be concerned? Why or why not?

Answer: Glucose is not normally present in urine. Janice should be concerned if repeated testing shows elevated levels, and if she cannot attribute the elevated levels to recent glucose loading or stress, which increases glucose in the blood. Glucosuria generally indicates diabetes mellitus.

Page Ref: 944

5) Describe in detail the renin–angiotensin negative feedback loop that helps regulate blood pressure and glomerular filtration rate.

Answer: Stress causes a decrease in blood pressure, and thus, GFR. The JG cells of the juxtaglomerular apparatus sense decreased stretch and macula densa cells sense decreased NaCl and water. The JG cells secrete renin, which converts angiotensinogen in blood to angiotensin I, which is converted to angiotensin II by ACE in the lungs. Angiotensin II causes constriction of efferent arterioles, increased thirst, greater ADH secretion from the posterior pituitary, and increased secretion of aldosterone from the adrenal cortex. Blood volume is increased, which increases venous return, stroke volume, cardiac output, and blood pressure. GFR is also increased.

Page Ref: 936

6) Discuss the importance of countercurrent flow to the functioning of the nephron.

Answer: Countercurrent flow refers to the flow of fluid in opposite directions in parallel tubing (tubules and blood vessels). The arrangement allows gradients to develop between tubular fluid, blood, and interstitial fluid. Gradients allow for reabsorption of large amounts of water and ions from the tubular fluid.

Page Ref: 941

7) Describe the structural features of the renal corpuscle that enhance its blood filtering capacity.

Answer: Endothelial cells of the glomerular capillaries are fenestrated. Their basement membranes are part of the filtering mechanism. Podocytes with filtration slits between pedicels wrap the glomerular capillaries. The large surface area also contributes to filtering ability, as does the high glomerular hydrostatic pressure created by the arrangement of the afferent and efferent arterioles, in which the diameter of the efferent arteriole is smaller than that of the afferent arteriole.

Page Ref: 925

8) Predict the effect on reabsorption of sodium ions, bicarbonate ions, and water from the proximal convoluted tubule in an individual who has been given a drug to inhibit carbonic anhydrase activity. Explain your answer.

Answer: Carbonic anhydrase inhibitors block the conversion of bicarbonate ions to water and carbon dioxide for reabsorption. Thus, more bicarbonate ions are excreted. Sodium ions are excreted as they follow bicarbonate ions for electrical balance, and water follows sodium for osmotic balance.

Page Ref: 932–936

9) Predict the effect on GFR and net filtration pressure of each of the following: 1) hemorrhage; 2) increased permeability of the endothelial–capsular membrane; 3) constriction of the lumen of the proximal convoluted tubule. Explain your reasoning in each case.

Answer: 1) Ultimately GFR and NFP decrease as blood volume decreases, since the decreased volume will ultimately decrease blood pressure.
2) NFP increases as proteins escape into the glomerular capsule, increasing capsular colloid osmotic pressure. Water follows the proteins, ultimately decreasing blood volume and blood pressure, which decreases GFR.
3) As capsular hydrostatic pressure increases, NFP decreases. As capsular hydrostatic pressure rises, GFR is reduced.

Page Ref: 927

10) Predict the effects on levels of aldosterone and antidiuretic hormone of each of the following: 1) hemorrhage; 2) increased permeability of the endothelial–capsular membrane; 3) excessive loss of body water by sweating. Explain your answer in each case.

Answer: 1) Both will increase as blood pressure drops and blood volume decreases.
2) Both will increase as water is lost with escaping proteins, reducing blood volume, blood concentration, and blood pressure.
3) Both will increase as both sodium and water are lost from the blood.

Page Ref: 936

CHAPTER 27   Fluid, Electrolyte, and Acid-Base Homeostasis

MULTIPLE CHOICE. Choose the one alternative that best completes the statement or answers the question.

1) The primary means of water movement between fluid compartments is:

A) osmosis.

B) primary active transport.

C) secondary active transport.

D) facilitated diffusion.

E) pinocytosis.

Answer: A
Page Ref: 956

2) The direction of water movement between fluid compartments is determined by:

A) the electrical gradient.

B) the solubility of water in membrane lipids.

C) the concentration of solutes.

D) the diameter of blood vessels.

E) differences in pH.

Answer: C
Page Ref: 956

3) Women generally have a lower amount of total body water than men because:

A) they are smaller than men.

B) estrogen causes greater water loss than testosterone.

C) they have a higher body temperature.

D) they have a higher percentage of body fat.

E) All of these are correct.

Answer: C
Page Ref: 957

4) The thirst center is stimulated by **ALL** of the following **EXCEPT**:

   A) osmoreceptors in the hypothalamus.

   B) peripheral chemoreceptors.

   C) baroreceptors.

   D) dry mouth.

   E) angiotensin II.

   Answer: B
   Page Ref: 958

5) Natriuresis causes:

   A) reabsorption of sodium ions from renal tubules.

   B) reabsorption of water from renal tubules.

   C) increased release of ANP.

   D) increased water loss via the kidneys.

   E) Both A and B are correct.

   Answer: D
   Page Ref: 958

6) The primary determinant of body fluid volume is the:

   A) concentration of potassium ions inside cells.

   B) level of physical activity.

   C) amount of water ingested.

   D) body weight.

   E) number of sodium and chloride ions lost from the kidney.

   Answer: E
   Page Ref: 958

7) The stimulus for release of ANP is:

   A) renin.

   B) ADH.

   C) aldosterone.

   D) stretching of the atrial wall.

   E) osmoreceptors.

   Answer: D
   Page Ref: 958

8) A decrease in angiotensin II leads to:

   A) increased blood volume due to decreased GFR.

   B) decreased blood volume due to increased GFR.

   C) decreased blood volume due to decreased GFR.

   D) increased blood volume due to increased GFR.

   E) no changes in blood volume.

   Answer: B
   Page Ref: 959

9) An increase in ADH leads to:

   A) insertion of aquaporin–2 channels into principal cell membranes.

   B) an increase in aldosterone.

   C) stimulation of the thirst center.

   D) excretion of bicarbonate ions.

   E) Both A and C are correct.

   Answer: A
   Page Ref: 960

10) Drinking plain water after excessive sweating leads to:

    A) shut–down of sweat glands.

    B) hypernatremia.

    C) water intoxication.

    D) dehydration of cells.

    E) both C and D are correct.

    Answer: C
    Page Ref: 960

11) Hydrogen ions are normally eliminates from the body:

    A) by excretion in urine.

    B) via insensible perspiration.

    C) in expired air.

    D) both A and B are correct.

    E) both A and C are correct.

    Answer: A
    Page Ref: 967

12) The primary intracellular ions are:

    A) potassium and chloride ions and protein anions.

    B) sodium and phosphate ions.

    C) potassium and phosphate ions and protein anions.

    D) sodium and chloride ions.

    E) potassium, phosphate, and calcium ions.

Answer: C
Page Ref: 962

13) Protein anions are most abundant in:

    A) plasma.

    B) interstitial fluid.

    C) the cytosol.

    D) urine.

    E) glomerular filtrate.

Answer: C
Page Ref: 962

14) A person who has not eaten for a week is probably:

    A) generating ketone bodies.

    B) excreting excess hydrogen ions.

    C) generating new bicarbonate ions.

    D) breathing more rapidly than normal.

    E) All of these are correct.

Answer: E
Page Ref: 969

15) Bicarbonate ion acts as a:

    A) nonelectrolyte.

    B) strong acid.

    C) strong base.

    D) weak acid.

    E) weak base.

Answer: E
Page Ref: 966

16) ADH saves water by:

   A) promoting the excretion of sodium ions.

   B) stimulation the secretion of renin.

   C) enhancing passive movement of water out of the collecting ducts.

   D) stimulating constriction of the lumen of the distal convoluted tubules.

   E) lowering the glomerular filtration rate.

   Answer: C
   Page Ref: 960

17) The area that stimulates the conscious desire to drink water is located in the:

   A) adrenal cortex.

   B) kidney.

   C) medulla oblongata.

   D) hypothalamus.

   E) lumbar region of the spinal cord.

   Answer: D
   Page Ref: 959

18) Levels of sodium ions in the extracellular fluid are regulated primarily by:

   A) ADH.

   B) aldosterone.

   C) parathyroid hormone.

   D) epinephrine.

   E) insulin.

   Answer: B
   Page Ref: 961

19) Levels of potassium ions in the extracellular fluid are regulated primarily by:

   A) ADH.

   B) aldosterone.

   C) parathyroid hormone.

   D) epinephrine.

   E) insulin.

   Answer: B
   Page Ref: 962

20) Which of the following would serve to buffer H^+?

    A) NaH_2PO_4

    B) the –COOH end of a protein

    C) HCO_3^-

    D) any strong acid

    E) any weak acid

Answer: C
Page Ref: 966

21) Which of the following would serve to buffer OH–?

    A) NaH_2PO_4.

    B) HCO_3.

    C) the amine end of a protein.

    D) a monohydrogen phosphate ion.

    E) any strong base.

Answer: A
Page Ref: 966

22) In order for H^+ to be excreted, it must combine with other substances, including:

    A) HCO_3^-

    B) CO_2

    C) $H_2PO_4^-$

    D) hemoglobin

    E) HPO_4^{2-}

Answer: E
Page Ref: 966

23) In compensating for respiratory alkalosis, the body excretes more:

    A) ammonium ions.

    B) bicarbonate ions.

    C) dihydrogen phosphate ions.

    D) carbonic acid.

    E) hydrogen ions.

Answer: B
Page Ref: 969

24) In compensating for metabolic acidosis, the body:

A) increases respiratory rate.

B) excretes more bicarbonate ions.

C) excretes more monohydrogen phosphate ions.

D) decreases respiratory rate.

E) slows the rate of conversion of ammonia to urea.

Answer: A
Page Ref: 969

25) If the pH of blood plasma becomes 7.49 due to ingested substances, **ALL** of the following would happen to compensate **EXCEPT:**

A) respiratory rate decreases.

B) the kidney increases excretion of bicarbonate ions.

C) tubule cells produce more ammonia from glutamate.

D) the partial pressure of carbon dioxide in blood would begin to rise.

E) the kidney excretes fewer dihydrogen phosphate ions.

Answer: C
Page Ref: 969

26) Which of the following ions is most abundant in extracellular fluid?

A) Na^+

B) K^+

C) H^+

D) HPO_4^{2-}

E) Ca^{2+}

Answer: A
Page Ref: 961

27) Which of the following would be able to buffer a strong base?

A) HCO_3^-

B) NH_3

C) $H_2PO_4^-$

D) hemoglobin

E) another strong base

Answer: C
Page Ref: 966

28) Which of the following values is within homeostatic range for bicarbonate ions in arterial blood?

   A) 136–142 mEq/liter

   B) 3.8–5.0 mEq/liter

   C) 22–26 mEq/liter

   D) 4.6–5.5 mEq/liter

   E) 1.7–2.6 mEq/liter

   Answer: C
   Page Ref: 966

29) Which of the following falls within homeostatic range for levels of sodium ions in plasma?

   A) 136–142 mEq/liter

   B) 3.8–5.0 mEq/liter

   C) 22–26 mEq/liter

   D) 4.6–5.5 mEq/liter

   E) 1.7–2.6 mEq/liter

   Answer: A
   Page Ref: 961

30) Calculate the number of mEq/liter of cations of a 3 mmol/liter solution of Na_2SO_4. Assume complete ionization.

   A) To calculate the answer, the molecular weight is required.

   B) 57.9 mEq/liter

   C) 3 mEq/liter

   D) 6 mEq/liter

   E) 12 mEq/liter

   Answer: D
   Page Ref: 961

31) The cation that is necessary for generation and conduction of action potentials and that contributes nearly half of the osmotic pressure of extracellular fluid is:

   A) sodium ion.

   B) potassium ion.

   C) calcium ion.

   D) chloride ion.

   E) phosphate ion.

   Answer: A
   Page Ref: 961

32) Which of the following would you expect to see in response to an extracellular fluid calcium ion level of 5.7 mEq/liter?

   A) increased secretion of aldosterone.

   B) increased secretion of PTH.

   C) increased secretion of CT.

   D) decreased secretion of ANP.

   E) increased secretion of ADH.

   Answer: C
   Page Ref: 963

33) Aldosterone regulates the level of chloride ions in body fluids by:

   A) opening chloride channels in principal cells of distal convoluted tubules.

   B) reabsorbing chloride ions for electrical balance as bicarbonate ions are secreted from renal tubules.

   C) altering the permeability of glomerular capillaries.

   D) regulating secretion from gastric mucosal glands.

   E) controlling reabsorption of sodium ions, which chloride ions follow due to electrical attraction.

   Answer: E
   Page Ref: 962

34) When bicarbonate ion diffuses out of red blood cells into plasma, it is usually exchanged with which anion?

   A) sodium

   B) potassium

   C) phosphate

   D) hydrogen

   E) chloride

   Answer: E
   Page Ref: 963

35) Why are levels of bicarbonate ion higher in arterial blood than in venous blood?

   A) because the partial pressure of carbon dioxide is higher in arterial blood

   B) because more bicarbonate ions are used up in venous blood to buffer hydrogen ions

   C) because the higher oxygen levels in arterial blood promote dissociation of carbonic acid

   D) because cells in the pulmonary capillaries actively secrete bicarbonate ions into the plasma

   E) because the higher oxygen levels in arterial blood increase the activity of carbonic anhydrase

   Answer: B
   Page Ref: 963

36) Which of the following is **NOT** an effect of increased levels of parathyroid hormone?

   A) increased absorption of calcium ions from the gastrointestinal tract

   B) increased reabsorption of calcium ions by renal tubule cells

   C) increased reabsorption of phosphate ions by renal tubule cells

   D) increased release of calcium ions from mineral salts in bone matrix

   E) increased release of phosphate ions from mineral salts in bone matrix

   Answer: C
   Page Ref: 963

37) In studies of fluid balance, the term **water intoxication** refers to:

   A) poisoning of the body's water due to buildup of toxic substances during renal failure.

   B) increased blood hydrostatic pressure created by high total blood volume.

   C) movement of water from interstitial fluid into intracellular fluid due to osmotic gradients created by ion loss.

   D) any situation in which edema develops.

   E) failure of the neurohypophysis to secrete sufficient ADH.

   Answer: C
   Page Ref: 960

38) The carboxyl group of an amino acid acts as a buffer for:

   A) excess hydrogen ions.

   B) excess hydroxide ions.

   C) other carboxyl groups.

   D) carbonic acid in red blood cells.

   E) hydrochloric acid in gastric juice.

   Answer: B
   Page Ref: 965

39) Hemoglobin picks up a hydrogen ion when:

   A) it releases oxygen to tissues.

   B) it binds oxygen in pulmonary capillaries.

   C) chloride ions enter red blood cells.

   D) the intracellular concentration of monohydrogen phosphate ions is too low to be effective.

   E) chloride ions leave red blood cells.

   Answer: A
   Page Ref: 966

40) Which of the following does **NOT** act as a weak base?

   A) bicarbonate ion

   B) the $-NH_2$ end of an amino acid

   C) monohydrogen phosphate ion

   D) deoxyhemoglobin

   E) $H_2PO_4^-$

   Answer: E
   Page Ref: 966

41) The ratio of bicarbonate ions to carbonic acid molecules in extracellular fluid is normally about:

   A) 1:20.

   B) 1:1.

   C) 2:1.

   D) 20:1.

   E) 100:1.

   Answer: D
   Page Ref: 966

42) Which of the following cannot help protect against pH changes caused by respiratory problems in which there is an excess or shortage of carbon dioxide?

   A) plasma protein buffers

   B) hemoglobin

   C) bicarbonate ion/carbonic acid buffers

   D) phosphate buffers

   E) only phosphate buffers can help protect against such pH changes

   Answer: C
   Page Ref: 966

43) Which of the following statements is correct?

   A) A strong acid plus a weak acid yields water plus a weak base.

   B) A strong acid plus a weak base yields a salt plus a weak acid.

   C) A strong acid plus a weak base yields a weak base plus a weak acid.

   D) A strong acid plus a strong base yields a weak acid plus a weak base.

   E) A strong acid plus a weak acid yields a strong base plus a weak base.

   Answer: B
   Page Ref: 965

44) Which of the following statements is correct?

   A) A strong base plus a weak base yields a salt plus a weak base.

   B) A strong base plus a weak acid yields a strong acid and a weak base.

   C) A strong base plus a strong acid yields a weak base plus a weak acid.

   D) A strong base plus a weak acid yields water plus a weak base.

   E) A strong base plus a weak base yields a strong acid plus a weak acid.

   Answer: D
   Page Ref: 965

45) Increasing respiratory rate will:

   A) add more hydrogen ions to the extracellular fluid.

   B) result in an increase in excretion of excess bicarbonate ions in urine.

   C) result in an increase in excretion of dihydrogen phosphate ions in urine.

   D) lower the pH of extracellular fluid.

   E) cause a decrease in the affinity of hemoglobin for oxygen.

   Answer: B
   Page Ref: 969

46) The inspiratory center in the medulla oblongata triggers more forceful and frequent contractions of the diaphragm if:

   A) a decrease in pCO_2 is detected by peripheral chemoreceptors.

   B) a large quantity of an alkaline drug is ingested.

   C) levels of ketone bodies become elevated.

   D) hydrochloric acid is lost via severe vomiting.

   E) blood pressure is increased.

   Answer: C
   Page Ref: 968

47) Uncontrolled diabetes mellitus may lead to metabolic acidosis because:

   A) high glucose levels depress the respiratory centers in the medulla.

   B) glucose is an acidic substance.

   C) glucose is osmotically active, and for every water molecule retained, a hydrogen ion is also retained.

   D) most diabetics have chronic diarrhea, which leads to excessive loss of bicarbonate ions.

   E) increased rated of lipolysis and ketogenesis occur.

   Answer: E
   Page Ref: 969

48) Which of the following might trigger an increase in the rate of deamination of glutamine by renal tubule cells as a form of compensation for a pH imbalance?

A) an abrupt move to a high altitude

B) ingestion of alkaline drugs

C) plasma levels of bicarbonate ion at 30 mEq/liter

D) pulmonary edema

E) severe, prolonged vomiting

Answer: D
Page Ref: 969

49) A patient whose blood pH is 7.47, whose pCO_2 is 31 mmHg in arterial blood, and whose levels of bicarbonate ion in arterial blood are 23 mEq/liter is in:

A) compensated metabolic alkalosis.

B) uncompensated respiratory acidosis.

C) uncompensated respiratory alkalosis.

D) uncompensated metabolic acidosis.

E) uncompensated metabolic alkalosis.

Answer: C
Page Ref: 969

50) A patient whose blood pH is 7.47, whose pCO_2 in arterial blood is 40 mm Hg, and whose levels of bicarbonate ion in arterial blood are 28 mEq/liter is in:

A) compensated metabolic alkalosis.

B) uncompensated respiratory acidosis.

C) uncompensated respiratory alkalosis.

D) uncompensated metabolic acidosis.

E) uncompensated metabolic alkalosis.

Answer: E
Page Ref: 969

MATCHING. Choose the item in column 2 that best matches each item in column 1.

Choose the item from column 2 that best matches each item in column 1.

1) Column 1: hyponatremia

Column 2: muscle weakness, hypotension, tachycardia, shock

Answer: muscle weakness, hypotension, tachycardia, shock

Page Ref: 964

2) Column 1: hypernatremia

   Column 2: intense thirst, hypertension,
             edema, convulsions

   Answer: intense thirst, hypertension, edema, convulsions

   Page Ref: 964

3) Column 1: hypokalemia

   Column 2: flaccid paralysis, flattening of
             T wave on ECG

   Answer: flaccid paralysis, flattening of T wave on ECG

   Page Ref: 964

4) Column 1: hyperkalemia

   Column 2: anxiety, nausea, vomiting,
             diarrhea, ventricular
             fibrillation

   Answer: anxiety, nausea, vomiting, diarrhea, ventricular fibrillation

   Page Ref: 964

5) Column 1: hypocalcemia

   Column 2: hyperactive reflexes, tetany,
             bone fractures, laryngospasm

   Answer: hyperactive reflexes, tetany, bone fractures, laryngospasm

   Page Ref: 964

6) Column 1: hypercalcemia

   Column 2: bone pain, paresthesia, coma

   Answer: bone pain, paresthesia, coma

   Page Ref: 964

7) Column 1: hyperchloremia

   Column 2: lethargy, metabolic acidosis

   Answer: lethargy, metabolic acidosis

   Page Ref: 964

8) Column 1: hypochloremia

   Column 2: muscle spasms, tetany,
             metabolic alkalosis

   Answer: muscle spasms, tetany, metabolic alkalosis

   Page Ref: 964

MATCHING. Choose the item in column 2 that best matches each item in column 1.

Choose the item from column 2 that best matches each item in column 1.

1) Column 1: Na^+

Column 2: accounts for 50% of osmotic pressure in ECF; important for establishing resting potential and depolarization

Answer: accounts for 50% of osmotic pressure in ECF; important for establishing resting potential and depolarization

Page Ref: 961

2) Column 1: Cl^-

Column 2: important for anion balance between plasma and red blood cells; secreted by gastric mucosal cells

Answer: important for anion balance between plasma and red blood cells; secreted by gastric mucosal cells

Page Ref: 962

3) Column 1: $H_2PO_4^-$

Column 2: anion that is an important intracellular and urinary buffer

Answer: anion that is an important intracellular and urinary buffer

Page Ref: 963

4) Column 1: Ca^{2+}

Column 2: cation that is an important clotting factor and that is involved in release of neurotransmitters

Answer: cation that is an important clotting factor and that is involved in release of neurotransmitters

Page Ref: 963

5) Column 1: Mg^{2+}

Column 2: important cofactor for functioning of the Na^+/K^+ pump

Answer: important cofactor for functioning of the Na^+/K^+ pump

Page Ref: 963

6) Column 1: HCO_3^-

Column 2: important buffer for acids in
blood

Answer: important buffer for acids in blood

Page Ref: 963

7) Column 1: K^+

Column 2: intracellular cation important
in establishing resting
potential and repolarization

Answer: intracellular cation important in establishing resting potential and repolarization

Page Ref: 962

TRUE/FALSE. Write 'T' if the statement is true and 'F' if the statement is false.

1) The largest percentage of extracellular fluid is interstitial fluid.

Answer: TRUE
Page Ref: 956

2) People with a higher percentage of body fat have a lower percentage of body water than lean
people.

Answer: TRUE
Page Ref: 957

3) The tunica intima is the barrier between extracellular fluid and intracellular fluid.

Answer: FALSE
Page Ref: 956

4) Metabolic water is produced mainly by aerobic cellular respiration.

Answer: TRUE
Page Ref: 957

5) The so-called thirst center is located in the hypothalamus.

Answer: TRUE
Page Ref: 958

6) Aldosterone promotes natriuresis.

Answer: FALSE
Page Ref: 958

7) An increase in osmolarity of extracellular fluid stimulates release of ADH.

Answer: TRUE
Page Ref: 960

8) Intracellular fluid and interstitial fluid normally have the same osmolarity.

Answer: TRUE
Page Ref: 960

9) Chloride is the most abundant anion in intracellular fluid.

Answer: FALSE
Page Ref: 962

10) Low sodium ion levels cause ADH secretion to cease.

Answer: TRUE
Page Ref: 961

11) The amine end of a protein acts as a weak acid.

Answer: FALSE
Page Ref: 965

12) An increase in ventilation rate causes pH of extracellular fluid to decrease.

Answer: FALSE
Page Ref: 966

13) The Na^+/K^+ ATPase cannot function properly without magnesium ions.

Answer: TRUE
Page Ref: 963

14) The major physiological effect of acidosis is overexcitability of the nerves.

Answer: FALSE
Page Ref: 967

15) A person whose pH is 7.32, whose partial pressure of carbon dioxide is 47 mm Hg, and whose bicarbonate ions measure 24 mEq/liter is in uncompensated respiratory acidosis.

Answer: TRUE
Page Ref: 969

SHORT ANSWER. Write the word or phrase that best completes each statement or answers the question.

1) Severe diarrhea leads to the pH imbalance _____ due to loss of _____.
Answer: metabolic acidosis; bicarbonate ions
Page Ref: 969

2) Chronic obstructive pulmonary disease leads to the pH imbalance _____ due to _____.

Answer: respiratory acidosis; increased partial pressure of carbon dioxide (hypoventilation)
Page Ref: 969

3) Severe vomiting leads to the pH imbalance _____ due to loss of _____.

Answer: metabolic alkalosis; gastric acids

Page Ref: 969

4) Aspirin overdose leads to the pH imbalance _____ due to _____.

Answer: respiratory alkalosis; hyperventilation (decreased partial pressure of carbon dioxide)

Page Ref: 969

5) You would expect a person with chronic obstructive pulmonary disease to be excreting more _____ in urine than a healthy person.

Answer: hydrogen ions

Page Ref: 969

6) The physiological response to an acid–base imbalance that acts to normalize arterial blood pH is called _____.

Answer: compensation

Page Ref: 967

7) In the phosphate buffer system, the weak acid is _____ and the weak base is _____.

Answer: dihydrogen phosphate; monohydrogen phosphate

Page Ref: 966

8) The most abundant buffer in intracellular fluid and plasma is the _____ system.

Answer: protein buffer

Page Ref: 965

9) The _____ group of an amino acid acts as an acid.

Answer: carboxyl

Page Ref: 965

10) Hydrogen ions are buffered inside red blood cells by _____.

Answer: reduced hemoglobin

Page Ref: 965

11) Bone resorption is stimulated by the hormone _____ to raise the blood levels of _____ ions.

Answer: parathyroid hormone; calcium

Page Ref: 963

12) The normal range of plasma concentration of bicarbonate ions is _____ in arterial blood; it is slightly _____ in venous blood.

Answer: 22–26 mEq/liter; higher

Page Ref: 963

13) PTH stimulates _____ of calcium ions from kidney tubules, _____ of phosphate ions, and _____ of magnesium ions.

Answer: reabsorption; excretion; reabsorption

Page Ref: 963

14) The level of sodium ions in the blood is controlled by the hormones _____ , _____ , and _____ .

Answer: aldosterone; ANP; ADH

Page Ref: 963

15) The condition resulting when water intake exceeds the kidneys' excretory ability is called _____ .

Answer: water intoxication

Page Ref: 960

16) The thirst center is stimulated by _____ , _____ , and _____ .

Answer: dry mouth; angiotensin II; osmoreceptors in the hypothalamus

Page Ref: 959

17) In a healthy, resting person the greatest loss of water other than urinary loss is by _____ .

Answer: evaporation from the skin

Page Ref: 957

18) The major extracellular fluid compartments are the _____ and _____ .

Answer: interstitial fluid; plasma

Page Ref: 956

19) Plasma levels of potassium ions are regulated primarily by the hormone _____ .

Answer: aldosterone

Page Ref: 962

20) As age increases, the percentage of body weight that is water _____ ; as the amount of adipose tissue increases, the percentage of body weight that is water _____ .

Answer: decreases; decreases

Page Ref: 969–970

21) The positive or negative charge equal to the amount of charge in one mole of hydrogen ions is called one _____.
Answer: equivalent
Page Ref: 961

22) In intracellular fluid, the most abundant cation is _____ and the most abundant inorganic anion is _____.
Answer: potassium; monohydrogen phosphate
Page Ref: 962

23) The most abundant extracellular anion is _____.
Answer: chloride ion
Page Ref: 962

24) As blood passes through the pulmonary capillaries, the plasma level of bicarbonate ion _____.
Answer: decreases
Page Ref: 963

25) The homeostatic range of pH for extracellular fluid is _____ to _____.
Answer: 7.35; 7.45
Page Ref: 965

26) When respiratory rate increases, pH of extracellular fluid _____.
Answer: increases
Page Ref: 966

27) A strong acid combined with a weak base yields _____ and _____.
Answer: water; a weak acid
Page Ref: 966

28) The part of a protein buffer that acts as a weak base is _____.
Answer: the amine group
Page Ref: 965

29) If blood pH becomes 7.32, respiratory rate will _____ as a compensatory mechanism.
Answer: increase
Page Ref: 967

30) The three values needed in order to determine the cause of an acid–base imbalance are
_____ , _____ , and _____ .

Answer: pH; partial pressure of carbon dioxide; bicarbonate ion levels
Page Ref: 969

ESSAY. Write your answer in the space provided or on a separate sheet of paper.

1) Describe the fluid and electrolyte disorders to which the elderly are particularly susceptible.

Answer: 1) Dehydration and hypernatremia due to inadequate fluid intake or loss of more water than sodium in vomit, feces, or urine
2) Hyponatremia due to inadequate intake of sodium, impaired kidney function, or excessive sodium loss
3) Hypokalemia due to excessive laxative use or potassium–depleting diuretics
4) Acidosis due to lung or kidney disease
Page Ref: 970

2) Explain why aspirin overdose leads to respiratory alkalosis rather than acidosis.

Answer: Aspirin alters the respiratory centers in the brain stem, triggering hyperventilation. Loss of carbon dioxide reduces its partial pressure and raises pH.
Page Ref: 969

3) Explain how it is possible for a patient with chronic obstructive pulmonary disease to have a normal extracellular pH while having an elevated partial pressure of carbon dioxide.

Answer: Elevated partial pressure of carbon dioxide causes respiratory acidosis, which is compensated by an increase in plasma levels of bicarbonate ion. Because the patient cannot breathe off the excess carbon dioxide due to structural changes in the respiratory system, the partial pressure of carbon dioxide stays high, but compensated by bicarbonate.
Page Ref: 969

4) Cindy is on an extremely low calorie diet. What would you expect to see in terms of pH balance and any compensatory mechanisms? Explain your answer.

Answer: The effects of starvation would be seen—particularly increased lipolysis leading to ketogenesis. The ketones decrease pH to cause metabolic acidosis. This would trigger renal loss of excess hydrogen ions and increased respiratory rate to reduce partial pressure of carbon dioxide and raise pH of ECF.
Page Ref: 969

5) A patient's blood pH is 7.48; partial pressure of carbon dioxide is 32 mm Hg and levels of bicarbonate in the blood are 20 mEq/liter. What can you tell about this patient's condition? Explain your answer.

Answer: The patient is in respiratory alkalosis (high pH, low carbon dioxide), which is partially compensated (low bicarbonate).
Page Ref: 969

6) Patients with cholera may lose more than five liters of fluid per day from severe diarrhea. What effects on electrolyte balance and acid–base balance might this produce? What compensatory mechanisms (other than immune function) might be activated as a result of this disease?

Answer: Hyponatremia and loss of bicarbonate ions, leading to metabolic acidosis and depression of the CNS. There would also be an increase in aldsoterone, increased respiratory rate, renal generation of new bicarbonate, increased renal excretion of hydrogen ion via ammonium and dihydrogen phosphate. All feedback loops that raise blood pressure would be activated due to water loss.

Page Ref: 964

7) Describe the negative feedback loop that stimulates thirst as a result of dehydration.

Answer: Dehydration causes 1) decreased flow of saliva, which dries the mouth and pharynx, 2) increased blood osmotic pressure, which stimulates osmoreceptors in the hypothalamus, and 3) decreased blood volume, which lowers blood pressure, increasing release of renin from JG cells, increasing levels of angiotensin II. All of these stimulate the thirst center in the hypothalamus, which increases fluid intake via thirst, thus increasing body water.

Page Ref: 959

8) Identify four reasons why infants experience more fluid and electrolyte and acid–base imbalances than adults.

Answer: Compared with adults, babies have: 1) a greater percentage of body water; more water in ECF than ICF; rapid changes in ECF volume due to higher intake/output; 2) a higher metabolic rate generating more metabolic acids and wastes; 3) less efficient kidneys; 4) greater water loss through skin due to relatively high proportion of surface are to volume; 5) higher respiratory rate leading to increased water loss and higher pH; 6) higher levels of potassium and chloride ions causing a tendency toward acidosis.

Page Ref: 969–970

9) Explain how buffer systems work using generic formulas.

Answer: A strong acid is buffered by a weak base to yield a salt and a weak acid. A strong base is buffered by a weak acid to form water and a weak base. Conversion of strong acids/bases to weak acids/bases minimizes the stress on the pH of ECF by reducing the number of new hydrogen or hydroxide ions added by strong acids/bases.

Page Ref: 966

10) What are acidosis and alkalosis, and how do they develop? What are the primary effects of each?

Answer: Acidosis is blood pH under 7.35, which causes depression of the CNS via reduced synaptic transmission. Alkalosis is blood pH over 7.45, which causes overexcitability of the nervous system. Anything that causes partial pressure of carbon dioxide to rise or causes loss of bicarbonate ions or causes buildup of metabolic acids leads to acidosis. Anything that lowers partial pressure of carbon dioxide or causes loss of acids or any ingestion of alkaline substances leads to alkalosis.

Page Ref: 967

CHAPTER 28   The Reproductive Systems

MULTIPLE CHOICE. Choose the one alternative that best completes the statement or answers the question.

1) Testosterone is produced by:
   A) spermatozoa.
   B) sustentacular cells.
   C) interstitial cells.
   D) the hypothalamus.
   E) all cells in the male.

   Answer: C
   Page Ref: 978

2) The acrosome of a sperm cell contains:
   A) the chromosomes.
   B) mitochondria for energy production.
   C) testosterone.
   D) hyaluronidase for egg penetration.
   E) the flagellum.

   Answer: D
   Page Ref: 983

3) During the menstrual cycle, LH is at its highest levels:
   A) during the menstrual phase.
   B) just prior to ovulation.
   C) just after ovulation.
   D) just before menstruation begins.
   E) Levels of LH never change.

   Answer: B
   Page Ref: 1004

4) During the menstrual cycle, progesterone would be at its highest levels:
   A) during the menstrual phase.
   B) just prior to ovulation.
   C) just after ovulation.
   D) late in the postovulatory phase.
   E) levels of progesterone never change.

   Answer: D
   Page Ref: 1004

5) During the menstrual cycle, the endometrium would be at its thickest:

A) during the menstrual phase.

B) just prior to ovulation.

C) just after ovulation.

D) late in the postovulatory phase.

E) the thickness never changes.

Answer: D
Page Ref: 1003

6) Maintenance of the male secondary sex characteristics is the direct responsibility of:

A) estrogen.

B) testosterone.

C) FSH.

D) progesterone.

E) LH.

Answer: B
Page Ref: 983

7) Which of the following cells are diploid?

A) secondary oocytes.

B) secondary spermatocytes.

C) primary spermatocytes.

D) spermatids.

E) All of the above except spermatids.

Answer: C
Page Ref: 982

8) A function of FSH in the male is to:

A) inhibit progesterone.

B) initiate testosterone production.

C) increase protein synthesis.

D) inhibit estrogen.

E) initiate spermatogenesis.

Answer: E
Page Ref: 983

9) Final maturation of sperm cells occurs in the:

   A) epididymis.

   B) seminiferous tubules.

   C) prostate gland.

   D) urethra.

   E) female reproductive tract.

Answer: A
Page Ref: 982

10) Seminal vesicles produce:

   A) sperm cells.

   B) testosterone.

   C) fructose-rich fluid.

   D) estrogen.

   E) mucus.

Answer: C
Page Ref: 987

11) Sertoli cells produce:

   A) testosterone.

   B) androgen-binding protein.

   C) estrogen.

   D) FSH.

   E) LH.

Answer: B
Page Ref: 978

12) The normal number of spermatozoa per milliliter of semen is:

   A) 50–100.

   B) fewer than 20,000,000.

   C) more than 200,000,000.

   D) 50,000,000 –150,000,000.

   E) about 5 million.

Answer: D
Page Ref: 987

13) Repair of the endometrium during the preovulatory phase of menstruation is due to rising levels of:

A) FSH.

B) estrogen.

C) hCG.

D) progesterone.

E) inhibin.

Answer: B
Page Ref: 1004

14) During the menstrual cycle, progesterone is produced by:

A) the secondary oocyte.

B) the corpus luteum.

C) the stroma of the ovary.

D) primary follicles.

E) the endometrium

Answer: B
Page Ref: 1005

15) Which of the following does **NOT** produce estrogens?

A) adrenal cortex

B) placenta

C) ovarian follicle cells

D) testes

E) hypothalamus

Answer: E
Page Ref: 1002

16) During spermatogenesis, which of the following undergoes a meiotic division to produce haploid cells?

A) spermatids

B) secondary spermatocytes

C) primary spermatocytes

D) spermatogonia

E) spermatozoa

Answer: C
Page Ref: 982

17) The first meiotic division in oogenesis occurs:

  A) before birth.

  B) only if the egg is fertilized.

  C) after ovulation.

  D) monthly after puberty in response to FSH and LH.

  E) when adrenal gonadocorticoids begin to rise at the start of puberty.

Answer: A
Page Ref: 991

18) In the male, LH causes:

  A) initiation of spermatogenesis.

  B) development of secondary sex characteristics.

  C) testosterone production.

  D) ejaculation.

  E) release of GnRH.

Answer: C
Page Ref: 983

19) The part of the female reproductive system that is shed during menstruation is the:

  A) myometrium.

  B) mucosa of the vagina.

  C) tunica albuginea.

  D) stratum functionalis of the endometrium.

  E) germinal epithelium.

Answer: D
Page Ref: 1003

20) The main function of progesterone during the menstrual cycle is to:

  A) initiate ovulation.

  B) initiate menstruation.

  C) thicken the endometrium.

  D) repair the surface of the ovary after ovulation.

  E) stimulate the release of FSH and LH.

Answer: C
Page Ref: 1005

21) The function of the cremaster muscle is to:

   A) elevate the testes during sexual arousal and exposure to cold.

   B) generate peristaltic waves in the ductus deferens.

   C) control the release of secretions from the seminal vesicles.

   D) control the release of sperm cells from the testes into the epididymis.

   E) prevent urine from entering the urethra during ejaculation.

   Answer: A
   Page Ref: 976

22) The form (stage) of developing male gamete located nearest to the basement membrane of a seminiferous tubule is the:

   A) spermatid.

   B) primary spermatocyte.

   C) secondary spermatocyte.

   D) primordial germ cell.

   E) spermatogonium.

   Answer: E
   Page Ref: 982

23) Leydig cells are located:

   A) in all the male accessory reproductive organs.

   B) interspersed among developing sperm cells in seminiferous tubules.

   C) lining the epididymis and ductus deferens.

   D) within the tunica albuginea.

   E) in spaces between adjacent seminiferous tubules.

   Answer: E
   Page Ref: 978

24) The immune system does not normally attack spermatogenic cells because:

   A) they are recognized as "self" structures.

   B) they do not have any antigens on their cell membranes.

   C) spermatogenic cells are protected by the blood–testis barrier.

   D) the acrosome covers any antigens that would be recognized as foreign.

   E) spermatogenic cells are release chemicals that repel antigen-presenting cells.

   Answer: C
   Page Ref: 978

25) The process of crossing-over, or recombination, of genes occurs during:

A) meiosis I.

B) meiosis II.

C) spermiogenesis.

D) spermiation.

E) fertilization.

Answer: A
Page Ref: 982

26) Primordial germ cells arise from the:

A) mesonephric ducts.

B) yolk sac endoderm.

C) genital tubercle.

D) urethral folds.

E) paramesonephric ducts.

Answer: B
Page Ref: 978

27) The cells that result from the equatorial division of spermatogenesis are called:

A) spermatogonia.

B) primary spermatocytes.

C) secondary spermatocytes.

D) primordial germ cells.

E) spermatids.

Answer: E
Page Ref: 982

28) The process of spermiation is the:

A) reduction division of male gamete production.

B) equatorial division of male gamete production.

C) process producing the liquid portion of semen.

D) release of a sperm cell from its connection to a sustentacular cell.

E) change that occurs in the sperm cell following penetration of the egg.

Answer: D
Page Ref: 982

29) The principal androgen is:

A) ABP.

B) FSH.

C) testosterone.

D) hCG.

E) estradiol.

Answer: C
Page Ref: 983

30) **ALL** of the following are part of the spermatic cord **EXCEPT** the:

A) testicular artery.

B) lymphatic vessels.

C) cremaster muscle.

D) ductus deferens.

E) ejaculatory duct.

Answer: E
Page Ref: 976

31) The function of fructose in semen is to:

A) provide an energy source for ATP production by sperm.

B) promote coagulation of semen in the female reproductive tract.

C) buffer acids in the female reproductive tract.

D) inhibit the growth of bacteria in semen and the female reproductive tract.

E) provide an energy source for the zygote.

Answer: A
Page Ref: 987

32) The seminal vesicles are located:

A) inferior to the prostate within the urogenital diaphragm.

B) within the lobules of the testes.

C) within the spermatic cord.

D) posterior and inferior to the urinary bladder, in front of the rectum.

E) on the posterior surface of each testis.

Answer: D
Page Ref: 987

33) Which of the following does **NOT** manufacture products that become part of semen?

   A) seminiferous tubules.

   B) bulbourethral glands.

   C) penis.

   D) seminal vesicles.

   E) prostate gland.

   Answer: C
   Page Ref: 987

34) The function of seminalplasmin is to:

   A) provide an energy source for sperm.

   B) act as an antibiotic to control bacterial numbers.

   C) cause semen to coagulate in the female reproductive tract.

   D) prevent destruction of spermatogenic cells by the immune system.

   E) buffer the acidity of the female reproductive tract.

   Answer: B
   Page Ref: 987

35) The female structure that is homologous to the testis is the:

   A) ovary.

   B) uterus.

   C) vagina.

   D) clitoris.

   E) Bartholin's gland.

   Answer: A
   Page Ref: 989

36) The glycoprotein layer between the oocyte and the granulosa cells of an ovarian follicle is called the:

   A) theca interna.

   B) theca externa.

   C) antrum.

   D) zona pellucida.

   E) corona radiata.

   Answer: D
   Page Ref: 991

37) The secretory cells of an ovarian follicle are called the:

A) theca interna.

B) theca externa.

C) antrum.

D) zona pellucida.

E) corona radiata.

Answer: A
Page Ref: 991

38) Which of the following help move the oocyte into and through the uterine tube?

A) peristalsis.

B) cilia.

C) flagella.

D) fimbriae.

E) All of the above except flagella.

Answer: E
Page Ref: 993

39) The uterus is located:

A) between the urinary bladder and the pubic symphysis.

B) between the rectum and the sacrum.

C) between the urinary bladder and the rectum.

D) between the kidneys in the same horizontal plane.

E) along the inferior surface of the urinary bladder.

Answer: C
Page Ref: 994

40) The opening between the cervical canal and the uterine cavity is called the:

A) internal os.

B) external os.

C) isthmus.

D) fornix.

E) vagina.

Answer: A
Page Ref: 994

41) The folds of the peritoneum attaching the uterus to either side of the pelvic cavity are called the:

A) uterosacral ligaments.

B) broad ligaments.

C) cardinal ligaments.

D) round ligaments.

E) suspensory ligaments.

Answer: B
Page Ref: 995

42) Which of the following lists the uterine blood vessels in the correct order of blood flow?

A) radial arteries, arcuate arteries, spiral arterioles, straight arterioles

B) spiral arterioles, straight arterioles, radial arteries, arcuate arteries

C) straight arterioles, radial arteries, arcuate arteries, spiral arterioles

D) arcuate arteries, radial arteries, straight arterioles, spiral arterioles

E) arcuate arteries, straight arterioles, spiral arterioles, radial arteries

Answer: D
Page Ref: 997

43) The uterine blood vessels that penetrate deep into the myometrium are the:

A) radial arteries.

B) arcuate arteries.

C) uterine arteries.

D) straight arterioles.

E) spiral arterioles.

Answer: A
Page Ref: 997

44) The epithelium of the vaginal mucosa is:

A) simple squamous.

B) simple cuboidal.

C) simple columnar.

D) transitional.

E) stratified squamous.

Answer: E
Page Ref: 998

45) The female structure that is homologous to the scrotum is the:

A) mons pubis.

B) labia majora.

C) labia minora.

D) clitoris.

E) hymen.

Answer: B
Page Ref: 998

46) The perineum is bounded by the:

A) pubic symphysis, iliac crests, and sacral promontory.

B) anterior and posterior inferior iliac spines, and pubic symphysis.

C) pubic symphysis, ischial tuberosities, and coccyx.

D) pubic symphysis, posterior inferior iliac spines, and coccyx.

E) ischial tuberosities, iliac crests, and anterior inferior iliac spines.

Answer: C
Page Ref: 999

47) Mild production is stimulated primarily by the hormone:

A) FSH.

B) oxytocin.

C) DHT.

D) relaxin.

E) PRL.

Answer: E
Page Ref: 999

48) ALL of the following are functions of estrogens EXCEPT:

A) help control fluid and electrolyte balance.

B) promote protein anabolism.

C) help regulate secretion of FSH.

D) promote development and maintenance of female secondary sex characteristics.

E) raise blood cholesteol.

Answer: E
Page Ref: 1002

49) If fertilization does not occur, the corpus luteum:

   A) is expelled into the pelvic cavity.

   B) begins to secrete low levels of FSH.

   C) degenerates into the corpus albicans.

   D) continues to secrete progesterone until the next ovulation.

   E) Both A and C are correct.

Answer: C
Page Ref: 1005

50) The process by which sperm are deposited into the vagina is called:

   A) fertilization.

   B) spermiation.

   C) spermiogenesis.

   D) coitus.

   E) capacitation.

Answer: D
Page Ref: 1007

51) **ALL** of the following are **sympathetic** responses during sexual intercourse **EXCEPT**:

   A) peristalsis in the ductus deferens.

   B) increased blood pressure.

   C) contraction of perineal muscles.

   D) ejaculation of semen.

   E) erection of the penis/clitoris.

Answer: E
Page Ref: 1007

52) Oral contraceptives for women typically contain:

   A) human chorionic gonadotropin.

   B) progestin and estrogen.

   C) low levels of both FSH and LH.

   D) nonoxynol-9.

   E) testosterone.

Answer: B
Page Ref: 1008

53) Onset of puberty in both sexes is signaled by sleep-associated increases in levels of:
   A) estradiol.
   B) DHT.
   C) oxytocin.
   D) PRL.
   E) LH.

   Answer: E
   Page Ref: 1012

MATCHING. Choose the item in column 2 that best matches each item in column 1.

Choose the item from column 2 that best matches each item in column 1.

1) Column 1: oxytocin
   Column 2: stimulates ejection of milk
           from mammary glands
   Answer: stimulates ejection of milk from mammary glands
   Page Ref: 1000

2) Column 1: GnRH
   Column 2: produced by hypothalamus to
           promote secretion of FSH and
           LH
   Answer: produced by hypothalamus to promote secretion of FSH and LH
   Page Ref: 983

3) Column 1: LH
   Column 2: stimulates secretion of
           testosterone
   Answer: stimulates secretion of testosterone
   Page Ref: 983

4) Column 1: FSH
   Column 2: stimulates spermatogenesis
   Answer: stimulates spermatogenesis
   Page Ref: 983

5) Column 1: testosterone

Column 2: promotes protein anabolism; promotes musculoskeletal growth resulting in wide shoulders and narrow hips; contributes to libido in both sexes

Answer: promotes protein anabolism; promotes musculoskeletal growth resulting in wide shoulders and narrow hips; contributes to libido in both sexes

Page Ref: 983

6) Column 1: beta-estradiol

Column 2: lowers blood cholesterol; promotes fat distribution to abdomen, breasts, and hips

Answer: lowers blood cholesterol; promotes fat distribution to abdomen, breasts, and hips

Page Ref: 1002

7) Column 1: progesterone

Column 2: works synergistically with estrogens to prepare the endometrium for implantation of the fertilized egg and the mammary glands for milk secretion

Answer: works synergistically with estrogens to prepare the endometrium for implantation of the fertilized egg and the mammary glands for milk secretion

Page Ref: 1002

8) Column 1: hCG

Column 2: produced by the chorion of the embryo to maintain activity of the corpus luteum

Answer: produced by the chorion of the embryo to maintain activity of the corpus luteum

Page Ref: 1005

9) Column 1: inhibin

Column 2: secreted by Sertoli cells and corpus luteum; inhibits secretion of FSH

Answer: secreted by Sertoli cells and corpus luteum; inhibits secretion of FSH

Page Ref: 984

10) Column 1: relaxin

    Column 2: secreted by corpus luteum;
        softens pelvic connective
        tissues

    Answer: secreted by corpus luteum; softens pelvic connective tissues

Page Ref: 1002

MATCHING. Choose the item in column 2 that best matches each item in column 1.

Choose the item from column 2 that best matches each item in column 1.

1) Column 1: prostate gland

    Column 2: inferior to the urinary bladder;
        surrounds urethra; produces
        secretions making up about
        25% of seminal fluid

    Answer: inferior to the urinary bladder; surrounds urethra; produces secretions making up about
        25% of seminal fluid

Page Ref: 987

2) Column 1: bulbourethral glands

    Column 2: pea-sized glands that
        produce mucus and an acid-
        neutralizing substance for
        semen

    Answer: pea-sized glands that produce mucus and an acid-neutralizing substance for semen

Page Ref: 987

3) Column 1: seminal vesicles

    Column 2: located at the base of the
        bladder anterior to the rectum;
        produces fructose-rich
        secretion making up about
        60% of the volume of semen

    Answer: located at the base of the bladder anterior to the rectum; produces fructose-rich
        secretion making up about 60% of the volume of semen

Page Ref: 987

4) Column 1: epididymis

    Column 2: 20' of tubing packed onto the
        posterior borders of the testes;
        site of sperm maturation

    Answer: 20' of tubing packed onto the posterior borders of the testes; site of sperm maturation

Page Ref: 985

5) Column 1: ductus deferens

Column 2: 18" tube looping over posterior surface of the bladder between the epididymis and the urethra

Answer: 18" tube looping over posterior surface of the bladder between the epididymis and the urethra

Page Ref: 985

6) Column 1: scrotum

Column 2: external pouch enclosing the testes and epididymis

Answer: external pouch enclosing the testes and epididymis

Page Ref: 976

7) Column 1: testes

Column 2: male gonads; surrounded by capsule called the tunica albuginea

Answer: male gonads; surrounded by capsule called the tunica albuginea

Page Ref: 977

8) Column 1: corpora cavernosa

Column 2: dorsolateral masses of erectile tissue in the penis

Answer: dorsolateral masses of erectile tissue in the penis

Page Ref: 988

9) Column 1: corpus spongiosum

Column 2: erectile tissue in the penis surrounding the urethra

Answer: erectile tissue in the penis surrounding the urethra

Page Ref: 988

10) Column 1: ejaculatory duct

Column 2: tube leading from the seminal vesicle to the urethra

Answer: tube leading from the seminal vesicle to the urethra

Page Ref: 985

TRUE/FALSE. Write 'T' if the statement is true and 'F' if the statement is false.

1) Meiosis results in diploid cells.

   Answer: FALSE
   Page Ref: 975

2) Synapsis occurs in prophase I of meiosis, but not in mitosis.

   Answer: TRUE
   Page Ref: 976

3) Sperm are produced in seminiferous tubules.

   Answer: TRUE
   Page Ref: 977

4) The cremaster muscle contracts to cause erection of the penis.

   Answer: FALSE
   Page Ref: 976

5) Leydig cells are targets for FSH.

   Answer: FALSE
   Page Ref: 983

6) Sertoli cells form the blood–testis barrier.

   Answer: TRUE
   Page Ref: 978

7) Primary spermatocytes are diploid cells.

   Answer: TRUE
   Page Ref: 979

8) Spermiogenesis is the final stage of meiosis for male gametes.

   Answer: FALSE
   Page Ref: 982

9) Ovarian follicles are located in the ovarian cortex.

   Answer: TRUE
   Page Ref: 989

10) Oogonia begin to develop into primary oocytes at puberty.

   Answer: FALSE
   Page Ref: 991

11) The mammary glands are endocrine glands.

Answer: FALSE
Page Ref: 999

12) Fertilization normally occurs in the body of the uterus.

Answer: FALSE
Page Ref: 993

13) Estrogens are at their highest level in the late postovulatory phase.

Answer: FALSE
Page Ref: 1004

14) Estrogens promote protein anabolism.

Answer: TRUE
Page Ref: 1002

15) Progesterone is secreted mainly by the corpus luteum in the nonpregnant female.

Answer: TRUE
Page Ref: 1002

SHORT ANSWER. Write the word or phrase that best completes each statement or answers the question.

1) The drug Viagra enhances the effects of _____ in the penis.
Answer: nitric oxide
Page Ref: 1008

2) The role of nitric oxide in the erection of the penis is to _____.
Answer: relax smooth muscle in penile arteries
Page Ref: 1007

3) The corpus luteum is maintained following fertilization by a hormone called _____.
Answer: human chorionic gonadotropin
Page Ref: 1005

4) Ovulation is triggered by a surge in the level of the hormone _____.
Answer: LH
Page Ref: 1005

5) High levels of _____ in the late preovulatory phase exert a positive feedback effect on LH and GnRH.
Answer: estrogens
Page Ref: 1004

6) During the ovarian preovulatory phase, the uterus is in its _____ phase in which endometrial mass doubles under the influence of _____.

Answer: proliferative; estrogens

Page Ref: 1004

7) A decrease in levels of progesterone stimulates constriction of spiral arterioles by stimulating the release of _____.

Answer: prostaglandins

Page Ref: 1004

8) Inhibin primarily inhibits secretion of _____.

Answer: FSH

Page Ref: 1003

9) The three main estrogens are _____, _____, and _____.

Answer: beta–estradiol; estrone; estriol

Page Ref: 1002

10) Milk is stored near the nipples in spaces called _____.

Answer: lactiferous sinuses

Page Ref: 1000

11) Milk production is stimulated mainly by the hormone _____ and ejection of milk is stimulated mainly by the hormone _____.

Answer: prolactin; oxytocin

Page Ref: 1000

12) _____ in seminal fluid and _____ in prostate fluid are used by sperm for ATP production.

Answer: Fructose; citric acid

Page Ref: 987

13) About 60% of the volume of semen is contributed by the _____.

Answer: seminal vesicles

Page Ref: 987

14) The spermatic cord passes through an opening in the anterior abdominal wall called the _____.

Answer: inguinal canal

Page Ref: 985

15) Columnar cells in the epididymis have long, branching microvilli called _____ , which increase the surface area for _____ .

Answer: stercocilia; resorption of degenerated sperm

Page Ref: 985

16) The source of androgen–binding protein is the _____ ; the function of androgen–binding protein is to _____ .

Answer: Sertoli cells; keep testosterone levels high near seminiferous tubules

Page Ref: 983

17) In the prostate and seminal vesicles, 5 alpha–reductase converts testosterone to a more potent androgen called _____ .

Answer: dihydrotestosterone (DHT)

Page Ref: 983

18) The hyaluronidase–containing vesicle of a sperm cell is called the _____ .

Answer: acrosome

Page Ref: 983

19) The blood–testis barrier is formed just internal to the basement membrane of the seminiferous tubules by tight junctions between _____ cells.

Answer: Sertoli

Page Ref: 978

20) The cells in the seminiferous tubules that secrete testosterone are the _____ .

Answer: Leydig cells

Page Ref: 978

21) Division of each primary spermatocyte eventually produces _____ spermatids.

Answer: four

Page Ref: 982

22) The testicular artery, veins, autonomic nerves, lymphatic vessels, and the cremaster muscle together constitute the _____ .

Answer: spermatic cord

Page Ref: 985

23) The average volume of semen in an ejaculation is _____ with a sperm count of _____ per milliliter.

Answer: 2.5–5 mL; 50–150 million

Page Ref: 987

24) The vascular changes resulting in an erection are the result of a _____ reflex.
Answer: parasympathetic
Page Ref: 989

25) The foreskin of the penis is also known as the _____.
Answer: prepuce
Page Ref: 989

26) Degeneration of primary germ cells during female fetal development is called _____.
Answer: atresia
Page Ref: 991

27) The inferior narrow portion of the uterus that opens into the vagina is called the _____.
Answer: cervix
Page Ref: 994

28) The layer of the endometrium nearest the uterine cavity that is shed during menstruation is the _____.
Answer: stratum functionalis
Page Ref: 996

29) The female structure that is homologous to the penis of the male is the _____.
Answer: clitoris
Page Ref: 998

30) During the postovulatory phase of the menstrual cycle, the endometrium is prepared to receive the fertilized ovum principally by the hormone _____ produced by the corpus luteum.
Answer: progesterone
Page Ref: 1005

ESSAY. Write your answer in the space provided or on a separate sheet of paper.

1) Describe the role of the autonomic nervous system in the human sexual response.
Answer: In arousal, the parasympathetic nervous system stimulates vasocongestion of sexual organs, secretion of lubricating fluids, and relaxation of vaginal smooth muscle. The sympathetic nervous system stimulates an increase in heart rate and force of contraction, an increase in vasomotor tone, and hyperventilation. During orgasm, the sympathetic nervous system stimulates rhythmic contractions of smooth muscle in genital organs, ejaculation of semen, and closing off of the male bladder.
Page Ref: 1007

2) Describe the functions of testosterone.

Answer: Testosterone promotes the development and maintenance of male secondary sex characteristics, protein anabolism, development of sexual function (behavior, libido, spermatogenesis), and the male pattern of development during prenatal life.
Page Ref: 983–984

3) Identify the glands contributing to the composition of semen, and describe their specific functions.

Answer: The testes contribute sperm. The seminal vesicles contribute seminal fluid containing fructose, prostaglandins, and clotting proteins. It is an alkaline substance making up about 60% of semen volume. The prostate gland contributes a fluid containing citrate, PSA and other proteolytic enzymes, and acid phosphatase. Bulbourethral glands produce alkaline mucus for lubrication and neutralization of vaginal secretions. These fluids contribute to the motility and viability of sperm.
Page Ref: 987

4) **Predict the effect of exogenous testosterone on hormone balance in males.**

Answer: Exogenous testosterone causes GnRH to decrease, which causes LH and FSH to decrease. Endogenous testosterone production will decrease and Leydig cells will decrease their functioning.
Page Ref: 983

5) Compare and contrast the processes of spermatogenesis and oogenesis.

Answer: Both processes result in formation of gametes (haploid cells). One female stem cells yields one functional gamete plus 2 –3 polar bodies; one male stem cell yields four functional gametes. Once spermatogenesis begins at puberty, it continues throughout life, producing 300 million sperm daily. Oogenesis begins during fetal life, resumes at puberty and produces one mature gamete monthly until menopause.
Page Ref: 979; 991

6) Describe the development and possible fates of an ovarian follicle in a woman of reproductive age.

Answer: A primordial follicle is a single layer of cells around an oocyte. A primary follicle is 6 –7 layers of cuboidal epithelial cells around the oocyte. A secondary follicle has the theca externa, theca interna, and follicular fluid filling the antrum. The mature follcile (larger) ovulates the secondary oocyte, then collapses to form the corpus hemorrhagicum (clot inside). The clot is absorbed and the cells enlarge to form the corpus luteum, which either degenerates into the corpus albicans or is maintained by hCG depending on whether fertilization occurs.
Page Ref: 1006

7) Describe the role of cervical mucus in the female reproductive tract.

Answer: Mucus forms a plug to impede penetration of sperm except at ovulation. It also supplements the energy needs of the sperm, serves as a sperm reservoir, and protects the sperm from pH damage and phagocytosis. Mucus also plays a role in capacitation.
Page Ref: 996

8) Explain how bacteria entering the vagina could ultimately cause peritonitis.

Answer: Motile bacteria can move unaided into the reproductive tract. Others can be carried by sperm cells. Bceause the uterine tubes are open to the pelvic cavity, bacteria can easily enter the pelvic cavity and come in contact with folds of the peritoneum. Some bacteria may enter the blood or lymph and travel directly to the peritoneum.

Page Ref: 993

9) Identify the factors that increase a woman's risk of developing breast cancer.

Answer: Presence of certain genes; family history (especially mother or sister); no children or first child after age 34; previous cancer in one breast; exposure to ionizing radiations; excess intake of fat and/or alcohol; cigarette smoking.

Page Ref: 1015

10) Describe the positive feedback loop involved in ovulation.

Answer: FSH and LH promote follicular development, thus increasing estrogen production. High levels of estrogen during the late preovulatory phase stimulate release of GnRH from the hypothalamus. GnRH promotes release of more FSH and LH from the anterior pituitary.

Page Ref: 1004

CHAPTER 29   Development and Inheritance

MULTIPLE CHOICE. Choose the one alternative that best completes the statement or answers the question.

1) The observable characteristics of a person's genetic makeup are known as the:

   A) genotype.

   B) phenotype.

   C) gene pool.

   D) karyotype.

   E) autosomes.

   Answer: B
   Page Ref: 1045

2) During early pregnancy, the main function of hCG is to:

   A) nourish the embryo.

   B) stimulate placental growth.

   C) maintain the corpus luteum.

   D) depress estrogen production.

   E) prevent passage of testosterone to the developing embryo.

   Answer: C
   Page Ref: 1036

3) How many days after fertilization does implantation of the blastocyst occur?

   A) 2 days.

   B) 6 days.

   C) 14 days.

   D) 28 days.

   E) 120 days.

   Answer: B
   Page Ref: 1024

4) The chorion develops from the:

   A) inner cell mass.

   B) blastocele.

   C) trophoblast.

   D) yolk sac.

   E) corpus luteum.

   Answer: C
   Page Ref: 1027

5) The embryonic disc develops from the:
   A) inner cell mass.
   B) blastocele.
   C) trophoblast.
   D) yolk sac.
   E) corpus luteum.

   Answer: A
   Page Ref: 1027

6) The fetus is protected from mechanical injury by fluid contained within the:
   A) allantois.
   B) yolk sac.
   C) blastocele.
   D) amnion.
   E) decidua.

   Answer: D
   Page Ref: 1027

7) Human chorionic gonadotropin is produced by the:
   A) corpus luteum.
   B) embryo.
   C) endometrium.
   D) trophoblast cells of the chorion.
   E) blastocele.

   Answer: D
   Page Ref: 1035

8) Human chorionic gonadotropin is at its highest levels during:
   A) ovulation.
   B) fertilization.
   C) implantation.
   D) the ninth week of pregnancy.
   E) the third month of pregnancy.

   Answer: D
   Page Ref: 1036

9) How many pairs of autosomes does a normal human have?

   A) 22

   B) 23

   C) 44

   D) 46

   E) one

   Answer: A
   Page Ref: 1047

10) **ALL** of the following are **TRUE** for the placenta **EXCEPT**:

   A) it makes estrogen

   B) it allows for mixing of maternal and fetal blood

   C) it makes progesterone

   D) it allows for exchange of nutrients, wastes, and gases

   E) it develops in part from the trophoblast

   Answer: B
   Page Ref: 1029

11) An individual whose alleles for a particular trait are the same is said to be:

   A) dominant.

   B) recessive.

   C) homologous.

   D) homozygous.

   E) heterozygous.

   Answer: D
   Page Ref: 1044

12) What percentage of sperm cells introduced into the vagina normally reach the oocyte?

   A) less than 1%

   B) about 10%

   C) 25–30%

   D) 50%

   E) close to 100%

   Answer: A
   Page Ref: 1022

13) The term capacitation refers to:

    A) union of the male and female pronuclei.

    B) equatorial division of the secondary oocyte following penetration by a sperm cell.

    C) functional changes that sperm undergo in the female reproductive tract that allow them to fertilize the secondary oocyte.

    D) functional changes in the zona pellucida caused by release of calcium ions.

    E) a sperm cell's penetration of the zona pellucida and entry into a secondary oocyte.

Answer: C
Page Ref: 1022

14) The term **syngamy** refers to the:

    A) union of male and female pronuclei.

    B) equatorial division of the secondary oocyte following penetration by a sperm cell.

    C) functional changes that sperm undergo in the female reproductive tract that allow them to fertilize a secondary oocyte.

    D) functional changes in the zona pellucida and entry into a secondary oocyte.

    E) a sperm cell's penetration of the zona pellucida and entry into a secondary oocyte.

Answer: E
Page Ref: 1023

15) At day 4 after fertilization, the solid ball of cells that has formed is called the:

    A) zygote.

    B) blastocyst.

    C) gastrula.

    D) morula.

    E) embryo.

Answer: D
Page Ref: 1024

16) What is the next event following syngamy?

    A) penetration of the zona pellucida by a sperm cell

    B) depolarization and release of calcium ions by the oocyte

    C) cleavage

    D) meiosis II

    E) implantation.

Answer: B
Page Ref: 1023

17) Implantation usually occurs in the:

   A) uterine tube.

   B) myometrium.

   C) cervix adjacent to the internal os.

   D) posterior fornix.

   E) posterior wall of the body or fundus of the uterus.

   Answer: E
   Page Ref: 1024

18) The enzymes that allow implantation to occur are produced by the:

   A) syncytiotrophoblast.

   B) cytotrophoblast.

   C) blastocele.

   D) inner cell mass.

   E) acrosome.

   Answer: A
   Page Ref: 1025

19) The reason the corpus luteum is maintained in early pregnancy is to:

   A) continue production of hCG.

   B) produce ATP for the developing embryo.

   C) keep levels of estrogen and progesterone high enough to maintain the endometrium.

   D) produce the enzymes necessary for implantation.

   E) serve as the connection between the developing embryo and the endometrium.

   Answer: C
   Page Ref: 1035

20) The embryonic period of development covers what time period?

   A) the time between fertilization and implantation

   B) the first two months following fertilization

   C) the first trimester of pregnancy

   D) the first two trimesters of pregnancy

   E) the time between the appearance

   Answer: B
   Page Ref: 1027

21) The process by which an embryonic structure composed of the primary germ layers is formed is called:

   A) meiosis II.

   B) blastogenesis.

   C) capacitation.

   D) gastrulation.

   E) syngamy.

   Answer: D
   Page Ref: 1027

22) The amnion forms from the:

   A) syncytiotrophoblast.

   B) blastocele.

   C) cytrotrophoblast.

   D) decidua.

   E) inner cell mass.

   Answer: C
   Page Ref: 1027

23) The yolk sac forms from the :

   A) ectoderm of the inner cell mass.

   B) fluid within the amniotic cavity.

   C) allantois.

   D) decidua.

   E) endoderm of the inner cell mass.

   Answer: E
   Page Ref: 1027

24) The extraembryonic coelom becomes the:

   A) ectoderm.

   B) endoderm.

   C) amniotic cavity.

   D) ventral body cavity.

   E) blastocele.

   Answer: D
   Page Ref: 1027

25) The "water" referred to when a woman's "water breaks" prior to delivery is:

   A) amniotic fluid released when the amnion ruptures.

   B) maternal plasma leaking from weakened blood vessels.

   C) maternal urine expelled as compression of the bladder occurs.

   D) interstitial fluid released by separation of the layers of the placenta.

   E) mucus from stimulated glands in the cervix and vagina.

   Answer: A
   Page Ref: 1027

26) Exchange of gases, nutrients, and wastes between maternal and fetal blood takes place between the:

   A) amnion and chorion.

   B) decidua capsularis and chorion.

   C) decidua basalis and yolk sac.

   D) decidua basalis and chorionic villi.

   E) decidua capsularis and decidua basalis.

   Answer: D
   Page Ref: 1030

27) The portion of the endometrium that covers the embryo and is located between the embryo and the uterine cavity is the:

   A) decidua parietalis.

   B) decidua basalis.

   C) decidua capsularis.

   D) stratum basalis.

   E) amnion.

   Answer: C
   Page Ref: 1030

28) The portion of the endometrium that becomes the maternal portion of the placenta is the:

   A) decidua parietalis.

   B) decidua basalis.

   C) decidua capularis.

   D) stratum basalis.

   E) amnion.

   Answer: B
   Page Ref: 1030

29) What fills intervillous spaces?

   A) amniotic fluid.

   B) maternal blood only.

   C) fetal blood only.

   D) interstitial fluid.

   E) both fetal and maternal blood.

   Answer: B
   Page Ref: 1030

30) Most materials cross the placenta by:

   A) primary active transport.

   B) filtration.

   C) phagocytosis.

   D) diffusion.

   E) exocytosis.

   Answer: D
   Page Ref: 1030

31) Deoxygenated fetal blood is carried to the placenta via the:

   A) uterine arteries.

   B) uterine veins.

   C) umbilical arteries.

   D) umbilical vein.

   E) decidua basalis.

   Answer: C
   Page Ref: 1031

32) Peak secretion of hCS occurs:

   A) between fertilization and implantation.

   B) during the second trimester.

   C) late in the third trimester.

   D) just after delivery.

   E) at about the ninth week of pregnancy.

   Answer: C
   Page Ref: 1037

33) Once hCG levels decrease, estrogen and progesterone are secreted mainly by the:

A) placenta.

B) embryo.

C) corpus luteum.

D) hypothalamus.

E) stratum basalis.

Answer: A
Page Ref: 1036

34) Which of the following has occurred by the end of the first month of development?

A) The placenta has developed.

B) The eyes have formed and are open.

C) Ossification has begun.

D) Urine has begun to form.

E) The heart has formed and begun beating.

Answer: E
Page Ref: 1034

35) In a pregnant woman, decreased utilization of glucose and increased release of fatty acids from adipose tissue are promoted by the hormone:

A) estrogen.

B) progesterone.

C) inhibin.

D) hCS.

E) relaxin.

Answer: D
Page Ref: 1037

36) Early pregnancy tests are based on detection of what substance in the urine?

A) amniotic fluid.

B) blastomeres.

C) hCG.

D) high levels of progesterone.

E) hCS.

Answer: C
Page Ref: 1037

37) The human gestation period is about:

   A) 9 weeks.

   B) 24 weeks.

   C) 32 weeks.

   D) 38 weeks.

   E) 48 weeks.

   Answer: D
   Page Ref: 1027

38) Colostrum is different from true milk because it contains less lactose and virtually no:

   A) fat.

   B) protein.

   C) sodium.

   D) iron.

   E) antibodies.

   Answer: A
   Page Ref: 1043

39) The two alternative forms of a gene that code for the same trait and are at the same locus on homologous chromosomes are called:

   A) alleles.

   B) autosomes.

   C) Barr bodies.

   D) blastomeres.

   E) chromatids.

   Answer: A
   Page Ref: 1044

40) A person is heterozygous for a particular trait if he/she has:

   A) more than two copies of a particular gene.

   B) genes for the trait on both sex chromosomes and autosomes.

   C) one dominant allele and one recessive allele for the trait.

   D) two dominant alleles for the trait.

   E) two recessive alleles for the trait.

   Answer: C
   Page Ref: 1044

41) One person is homozygous dominant for a particular trait, and another person is heterozygous for the same trait. Which of the following statements is **TRUE** regarding these two people?

A) The homozygous person is female and the heterozygous person is male.

B) The homozygous person exhibits the trait, but the heterozygous person does not.

C) The heterozygous person exhibits the trait, but the homozygous person does not.

D) Neither person exhibits the trait.

E) The two people both exhibit the trait.

Answer: E
Page Ref: 1044

42) If a person's phenotype is intermediate between homozygous dominant and homozygous then inheritance of this trait is an example of:

A) codominance.

B) sex-linked inheritance.

C) incomplete dominance.

D) nondisjunction.

E) lyonization.

Answer: C
Page Ref: 1045

43) Inheritance of the ABO blood type is an example of:

A) codominance.

B) sex-linked inheritance.

C) incomplete dominance.

D) nondisjunction.

E) lyonization.

Answer: A
Page Ref: 1046

44) What would be the possible blood phenotypes of the offspring of parents whose genotype **ii** and I^{A}I^B?

A) type O only.

B) type AB only.

C) types A or B only.

D) types A, B, or O only.

E) all ABO types are possible.

Answer: C
Page Ref: 1046

45) A person who expresses the SRY gene is:

   A) exhibiting sickle–cell anemia.

   B) expressing a recessive trait.

   C) expressing DNA that was originally part of a virus.

   D) phenotypically female.

   E) phenotypically male.

   Answer: E
   Page Ref: 1048

46) Teratogens are:

   A) traits carried only on sex chromosomes.

   B) agents that induce physical defects in developing embryos.

   C) cells with an abnormal number of chromosomes.

   D) all of the alleles that contribute to a particular trait.

   E) genes that are inactivated during fetal development.

   Answer: B
   Page Ref: 1049

47) What event marks the beginning of the stage of expulsion in true labor?

   A) when the woman's water breaks

   B) appearance of lochia

   C) complete cervical dilation

   D) severing of the umbilical cord

   E) completion of two hours of rhythmic uterine contractions

   Answer: C
   Page Ref: 1040

48) A couple who are both phenotypically normal have a child who expresses a sex-linked recessive trait. Which of the following represents this child's genotype? [Let the trait be designated T (dominant) or t (recessive).]

   A) Tt

   B) tt

   C) X^tX^t

   D) X^tY

   E) Both C and D could be correct.

   Answer: D
   Page Ref: 1044

49) A child expresses an autosomal recessive trait. Which of the following are NOT possible genotypes for the parents?

   A) Both father and mother are homozygous recessive.

   B) Both father and mother are heterozygous.

   C) The father is heterozygous and the mother is homozygous recessive.

   D) The mother is heterozygous and the father is homozygous recessive.

   E) The father is heterozygous and the mother is homozygous dominant.

Answer: E
Page Ref: 1047

50) By doing karyotyping, one can determine the gender of the child because:

   A) the external genitalia can be seen on the screen.

   B) the total number of chromosomes would be different between the sexes.

   C) the Y chromosome is much smaller than the X chromosome.

   D) levels of testosterone are higher in the amniotic fluid of male embryos.

   E) the embryonic membranes are thicker around male embryos.

Answer: C
Page Ref: 1047

MATCHING. Choose the item in column 2 that best matches each item in column 1.

Choose the item from the column 2 that best matches each item in column 1.

   1) Column 1: ZP3

   Column 2: sperm receptor

   Answer: sperm receptor

   Page Ref: 1023

   2) Column 1: hCG

   Column 2: secreted by trophoblast to
   maintain corpus luteum

   Answer: secreted by trophoblast to maintain corpus luteum

   Page Ref: 1035

   3) Column 1: alphafetoprotein

   Column 2: substance in amniotic fluid
   indicative of congenital neural
   defects

   Answer: substance in amniotic fluid indicative of congenital neural defects

   Page Ref: 1033

4) Column 1: relaxin
   Column 2: increases flexibility of pubic
             symphysis
   Answer: increases flexibility of pubic symphysis
   Page Ref: 1037

5) Column 1: hCS
   Column 2: causes decreased glucose
             utilization and increased fatty
             acid utilization by mother
   Answer: causes decreased glucose utilization and increased fatty acid utilization by mother
   Page Ref: 1037

6) Column 1: progesterone
   Column 2: inhibits uterine contractility
             and prepares breasts for milk
             production
   Answer: inhibits uterine contractility and prepares breasts for milk production
   Page Ref: 1035

7) Column 1: CRH
   Column 2: "clock" that establishes the
             timing of birth
   Answer: "clock" that establishes the timing of birth
   Page Ref: 1037

8) Column 1: DHEA
   Column 2: secreted by fetal adrenal
             cortex and converted to
             estrogen by the placenta
   Answer: secreted by fetal adrenal cortex and converted to estrogen by the placenta
   Page Ref: 1039

9) Column 1: oxytocin
   Column 2: stimulates uterine
             contractility
   Answer: stimulates uterine contractility
   Page Ref: 1039

10) Column 1: prolactin
    Column 2: promotes milk production
    Answer: promotes milk production
    Page Ref: 1042

MATCHING. Choose the item in column 2 that best matches each item in column 1.

Choose the item from the column 2 that best matches each item in column 1.

1) Column 1: zygote

   Column 2: a segmentation nucleus, cytoplasm, and the zona pellucida

   Answer: a segmentation nucleus, cytoplasm, and the zona pellucida

   Page Ref: 1023

2) Column 1: morula

   Column 2: solid mass of cells called blastomeres

   Answer: solid mass of cells called blastomeres

   Page Ref: 1024

3) Column 1: blastocyst

   Column 2: hollow ball of cells that implants into the uterine wall

   Answer: hollow ball of cells that implants into the uterine wall

   Page Ref: 1024

4) Column 1: trophoblast

   Column 2: part of the blastocyst that secretes hCG

   Answer: part of the blastocyst that secretes hCG

   Page Ref: 1024

5) Column 1: amnion

   Column 2: embryonic membrane nearest to the embryo

   Answer: embryonic membrane nearest to the embryo

   Page Ref: 1027

6) Column 1: chorion

   Column 2: embryonic membrane that becomes the principal embryonic part of the placenta

   Answer: embryonic membrane that becomes the principal embryonic part of the placenta

   Page Ref: 1027

7) Column 1: decidua basalis
   Column 2: portion of the endometrium
           that becomes the maternal
           part of the placenta
   Answer: portion of the endometrium that becomes the maternal part of the placenta
   Page Ref: 1030

8) Column 1: allantois
   Column 2: embryonic membrane that
           forms the vascular portion of
           the umbilical cord
   Answer: embryonic membrane that forms the vascular portion of the umbilical cord
   Page Ref: 1027

9) Column 1: decidua capsularis
   Column 2: portion of the endometrium
           that covers the embryo
   Answer: portion of the endometrium that covers the embryo
   Page Ref: 1030

10) Column 1: inner cell mass
    Column 2: part of the blastocyst that
            becomes the embryo
    Answer: part of the blastocyst that becomes the embryo
    Page Ref: 1025

TRUE/FALSE. Write 'T' if the statement is true and 'F' if the statement is false.

1) About 50% of sperm introduced into the vagina reach the secondary oocyte.

   Answer: FALSE
   Page Ref: 1022

2) Dizygotic twins are produced from the independent release of two secondary oocytes and subsequent fertilization by different sperm.

   Answer: TRUE
   Page Ref: 1023

3) The morula is a hollow ball of cells.

   Answer: FALSE
   Page Ref: 1024

4) The layer of cells of the inner cell mass that is closer to the amniotic cavity develops into the ectoderm.

Answer: TRUE
Page Ref: 1027

5) The yolk sac develops from endoderm.

Answer: TRUE
Page Ref: 1027

6) The chorion is the principal maternal part of the placenta.

Answer: FALSE
Page Ref: 1027

7) Maternal and fetal blood mix in spaces called intervillous spaces.

Answer: FALSE
Page Ref: 1030

8) The allantois is an early site of blood formation.

Answer: TRUE
Page Ref: 1027

9) CRH produced by the placenta is thought to be the "clock" that establishes the timing of birth.

Answer: TRUE
Page Ref: 1037

10) Peak hCG secretion occurs just before parturition.

Answer: FALSE
Page Ref: 1036

11) The rise in CRH levels near the end of pregnancy results in a sharp increase in progesterone and a decrease in estrogen.

Answer: FALSE
Page Ref: 1037

12) Estrogen causes myometrial cells to display oxytocin receptors near the time of parturition.

Answer: TRUE
Page Ref: 1035

13) In an error of meiosis called translocation, a chromosome is left out of a gamete.

Answer: FALSE
Page Ref: 1045

14) In incomplete dominant, a heterozygote has a phenotype intermediate between homozygous dominant and homozygous recessive.

Answer: FALSE
Page Ref: 1045

15) Nondisjunction of chromosomes results in an abnormal number of chromosomes.

Answer: TRUE
Page Ref: 1045

SHORT ANSWER. Write the word or phrase that best completes each statement or answers the question.

1) Fusion of a sperm with a secondary oocyte is called _____.
Answer: syngamy
Page Ref: 1023

2) Smaller cells produced by cleavage of the zygote are called _____.
Answer: blastomeres
Page Ref: 1024

3) In the region of contact between the blastocyst and the endometrium, the trophoblast develops two layers: the _____ and the _____.
Answer: syncytiotrophoblast; cytotrophoblast
Page Ref: 1025

4) The inner cell mass is called the _____ once the amniotic cavity develops.
Answer: embryonic disc
Page Ref: 1027

5) The organ that is the site of exchange of nutrients and wastes between mother and fetus is the _____.

Answer: placenta
Page Ref: 1027

6) During the first three to four months of pregnancy the lining of the uterus is maintained by progesterone and estrogen secreted by the _____.
Answer: corpus luteum
Page Ref: 1035

7) Early pregnancy tests detect the hormone _____.
Answer: hCG
Page Ref: 1037

8) The postpartum discharge of blood and serous fluid is called _____.

Answer: lochia

Page Ref: 1041

9) A cell that has one or more chromosomes of a set added or deleted is called _____.

Answer: aneuploid

Page Ref: 1045

10) The prime male–determining gene is called _____ and is located on the _____ chromosome.

Answer: SRY; Y

Page Ref: 1048

11) An agent that causes developmental defects in the embryo is called a(n) _____.

Answer: teratogen

Page Ref: 1049

12) If two genes for a trait are expressed equally in a heterozygote they are said to be _____.

Answer: codominant

Page Ref: 1046

13) A permanent, heritable change in a gene that causes it to have a different effect than it previously had is called a(n) _____.

Answer: mutation

Page Ref: 1044

14) The phenomenon in which the phenotype is dramatically different depending on the parental origin is called _____.

Answer: genomic imprinting

Page Ref: 1045

15) At parturition the androgen _____ is secreted from the fetal adrenal cortex and converted to _____ by the placenta.

Answer: DHEA; estrogen

Page Ref: 1039

16) The hormone _____ inhibits uterine contractions; the hormone _____ promotes uterine contractions.

Answer: progesterone; oxytocin

Page Ref: 1039

17) From the third to the ninth month of pregnancy, estrogen and progesterone levels are kept high enough to maintain the pregnancy by the _____.

Answer: placenta

Page Ref: 1036

18) The glycoprotein receptor for sperm called ZP3 is located in a glycoprotein layer around the oocytes called the _____.

Answer: zona pellucida

Page Ref: 1023

19) _____ is the term for the functional changes that sperm undergo in the female reproductive tract that allow them to fertilize a secondary oocyte.

Answer: Capacitation

Page Ref: 1022

20) The fertilized ovum is called a(n) _____.

Answer: zygote

Page Ref: 1023

21) The part of the female reproductive tract in which fertilization normally occurs is the _____.

Answer: uterine tube

Page Ref: 1022

22) By the end of the third day after fertilization, the fertilized egg has become a solid ball of cells called the _____.

Answer: morula

Page Ref: 1024

23) The hollow ball of cells that is implanted into the uterine wall is called the _____.

Answer: blastocyst

Page Ref: 1024

24) The primary germ layers are the _____, the _____, and the _____.

Answer: ectoderm; mesoderm; endoderm

Page Ref: 1024

25) The structure derived from the trophoblast of the blastocyst that becomes the principal embryonic part of the placenta is the _____.

Answer: chorion

Page Ref: 1027

26) The chorion of the placenta secretes the hormone _____ , which mimics the action of LH.
Answer: human chorionic gonadotropin
Page Ref: 1027

27) The complete genetic makeup of an organism is called the _____ .
Answer: genome
Page Ref: 1044

28) The physical or outward expression of a gene is called the _____ .
Answer: phenotype
Page Ref: 1045

29) A diploid human cell contains _____ pair(s) of autosomes and _____ pair(s) of sex chromosomes.
Answer: 22; one
Page Ref: 1047

30) The embryo develops from the layer of the blastocyst called the _____ .
Answer: inner cell mass
Page Ref: 1024

ESSAY. Write your answer in the space provided or on a separate sheet of paper.

1) Describe the composition and functions of amniotic fluid.
Answer: Initially amniotic fluid is a filtrate of maternal blood, then fetal urine is added daily. It acts as a shock absorber and fetal temperature regulator, and prevents adhesion of fetal skin to surrounding tissues.
Page Ref: 1033

2) Describe the structure and function of the umbilical cord.
Answer: The umbilical cord consists of two umbilical arteries that carry deoxygenated fetal blood to the placenta, one umbilical vein that carries oxygenated blood to the fetus, and supporting mucous connective tissue derived from the allantois called Wharton's jelly. The entire cord is surrounded by a layer of amnion.
Page Ref: 1040

3) Describe the process and purpose of amniocentesis.
Answer: The position of the fetus and placenta is identified via ultrasound and palpation, and the skin is prepared with antiseptic and local anesthetic. A hypodermic needle is inserted through the abdominal wall and uterus to withdraw 10 mL of amniotic fluid from the amniotic cavity. The fluid and cells are examined and biochemically tested for abnormal proteins and chromosome abnormalities that may signal fetal problems and congenital defects.
Page Ref: 1033

4) Describe the hormonal events surrounding parturition.

Answer: Fetal CRH secretion increases, which causes estrogen to increase as fetal ACTH triggers an increase in cortisol and DHEA, which is converted to estrogen by the placenta. Estrogen increases oxytocin receptors on uterine smooth muscle fibers and makes them form gap junctions. Oxytocin stimulates uterine contraction, and relaxin dilates the cervix and loosens the pubic symphysis. Estrogen also increases prostaglandins to digest collagen in the cervix. Oxytocin the cervix, and the hypothalamus maintain a positive feedback loop to maintain labor.

Page Ref: 1039

5) Describe the potential hazards to the embryo and fetus associated with alcohol consumption and cigarette smoking.

Answer: Acetaldehyde, a metabolic product of alcohol, causes fetal alcohol syndrome, which is characterized by slow growth, small head, unusual facial features, defective heart and other organs, malformed limbs, and CNS abnormalities that may lead to behavioral problems. Cigarette smoking leads to low birth weight and increased risk of fetal/infant mortality, cardiac problems, anencephaly, and cleft lip and cleft palate.

Page Ref: 1049

6) Describe the cardiovascular adjustments that occur in the infant at birth.

Answer: The foramen ovale closes first (between atria), then the ductus arteriosus closes. Both divert blood to the lungs. After severing of the umbilical cord, blood no longer travels through the ductus venosus (bypassing liver). Pulse rate is high (120 −160 bpm) then slows. Production of red blood cells and hemoglobin is increased. The very high leukocyte count decreases after about one week.

Page Ref: 1041

7) Describe the events of early development from fertilization through implantation.

Answer: At fertilization, the male and female pronuclei fuse into the segmentation nucleus, which, with cytoplasm and zona pellucida, form the zygote in the uterine tube. The zygote undergoes cleavage to form blastomeres, which are arranged as a solid ball of cells called the morula. By the fifth day after fertilization, the hollow blastocyst has formed (trophoblast, inner cell mass, and blastocele), which implants into the uterine wall oriented toward the endometrium.

Page Ref: 1022

8) Identify the embryonic/fetal membranes, and describe the location and functions of each.

Answer: The allantois is an outpouching from the yolk sac and is an early site of blood cell formation. It becomes the umbilical cord. The yolk sac extends between the amnion and chorion. It also is an early site of blood cell formation and is the source of cells that become primitive germ cells. The amnion covers the embryonic disc. It eventually surrounds the embryo/fetus and holds amniotic fluid (shock absorber, etc.). The chorion lies between the amnion and the decidua. Villi grow into the decidua. The chorion is the principal embryonic part of the placenta, where exchange of materials between mother and fetus occurs.

Page Ref: 1027

9) A child is born who is blood type O. The mother's blood type is A. The man the mother claims is the father of the baby is blood type B. Because he is blood type B, this man claims he cannot be the baby's father. Is he correct? Explain your answer. What, if anything, can you tell about the blood phenotypes and genotypes of the maternal grandparents?

Answer: The man is not correct. The woman could be genotype $I^A i$, and he could be $I^B i$. A Punnet square would show the possibility of an ii genotype. The woman's parents could have been phenotypes A ($I^A I^A$ of $I^A i$) and O (ii), A($I^A i$) and A ($I^A i$), or A ($I^A I^A$ or $I^A i$) and B ($I^B i$).

Page Ref: 1046

10) A woman who is a carrier of a sex (X)–linked trait marries a man who does not express the trait. What are the possible phenotypes and genotypes for male and female offspring? Explain your answer.

Answer: All girls will have a normal phenotype, because all will possess at least one dominant allele. Half will be homozygous dominant, half will be heterozygous carriers. Half of the boys will be of normal phenotype, because they will have the dominant allele on the X chromosome. Half of the boys will express the trait because they will have only one X chromosome, which has the recessive allele.

Page Ref: 1044